THE NEW FACE OF THE NHS
2nd edition

Edited by Peter Spurgeon,
Director of Research and Consultancy,
Health Services Management Centre, Birmingham

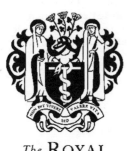

The ROYAL

SOCIETY *of*

MEDICINE

PRESS *Limited*

British Library Cataloguing in Publication Data
A catalogue record for this book is available from the British Library
ISBN 0-443-05969-1

Phototypeset by Saxon Graphics Ltd, Derby
Printed in Great Britain by Redwood Books

Contents

Foreword
Stuart Dickens

It is curious that a book entitled The New Face of the NHS should now be in its third edition within seven years. This is no mere updating either. As in previous editions there is much in the current scene to more than justify the word new in the title. Even before a landslide Labour victory in May 1997 there were signs of a changing mood amongst health managers motivated by the stress of budget pressures. Recognition that confrontational relationships were short on outcomes and the need to take devolved commissioning seriously. A decision to put back the publication date of this edition was clearly justified given the outcome of the election and the announcement of early policy decisions.

Taking a long term view of change over the last four decades we can chart the ebb and flow of centralising and decentralising policies. However the change sign wave appears to have flattened out, at least for the time being, as the voluntary movement towards devolved commissioning becomes the preferred organisational approach of the new Government. Once again Health Authorities, which have had to make more cultural changes in the 90s than in the previous thirty years, are asked to reinvent themselves.

Devolved commissioning to Primary Care Groups and the emergence of Primary Care Trusts requires new processes but, importantly, it demands new behaviours. The Health Authority that appears to use contracting as another means of command and control, as one Trust Chief Executive observed, is going to have real difficulty in coming to terms with a culture which will demand collaboration and alliance building; the sharing of health intelligence and the stitching together of diverse local agendas.

Diversity was a theme in the last edition of this book and it will continue to be a feature of a devolved commissioning environment. Locality commissioning involves the creation of local agendas with local priorities which reflect the differential needs of communities. The new strategically focused Health Authority will remain the conduit for the implementation of national and regional policies and priorities. Nevertheless, those priorities will have to be skilfully integrated with the local perspective on what is important, if the locality is to avoid being yet another management fashion victim.

During the last two years the polarisation of organisational cultures has been increasingly observable. Health Authorities staking out the moral high ground of their health gain strategic vision are to be found in endless contracting rounds with Trusts struggling to reshape (and retain) services within increasingly constrained resources. The purchaser : provider split is now even more obviously a division between strategic and operational management.

Many Health Authorities have had real difficulty in translating strategic thinking into a service reality. Trusts have found it equally hard to reconcile day to day business reality with the published aspirations of their main purchasers. There is very little high ground here only the prospect of more stressful meetings and uncomfortable compromises.

The advent of a new Government has provided the opportunity to take stock. Although there is an acceptance that the genie separating purchasers from providers is out of the bottle there is an apparent determination to create a one health system environment which will embrace the strategic and operational environments.

One of the causes of the perceived tension between some Authorities and Trusts is the determination to get beyond the ... *more of the same* ... scenario which was an inevitable feature of the early years of the reforms. Recurrent financial crises will have a number of different origins and some of them could undoubtedly be resolved with additional resources. Realistically, however, given the constraints of the national economy, they are much more likely to be resolved or ameliorated through joint action and collaborative working. Financial pressure has internal and external perspectives and you need both to understand the nature of the problem and the potential for resolution.

Seven years is long enough to discern organisational trends and there is certainly a discernible behavioural cycle which many Authorities and Trusts have been unable to avoid. The figure below demonstrates this:

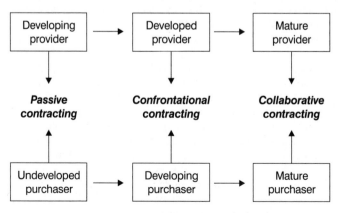

Purchaser: Provider Behavioural Cycle

As a contract is the means of mediating the relationship between purchaser and provider the contracting process is used here as the most tangible barometer of inter organisational health.

At the outset there was widespread recognition that the role of commissioners was underdeveloped with a consequent sense that providers were dominating the relationship. It is hardly surprising that emergent expertise within Authorities and the learned behaviour of an effective purchaser should manifest itself in what was seen as aggressive behaviour and hard nosed contract making. Confrontational contracting has proved stressful and undoubtedly produced sub optimal health care solutions. It is this realisation that has given the emphasis to collaborative working. We know that collaboration is most successful between mature organisations who are confident in their individual roles in the health system. Those of us who opined that it would be some five years before the new infrastructure would mature were not far out.

The mantra of the primary care led NHS is now heard less often. Health Authority managers and GPs alike are showing concern at the dangers of simplistic sloganising. The primary care role in the NHS has never been stronger and will be strengthened further as Primary Care Groups are established. Notwithstanding the Audit Commission's conclusions about the lack of real strategic impact by GP Fundholders, there will be few who have not observed some of the changes in clinical practice that many fundholders have been able to achieve. I suspect that it is not fundholding per se that should be credited for these developments but something about the quality of the relationship between clinicians. Ultimately change in clinical practice will be catalysed and achieved by clinicians rather than executive action – a conclusion reflected in the Governments decision to support devolved purchasing.

The emergence of locality commissioning has the capacity to embrace many of the desirable features of the late 90s NHS – devolved decision making collaborative behaviour, the most effective primary:secondary care relationship and an increased capacity to engage the communities served in decisions about health priorities and health care provision. The last of these features presents another of the long term challenges.

Tokenism is a common experience in user involvement despite the energy now being put into engaging patients and carers. Voluntary organisations are still learning how to get into the commissioning cycle to make an impact on decisions about the use of health and social care resources. Experience working with service users demonstrates that there is widespread ignorance about health care institutions – who does what and why. It is also clear that engaging individuals about health strategy is going to be problematical when their pressing concerns are most commonly about the availability and quality of services for themselves and their family. It is salutary to reflect on the concerns expressed by consultant clinicians about the unreasonable demands of purchasers of all kinds – is the perspective of the service user likely to have more credibility? The search for effective ways of involving the public continues.

The chapters of this book are a reminder of where the NHS has come from and how far there is yet to travel. Much of the change agenda in terms of a new Government has focused upon the role of the Health Authority and models of commissioning, the role of public health and as is now clear from the white paper, a move away from the internal market. These issues are addressed in the first three chapters by Chris Ham, Rod Griffiths & Bernard Crump, and Penelope Mullen.

The emphasis upon financial management and efficiency has been maintained, indeed some might argue it has been strengthened with the intended reduction in transactional costs. Chapters 4 (Tony Cook) and 5 (Mike Drummond) discuss this area of continuing debate. A new chapter on Information Management recognises the attention being given to this area and its link to effective management.

Quality issues have been highlighted as at the top of the new Government's agenda and contributions from John Øvretveit and Judith Smith (Managed Care) emphasise this focus upon clinical management. Also a new chapter on Evidence – based Medicine (Kieran Walshe) provides further focus to this burgeoning area.

There has been a significant strengthening of interest in good staff management and the three chapters on Human Resource Management (Flanagan) and Management Development (Thompson) and a new chapter on Managing Stress (Spurgeon) reflect this concern.

Finally the vital area of primary healthcare and its future development are discussed by Willis and Shapiro. A new chapter on public/consumer involvement in healthcare highlights the growing interest in involving the public in the health debate.

The spirit of learning through doing is still the prevailing mood. The notion of building from the last platform is a more welcome strategy than digging up and replacing the foundations. However there is one important lesson that has been learnt the hard way by some organisations. Too much concern for structure, the anatomy of the business, at the expense of process and behaviour, the physiology, will lead to dysfunctional organisations and unfulfilled aspirations. The one health system vision for the NHS, which is now openly espoused, is an important feature of local commissioning and collaborative working. Health authorities that were slow, or reluctant to change in 1991 will experience similar difficulties with the cultural shift that is demanded yet again. The prize however is one that continues to dominate the horizon – cost effective health services genuinely geared to local needs with tangible health gain for the communities which they serve.

Stuart Dickens
Dearden Management

During the preparation of the chapters in this text the new Labour government published a White Paper (The new NHS: Modern, Dependable) on the future of the NHS. Many of the proposals had been anticipated (correctly) by authors whose areas were likely to be affected by an alternative political perspective. Perhaps the most significant of the changes outlined are:

- a modified role for Health Authorities emphasising their strategic and monitoring functions.
- a move away from the internal market to a more collaborative framework.
- the establishment of Primary Care Groups to evolve later to Primary Care Trusts incorporating current and G.P. Commissioning Groups as both commissioners and providers of healthcare.
- a focus on quality of services reinforcing evidence-based medicine and creating an important new concept of clinical governance.
- an emphasis upon positive, supportive and participative management of health service staff.

The precise manner of implementation of these concepts is still to be determined. The strong emphasis upon local determination in the White Paper suggests a plurality of models and structures will ultimately emerge. The fascination for those interested in the NHS and its operations will be to observe this process over the coming months.

Peter Spurgeon

Contributors

Stuart Dickens	Dearden Management
Chris Ham	Director, Health Services Management Centre, Birmingham
Rod Griffiths	Regional Director of Public Health, NHS Executive (West Midlands)
Bernard Crump	Director of Public Health, Leicestershire Health
Penelope M Mullen	Senior Lecturer, Health Services Management Centre, Birmingham
Tony Cook	The Birmingham Business School, The University of Birmingham
Michael F Drummond	Centre for Health Economics, University of York
Fred Barwell	Honorary Research Fellow, Health Services Management Centre, Birmingham
John Øvretveit	Professor of Health Policy and Management, Nordic School of Public Health, Sweden
Judith Smith	Fellow, Health Services Management Centre, Birmingham
Hugh Flanagan	Visiting Senior Fellow, Health Services Management Centre/Ferndale Management Consultancy
David Thompson	Associate Professor, Department of Management, The Hong Kong Polytechnic University
Michael Tremblay	Managing Partner, Tremblay Consulting
Peter Spurgeon	Director of Research and Consultancy, Health Services Management Centre, Birmingham
Jonathan Shapiro	Senior Fellow, Health Services Management Centre, Birmingham

Andrew Willis   Northampton GP & Chairman of the
                           NACGPs (National Association of
                           Commissioning General Practitioners)

Stuart Cumella   Senior Research Fellow, Queen Elizabeth
                           Psychiatric Hospital

Kieran Walshe   Senior Research Fellow, Health Services
                           Management Centre, Birmingham

Shirley McIver   Senior Fellow, Health Services
                           Management Centre, Birmingham

1 Population centred and patient focused purchasing: the UK experience

Chris Ham

This is an edited and updated version of a paper which first appeared in *The Milbank Quarterly* 74 (2), 1996, and which is reproduced with kind permission.

Introduction

The reforms to the UK National Health Service (NHS) initiated by the Thatcher Government in 1989 have attracted interest around the world. These reforms seek to introduce market principles into a centrally planned and publicly financed health service. To use the conceptual framework proposed by the Organisation for Economic Co-operation and Development (OECD), they have transformed an integrated system in which Health Authorities both held the budget for health care and managed services directly to a contract system based on the separation of purchaser and provider functions (OECD 1992). This is consistent with reforms in other countries which are moving in a similar direction (Ham, Robinson and Benzeval 1990; Saltman and von Otter 1992). As Figure 1.1 illustrates, there are two types of purchaser in the new NHS: Health Authorities and general practitioner fundholders. Similarly, there are two types of provider: NHS trusts and general practitioners.

A private health care sector exists as a supplement to the NHS and is of growing importance in certain sectors of care. Private expenditure on health care comprises some 15 per cent of total health expenditure in the UK. The contribution of the private sector is particularly significant in relation to non-urgent hospital care. Estimates suggest some 16 per cent of common surgical procedures are performed in the private sector, with an even higher proportion being carried out in London and the South East (Nicholl, Beeby, and Williams 1989). The costs of care delivered in this way are met mainly by private medical insurance, which covers around 12 per cent of the population, and is provided principally as an employment benefit to white collar workers and their families.

Like the NHS, the private sector is divided into purchasers and providers. There has been increasing competition among private purchasers as new health insurers have entered the market. Private hospitals have also felt the force of competition as capacity has expanded and as NHS trusts have sought to increase their share of the market for private

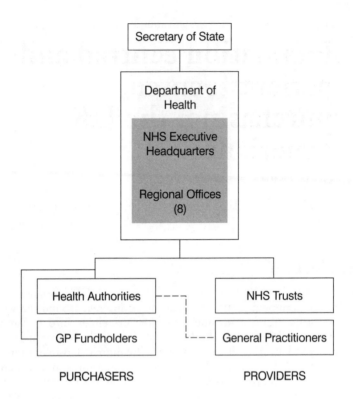

Figure 1.1   The organization of the NHS in England

patients. While private patients have always been treated in designated private beds in NHS hospitals, one of the effects of the Thatcher
Government's reforms has been to blur still further the distinction
between the public and private sectors. Thus, just as NHS trusts have
attempted to attract additional private patients, so private hospitals have
sought to win contracts from NHS purchasers to provide care to NHS
patients. While the effect of these developments has so far been marginal,
in the longer term they could extend still further the mixed economy of
health care provision in the UK, a point we return to below.

Privatisation or modernisation?

Critics of the Thatcher and Major Governments have maintained consistently that these changes are leading to the commercialisation of health care
and will eventually result in the privatisation of service provision (Labour
Party 1995). In assessing this claim, it is important to remember that the
reforms introduced in 1989 have not changed the way in which health care is
financed in the UK. The NHS continues to be funded primarily out of

resources raised through the tax system and there are limited incentives (in terms of tax relief) for people to take out private medical insurance. Furthermore, the government has increased the NHS budget annually to ease the process of implementing the reforms. The purpose of the reforms is less to control NHS spending, which governments have always been able to do, than to ensure that the resources available are used efficiently and that services provided are responsive to patients and service users.

It is this objective that explains the interest on the part of policy makers in introducing market principles into the NHS. Having examined alternative sources of finance for health care and decided to leave the single payer tax system in place, the Thatcher Government turned its attention to reforming the delivery of health care. Inspired partly by the ideas of Alain Enthoven (1985), an influence acknowledged by the Secretary of State for Health at the time of the Thatcher review (Kenneth Clarke quoted in Roberts 1990), and partly by similar reforms to other parts of the public sector like education, the Government came to the conclusion that an NHS based on centralised planning and without the stimulus of the market was inherently inefficient. Additionally, the system of allocating resources within the NHS created a number of perverse incentives. Foremost amongst these was the so-called 'efficiency trap' in which public hospitals funded through prospective global budgets were in effect penalised for treating additional patients because their income remained fixed while their expenditure rose as a result of the extra services these patients consumed.

In the light of this analysis, it was not surprising that the Government's proposals centred on the development of a system in which money would follow the patient. This was intended to overcome the efficiency trap and to reward providers who delivered well-managed care that was responsive to the demands of patients and those who purchased care on their behalf. In order to create a market, the functions of Health Authorities were separated. Those providing hospital and community health services were reconstituted as self-governing NHS trusts, enabling Health Authorities to concentrate on purchasing services for the populations they served. In this way, Health Authorities were free to negotiate contracts with the hospitals of their choice and not simply those they managed directly. Equally, of course, NHS trusts were able to increase their income by winning contracts from a range of Health Authorities.

Alongside these plans, proposals were formulated to give budgets to groups of general practitioners. These general practitioners, who became known as fundholders, received a sum of money with which to buy a defined range of services for their patients. Like other general practitioners, fundholders were also responsible for providing primary care to their patients, which in effect made them purchasers and providers. Initially, fundholding was confined to larger groups of general practitioners and to practices with the necessary management and professional capacity. The scope of fundholding was also limited to the cost of drugs prescribed by general practitioners, the staff they employed, and the purchase of a number of hospital services such as outpatient care, diagnostic tests and non-urgent surgical procedures. To avoid the risks of high cost patients, fundholders were responsible for paying for the cost of care up to a limit of £5,000 a year per patient, with Health Authorities having to pick up expenditure over this limit.

Whether these reforms to the NHS, involving the continuation of tax funding and the introduction of competition into the delivery of health care, justify the claim that health care is being privatised remains a matter of dispute. Government ministers have argued that they are committed to the preservation of a health service available to all, providing services on the basis of need and not ability to pay. This was stated clearly in the White Paper *Working for Patients* which launched the reforms. In her foreword to the White Paper, Thatcher noted that:

> The National Health Service will continue to be available to all, regardless of income, and to be financed mainly out of taxation. (Secretary of State for Health et al. 1989)

In essence, the Government has argued that the reforms are intended to modernise the structure of the NHS and are not a retreat from the principles on which it was established in 1948.

For their part, the Government's critics point not only to the impact of competition on the NHS but also to the effect of policies pursued throughout the 1980s to make the NHS more businesslike. These policies encompassed putting NHS services like catering, cleaning and laundry out to competitive bids; introducing general management into the NHS and giving hospital doctors budgets with which to manage their services; and encouraging Health Authorities to generate additional income through introducing car parking charges, retail developments and similar schemes at NHS hospitals. More recently, the Government's private finance initiative has required NHS trusts to seek funds from the private sector for major building projects before they will be considered for public funding. Taken together, it is argued that these changes are fundamentally altering the ethos and values of the NHS, transforming it from a public service into an organisation that has many of the features of the private sector (Mohan 1995).

In so far as there is agreement on the effects of recent changes, it is that the NHS has been progressively redefined. This was acknowledged by Virginia Bottomley, Secretary of State for Health between 1992 and 1995, in a newspaper article, in which she argued:

> We start by recognising that we have, in effect, redefined what we mean by the National Health Service. The service should not be defined by who provides it, but by the fundamental principle which underpin their work: to provide care on the basis of clinical need and regardless of ability to pay. The precise nature of the services provided should increasingly become a matter for local decision. In the NHS of the future we can expect to see much greater diversity of provision. (Bottomley 1994)

Put another way, the NHS has gradually shifted from being the more or less monolithic funder and provider of health care and is becoming a national health insurer guaranteeing access to necessary medical care for the population. Who provides this care is seen by the Government as of secondary importance and the logical (though not inevitable) outcome of current developments is that service provision will become the responsibility of a variety of public and private organisations. In this sense, the NHS is moving in the direction of other health care systems in which public finance is combined with alternative forms of service delivery: some public, some private, some for-profit, some not-for-profit. The key question is how fast this will occur and what will happen to the ownership and management of NHS trusts in the process.

In making this point it is relevant to note *en passant* that primary care has always been organised in this way within the NHS. General practitioners are independent contractors (in effect private practitioners) who deliver care to NHS patients under the terms of contracts negotiated nationally between the Government and the medical profession. This reflects the desire of general practitioners to preserve their autonomy and to resist salaried employment by the state. Patients do not pay to see a general practitioner, and general practitioners are not allowed to make charges for the provision of NHS services. It could be argued that the changes taking place in other parts of the NHS are simply moving these services in the direction of primary care and that there is no reason to believe that this in itself will undermine the principles on which the NHS is based.

Changing relationships in the NHS

Leaving on one side the intensity of the political debate surrounding the reforms and their ultimate outcome, the fascination for the health policy analyst is the impact of the separation of purchaser and provider roles on the power of different groups within the NHS. Whereas in the past those running hospital and specialist services exerted considerable influence and won the lion's share of resources to develop their services, in the new NHS this has begun to change. Doctors and managers in NHS trusts have been held more accountable for the use of resources by a combination of Health Authorities and general practitioner fundholders. General practitioners who are not fundholders work closely with Health Authorities in many places in setting priorities for the use of budgets and in this way have increased their leverage within the NHS. While it would be wrong to exaggerate either the extent or the pace of these changes, they have nevertheless had a discernible effect on the delivery of health care to patients. Of particular interest in this respect are the relative merits of Health Authorities and general practitioner fundholders as purchasers. There is a key distinction here between population centred purchasing and patient focused purchasing. A more detailed discussion follows.

Population centred purchasing

Health Authorities are responsible for purchasing health care for all citizens who reside within their boundaries. There are around 100 Health

Authorities in England and on average each authority serves a population of 500,000, although there are considerable variations around this average. Health Authorities are not elected by the people they serve but are appointed bodies nominated to act as agents of the Secretary of State for Health in purchasing services for their populations. They are governed by a board comprising a chairman, five non-executive members and a group of executives led by the chief executive. The accountability of Health Authorities is first and for most to the Secretary of State for Health, although they are expected to consult local people and take account of their views in deciding which services to purchase.

Health Authorities are allocated a budget by the Department of Health on the basis of a weighted capitation formula. This is meant to reflect the need for health care of the population served. With this budget, authorities are responsible for buying all services except those that are covered by general practitioner fundholders in their area. A critical task for Health Authorities is to improve the health of the population. They are expected to do this partly by purchasing health services and partly by assessing the health needs of populations and taking action to reduce major causes of morbidity and mortality. This work is led by directors of public health who are required to produce an annual report on the population's health. Furthermore, in 1992 the Government published a national health strategy for England, *The Health of The Nation* (Secretary of State for Health 1992), setting out targets for improving the nation's health. Health Authorities are responsible for translating these national objectives into local policies and for working with other agencies to address the conditions which give rise to ill health.

Health Authorities are also responsible for primary care services. In the past, there have been separate authorities in England and Wales for the management of hospital and community health services on the one hand and primary care services on the other, the latter being known as Family Health Services Authorities. The NHS reforms underlined the need to integrate these responsibilities; the two types of Health Authority formally merged in April 1996. In preparation for this event, however, considerable progress was made in bringing the two sets of functions together (Ham and Shapiro 1995b). This was supported by the policy, enunciated in 1994, of developing a primary care led NHS (NHS Executive 1994b). As with the priority given to public health, this policy was intended in part to restore the balance within the NHS and to counteract the emphasis traditionally attached to hospital and specialist services.

A further move in this direction came with the establishment of the NHS research and development programme. This included a series of initiatives concerned with health technology assessment and the promotion of evidence based medicine. These initiatives encompassed the establishment of the UK Cochrane Centre at Oxford, the NHS Centre for Reviews and Dissemination at York and the provision of information to Health Authorities to enable them to concentrate resources on services of proven clinical effectiveness. The aim of this policy is to create a culture in which clinicians in NHS trusts draw on evidence in deciding which services to provide and purchasers are given the ammunition to challenge providers and achieve the most health benefit with the budgets available.

The priority attached to public health, primary care and evidence based medicine promised to alter fundamentally the orientation and approach of Health Authorities. In fact, change was slow to occur in many places, chiefly because the staff in charge of the Health Authorities had developed their careers in the old NHS, where the main preoccupation was the management of health care institutions. With a few exceptions, it took time to break away from this tradition and to focus on the population and its health needs. The transition from a provider oriented health service to one centred on purchasing was not helped by the time consuming nature of the contracting arrangements introduced under the NHS reforms. The establishment of an annual contracting cycle between purchasers and providers meant that Health Authorities spent considerable amounts of time in negotiating and monitoring contracts for the provision of health care, which pre-empted resources for addressing the public health agenda.

Surveys of Health Authorities and their purchasing plans demonstrated, perhaps not surprisingly, that change was incremental rather than radical. This was illustrated by work carried out at the University of Bath. In a series of surveys, Klein and colleagues traced the development of purchasing plans and priorities in a selection of Health Authorities in England (Klein and Redmayne 1992, Redmayne, Klein and Day 1993, Redmayne 1995). They found that Health Authorities tended to spread their money around between services, and that authorities were reluctant to challenge established patterns of expenditure. Initially, acute hospital services received high priority but gradually the emphasis shifted to primary and community care and public health, in line with developments in national policy. Even so the shift in priorities was not dramatic. This conclusion was reinforced by a study of priority setting in six Health Authorities which found that purchasing decisions were strongly influenced by historical commitments and that attempts to set priorities on a more systematic basis were at an embryonic stage (Ham, Honigsbaum and Thompson 1994).

Yet if survey evidence that Health Authorities were making a difference as purchasers were lacking, reports by those leading the work of those authorities offered a different interpretation (James 1994). These reports suggested that, freed from the responsibility of managing health services, Health Authorities were beginning to question traditional patterns of expenditure and to behave in new ways. This was best illustrated by the effort many Health Authorities expended on consulting with general practitioners and on heeding their views when they made decisions. In fact, this trend was noted in the surveys of Health Authorities' purchasing plans (Klein and Redmayne 1992), as well as in other reports (Carruthers *et al.* 1995). A major effort was also made to involve the public in the work of Health Authorities (NHS Management Executive 1992). While their impact on resource allocation may have been limited, it was possible to detect in these developments a change in behaviour and a refocusing on previously overlooked aspects of health and health care.

In recognition of the need to develop the role of Health Authorities more rapidly, the Government committed resources to a development programme to support purchasing during 1993. This was aimed at helping Health Authorities to acquire the skills and expertise needed in their new role. The Minister of Health explained the importance of the programme in three high profile speeches on the subject and in this was supported by the NHS Chief Executive (Mawhinney and Nichol 1993). The Government's initiative in this area reflected recognition that, in a health service traditionally commanded by providers, Health Authorities needed extra support to assume their responsibilities as purchasers.

Patient focused purchasing

General practitioner fundholding also developed slowly at first and in the face of strongly held opposition from many doctors, who were concerned that trust between patients and general practitioners would be undermined by the introduction of the financial incentives contained within fundholding. To ameliorate the adverse effects of these incentives, general practitioners were not intended to benefit personally from any savings made in their budgets. Another safeguard was that budgets were set for fundholders on the basis of the use patients made of the services included in the fundholding scheme rather than by reference to a capitation formula. This was designed to ensure that general practitioners had sufficient resources in their budgets to meet the demands of patients on their lists and would not engage in risk selection. However, the Government did commit itself to move toward capitation based budgets for fundholders over a number of years, although no deadline was set for achieving this.

Fundholders typically purchase care for groups of around 10,000–12,000 patients and the average fundholding practice has a budget of around £1.7million. Established as a voluntary scheme, fundholding covered 7 per cent of the population in the first year in England, increasing to over 50 per cent in 1997. Coverage varied significantly, however, from place to place with some districts having 84 per cent of general practitioners involved in fundholding and others only 4 per cent. To assist with the costs involved in holding a budget, general practitioners were given additional funds to prepare for fundholding. They also received an annual management allowance. This enabled fundholding practices to employ staff to help in the management of the budget and to acquire computers and support systems.

Research into the impact of fundholding in the early phases appeared to suggest that there was little difference between fundholding and non-fundholding general practitioners in the way in which they provided care. For example, Coulter and Bradlow (1993) found no difference in referral behaviour in a study of fundholding and non-fundholding practices in the Oxford region. Yet, gradually, a mixture of evidence drawn from evaluative research and reports from fundholding practices suggested that the scheme was having an effect on the delivery of services. This was apparent in changes in prescribing policies (Bradlow and Coulter 1993,

Maxwell *et al.* 1993) which resulted in savings in drugs budgets. In many cases these savings were used to provide additional services to patients. Attitude surveys also suggested that general practitioners involved in fundholding were enthusiastic and that the scheme had changed relationships within the NHS (Newton *et al.* 1993). In particular, hospital specialists were more responsive to the needs of general practitioners, which was reflected in improved discharge summaries and better communication between general practitioners and specialists.

These positive findings were supported by work carried out in Scotland which also looked at the impact of fundholding on the quality of care (Howie, Heaney and Maxwell 1995a). This research found that the clinical care of patients had generally remained stable during the period in which fundholding was implemented. However, the proportion of patients with self diagnosed joint pain who were investigated or referred to hospital fell significantly (Howie, Heaney and Maxwell 1994). The Scottish research also found that patients with some conditions appeared to have benefited at the expense of patients with other conditions (Howie, Heaney and Maxwell 1995b). Nevertheless, patients reported that they were generally satisfied with the quality of the services they received from fundholders, and remained so as fundholding was implemented. The main concern arising from this and other studies was the workload that fundholding entailed for general practitioners and the additional burden this imposed on busy professionals.

The most powerful support for fundholding came from Glennerster and his colleagues, who, in a series of widely cited publications, argued that fundholders had proved more effective purchasers than Health Authorities (Glennerster, Matsaganis and Owens 1992 and 1994). In support of their thesis, they maintained that fundholders had achieved greater success in reducing the time patients had to wait for hospital outpatient appointment or to have an operation, had increased the efficiency of diagnostic services delivery, and had encouraged the hospital staff to be more responsive. In addition, they held that the incentives of fundholding had reduced the cost of prescribing, and the scheme had also encouraged general practitioners to offer a wider range of services in their own practices. Equally important, their research produced little evidence that the potential adverse effects of fundholding, such as risk selection, had materialised.

It was partly on the basis of these findings that the Government announced a major development of fundholding in 1994 (NHS Executive 1994b). This involved the expansion of the original scheme to include a longer list of services together with two new options: total purchasing, in which groups of practices would be allowed to purchase all services for their patients; and community fundholding in which general practitioners would receive a budget to cover only the costs of drugs, practice staff and community health services. And while fundholding remained a voluntary scheme for general practitioners, pressure was exerted on Health Authorities to persuade more practices to participate (Ham and Shapiro 1995a). In espousing this policy, ministers emphasised that Health Authorities would have a continuing role as fundholding expanded, although this would shift from the direct purchasing of care for patients to a more strategic and enabling function.

Notwithstanding the enthusiasm of the Government for fundholding, independent analysts were divided in their assessments (Coulter 1995). It was argued, for instance, that there had been no rigorous comparisons between fundholding and non-fundholding practices. This made it difficult to assess whether the achievements of fundholders were due solely to holding a budget or were the result of other changes introduced by the reforms. While systematic research into the impact of Health Authority purchasing was also lacking, a number of reports suggested that many of the changes brought about by fundholders had been achieved by Health Authorities working with general practitioners (Black, Birchall and Trimble 1994, Graffy and Williams 1994). Furthermore, there was evidence to suggest that one of the most widely quoted changes brought about by fundholding, the reduction in prescribing costs, may have been caused partly by general practitioners using the budget setting process to increase the resources available for this element of their spending, thereby making it easier to produce savings (Dowell, Snodden and Dunbar 1995).

Analysis was further complicated by the emergence of a range of hybrid approaches combining features of both population centred and patient-focused purchasing (Ham and Willis 1994, Mays and Dixon 1996, Smith *et al*. 1997). These approaches were established as some Health Authorities recognised the need to work with general practitioners and some fundholders acknowledged that Health Authorities could add value to their purchasing. The models pursued included locality based purchasing, formation by general practitioners of commissioning groups to advise Health Authorities, and the establishment of networks of fundholding practices that became known as multi-funds (Shapiro 1994). Consequently, the two approaches outlined in *Working for Patients* multiplied into a range of alternatives. Yet cooperation between Health Authorities and general practitioners in some parts of the NHS was paralleled by lukewarm relationships elsewhere as the different types of purchaser preferred to pursue a policy of competition rather than collaboration. The introduction by the Government of an accountability framework for fundholders in 1995 (NHS Executive 1995) was an attempt to ensure that there were effective links between fundholders and Health Authorities, but, as much depended on the quality of relationships at a local level, the strengths of these links varied widely across the NHS.

Analysis

Six years into the implementation of the reforms, the achievements of Health Authorities and fundholders continue to be debated. The strengths of the Health Authority approach include an ability to plan for whole communities and to assess the needs of these communities. Health Authorities are also well placed to bring together expertise in different fields, like public health, finance and general management in deciding which services to purchase. This has assisted in the development of alliances with other agencies and in accessing information and intelligence to support decision-making. A further advantage of Health Authorities is their ability to lead major changes in service configuration, especially in urban areas.

The strengths of fundholding include direct contact with patients on a day to day basis and an ability arising from this to respond quickly to patients' demands. Fundholders have also demonstrated, somewhat paradoxically, that they are able to negotiate favourable terms with providers even though they control a much smaller proportion of the budget than Health Authorities. In part this is because fundholders are smaller and more flexible than Health Authorities and can move rapidly to achieve improvements in the delivery of the services they purchase. It may also be attributable to the fact that the general practitioners involved in fundholding practices are amongst the best organised primary care physicians in the country. The rules on fundholding restricted entry to larger practices with the necessary management and professional expertise to maintain a budget, a 'selection effect' that should be borne in mind in evaluating the impact of the scheme.

In relation to fundholding, Dixon and Glennerster offer the following comment:

> *The financial incentives of fundholding seem to be curbing the upward trend in prescribing costs, but the effect on rates of referral to hospital is unclear. Fundholders are challenging the traditional interface of primary and secondary care and offering more services in-house. Significant improvements in access to and the process of care have been secured by some fundholders. Giving budgets to general practitioners has been associated with a noticeable change in their relationship with hospital consultants.*
>
> *Set against these important gains, some drawbacks are evident. The costs to the NHS of contracting with many fundholding practices are unknown but estimated to be high. While fundholders report greater access to care, there is a weight of anecdotal (though not yet hard) evidence that a two tier service is operating. Research suggests that fundholders have been funded more generously than non-fundholding practices. (Dixon and Glennerster, 1995, p. 729)*

As this comment indicates, the balance sheet on fundholding is evenly weighted.

In arguing that Health Authorities and fundholders have distinctive strengths, it is important not to overlook the drawbacks of introducing two models of purchasing and the hybrids they have spawned. Foremost among these is the risk of fragmentation in service delivery (Light 1994). Put simply, there is no guarantee that the sum of multiple purchasing decisions will add up to a pattern of service provision appropriate to the needs of the population concerned. This is linked to the impact of expanding the fundholding scheme on the ability of Health Authorities to plan strategically for the population's health needs. With an increase in the proportion of the NHS budget under the direct control of general practitioners, it is not easy to see how Health Authorities can exert influence to improve the population's health. At a time when policy is targeting improvements in the population's health through the national health strategy, it appears that the left hand of Government is not always aware of what the right hand is doing.

A further concern, acknowledged even by the advocates of fundholding (Glennerster, Matsaganis and Owens 1994), is that the Government's desire to move away from workload based budgets for general practitioners to capitation funding may create an incentive for general practitioners to discriminate against patients who are older and sicker. No doubt for this reason, capitation based budgets for fundholders have been established only slowly. And as research has demonstrated, there are a number of technical challenges in applying a capitation formula at the practice level (Sheldon *et al.* 1994). This has given rise to the claim that the achievements of fundholders are not the result of them being better purchasers but are a consequence of more generous funding. On this point the evidence is mixed, with some studies suggesting that fundholders have received more than their fair share of resources (Dixon *et al.* 1994), and others disputing this claim.

The method of setting budgets for fundholders has led to wide variations in the amount of resources available to different practices (Glennerster, Matsaganis, and Owens 1992, Audit Commission 1995). It has also resulted in most fundholders making savings in their budgets. The level of these savings and the uses to which they are put has received increasing attention (National Audit Office 1994, Public Accounts Committee 1995, Audit Commission 1995). While average savings comprised only 3.5 per cent of budgets in 1993 and 1994, 20 per cent of fundholders underspent by £100,000 or more. Studies into how these savings are deployed raised questions about the use of public resources and also cast doubts on the policy that general practitioners should not benefit personally from fundholding. In particular, the use of savings to improve the buildings from which general practitioners practise – the most common use of savings (Audit Commission 1995) – and thereby to increase their value opened up the clear possibility of financial gain, given that general practitioners as independent contractors usually own their own clinics and receive additional money when they sell their equity.

Yet another issue raised by fundholding is the transactions cost involved in a system in which budgets are controlled by a large number of small purchasers. These costs arise partly from the management allowances paid to fundholders and partly from the workload involved for NHS trusts in negotiating contracts with fundholders. Although the latter is difficult to quantify, it is undoubtedly one of the factors behind the increase in the share of the NHS budget allocated to administration as a consequence of the NHS reforms. In a series of answers to parliamentary questions, health ministers provided information which showed that the amount of money spent on managers and administration rose from £1.2bn in 1989/90 to £2.1bn in 1993/94 (Brindle 1995). While some of this increase was due to a reclassification of nurses and other professional staff as managers, the introduction of an annual contracting system between purchasers and providers was also a factor. Fundholding played a part, although it is difficult to estimate the proportion of the overall increase in management costs that can be attributed to patient focused purchasing.

The most comprehensive assessment of fundholding, that carried out by the Audit Commission, was published in 1996. In a wide ranging review, the Audit Commission noted that most fundholders had achieved some improvements for their patients, most notably improved communications with hospitals and more cost-effective prescribing. However, only the best managed practices had had a major impact on services. Overall, the costs of fundholding outweighed the efficiency savings achieved, and the Audit Commission made a series of proposals designed to strengthen the scheme and ensure its benefits were extended to other practices. These proposals included improving management skills and capacity within primary care and developing the role of Health Authorities in support of fundholders (Audit Commission 1996).

As this analysis indicates, there is little consensus in the UK health policy community on the respective merits of Health Authority purchasing and general practitioner fundholding. Each has strengths and weaknesses and as time went on the most interesting question became not whether one approach was superior to the other, but how the best elements of each could be combined. As one director of public health put it, the challenge was to join the 'leverage' of Health Authorities and the 'bite' of fundholders (Steve Watkins cited in Shapiro 1994). The hybrid approaches that were established reflected recognition of this among doctors and managers, and illustrated how the details of policy implementation were driven from the bottom up, not the top down.

The future

Evidence that management costs had increased led the Conservative Government to take action to streamline the structure of the NHS. This included a reduction in the number of civil servants in the Department of Health, cuts in the number of Regional Health Authorities and the staff they employed, the merger of District Health Authorities and Family Health Services Authorities, and controls over management costs in Health Authorities and NHS Trusts. Despite these measures, the increase in management costs was one of the factors which prompted a reappraisal of the impact of the reforms as a whole. This process was not helped by the lack of good data enabling comparisons to be made of the performance of the NHS before and after *Working for Patients*. Evaluation was further hampered by changes to the way in which information was collected within the NHS (Radical Statistics Health Group 1992 and 1995). With independent analysts arguing that more time was needed to make a proper assessment and that the jury was still out (Robinson and Le Grand 1994), it was not easy to reach agreement on whether a market oriented system based on a separation of purchaser and provider roles had brought more benefits than costs (Klein 1995). The assessment produced by the OECD (1994) may have reached positive conclusions, but these were immediately criticised for painting too rosy a picture and being based on inadequate evidence (Bloor and Maynard 1994).

What does emerge from experience is that the reforms contain within their design a number of self-correcting mechanisms. Unlike previous reorganisations, which were planned in great detail with little apparently left to chance, the changes which stem from *Working for Patients* are an example of an emergent strategy (Ham 1994). This is because the White Paper that launched the reforms set the broad framework for change but left out much of the detail. The sketchy nature of *Working for Patients* reflected the tight timetable set by Thatcher for carrying out the review and the fact that the resulting proposals had only been partially thought through. It follows that policy has been made as it has been implemented, leaving much of the responsibility with local staff in the NHS.

Political ideology has in this way been mediated by managerial pragmatism and an assessment of what was likely to be acceptable to the health care professions. As an example, the workload involved in annual contracting led purchasers and providers to move toward longer term service agreements, a move that received the support of health ministers. In parallel, the more radical aspirations of pro-market reformers were modified by the realisation that the competitive scope was limited in many parts of the NHS by the existence of monopoly or near monopoly providers. Even where purchasers had a choice of providers, they often chose to work in collaboration with those hospital and community health service organisations that were particularly significant in their areas. This led to the development of partnership and preferred provider relationships, a move justified in part by experience outside the health sector indicating that many of the most successful companies worked in this way with their suppliers.

A further example of the adjustments made to the reforms in the course of implementation concerned market regulation. The potential dangers of competition developing in an unregulated fashion quickly became clear, leading to the development of a number of rules for dealing with the consequences of competition. Many of these rules were brought together under the guidance of the Department of Health and were presented as a codification of existing practices and case law rather than the development of new procedures (NHS Executive 1994a). This guidance covered issues like provider mergers, purchaser mergers, arrangements for handling providers in difficulty and collusions. In parallel, the role of Regional Health Authorities and their successors, Regional Offices of the NHS Executive, came to include market regulation.

One area in which the reforms did not succeed was in enabling money to follow the patient. This was because most hospitals derived the bulk of their income from block contracts which offered little advantage over the global budgets they replaced. These contracts were largely insensitive to changes in the number of patients treated and they failed to provide the incentives that Thatcher and her advisers had desired. Given the importance of this goal in stimulating the reforms in the first place, the failure of money to follow the patient was a disappointment, not only to the Government, but also to NHS Trusts who continued to carry most of the risks of variations in patient workload.

The effect of these developments was to modify, in some cases significantly, the aspirations of the architects of the reforms. This was reinforced by changes among the politicians responsible for steering through their implementation. The replacement of Thatcher by Major, and the appointment as Secretary of State for Health of a succession of politicians who were more consensual in their approach and less convinced of the merits of competition than Clarke, the Secretary of State at the time *Working for Patients* was published, undoubtedly contributed to this process. By 1996, the impact of these changes was that the main structural elements set out in *Working for Patients* had been implemented but the way in which they were used departed from the original plan in a number of important respects. In particular, the merits of markets and competition were de-emphasised, and the priority shifted to cooperation between purchasers and providers in order to achieve greater responsiveness to patients and provide value for their money.

It was therefore not surprising that when the Labour Party published its policy on the health service in 1995 (Labour Party 1995), it exhibited a willingness to adopt a discriminating response to the reforms and to adapt key elements to suit Labour's own purposes. For example, the value of maintaining a distinction between purchaser and provider roles was accepted. On the other hand, Labour expressed its opposition to general practitioner fundholding and argued instead for a model of general practice commissioning involving general practitioners collaborating with Health Authorities in making purchasing decisions. Labour also committed itself to ending competition within the NHS. However, given that Conservative politicians were themselves emphasising the need for partnership within the NHS (Bottomley 1995), the differences between the two main political parties on this issue were not as great as they appeared. Indeed, what was striking was how much common ground there was between Labour and the Conservatives, particularly in relation to priorities for health policy. This included cross party support for a national health strategy, a primary care led NHS, evidence based medicine and a health service in which the needs of patients received greater attention. To be sure, there remained differences of emphasis and style, as well as lively debates within each party on the direction of reform, but on most of the critical policy questions these were far less important than the areas of agreement.

The election of a Labour Government in May 1997 confirmed these trends. As far as purchasing was concerned, the new Government delayed the establishment of the eighth wave of fundholding in 1998 rather than announcing its intention to abolish the scheme. It also made a commitment to move to common waiting lists within the NHS, thereby preventing fundholders from obtaining quicker appointments for their patients. In parallel, the Government decided that a number of GP commissioning pilots would be set up in which GPs would work together in a locality to influence the development of services. The long term future of fundholding, Health Authority commissioning and their various hybrids was encompassed in a programme of work initiated by the Government to determine what should be put in place of the market. The outcome of this was expected to be known in autumn 1997 when a White Paper on the Government's plans was promised.

This suggests that, after a decade or more of often acrimonious disagreement on the future of the NHS, there is the prospect of a new consensus. This will not involve a return to the pre-reformed NHS, nor will it entail a market driven system. Rather, the NHS will continue to evolve along the path of change that has been set and there are unlikely to be any further changes in the structure of the service beyond those already announced. The emphasis will be placed instead on collaboration between purchasers and providers (or whatever terminology is used to describe these roles) and the use of competition at the margins, if at all.

What this also indicates is that, following a period of activism in UK health policy, the prospects now are for consolidation and assimilation, not further major reforms. Having attracted interest from many countries for being a laboratory of reform, the NHS seems set for quieter times. This judgement is, of course, relative, since change in health care is permanent and is only partly the result of action by politicians. Nevertheless, the stance adopted by the Conservative and Labour parties indicates that the 'big bang' produced by *Working for Patients* is becoming an increasingly faint echo (Klein 1995).

Conclusion

After the shockwaves of recent changes, the NHS defies description in the terms which have traditionally been used to classify health systems. While it remains a national system in name, and in some ways is run in a more centralised manner than ever before, it is also the case that power has been devolved to a local level through both general practitioner fundholding and the establishment of self governing NHS Trusts. Similarly, although the NHS is mainly a public system, both in terms of financing and delivery, there is an increasing blurring of the distinction between the public and private sectors as the mixed economy of health care continues to evolve. And while a market has developed between providers in some parts of the NHS, competition is used alongside regulation in what is best described as a politically managed health care market. Consistent with trends in health care reforms elsewhere in Europe, the UK has moved in a similar direction to the Netherlands and Sweden (Ham and Brommels 1994, Saltman 1994, Ham 1997), as well as New Zealand (Salmond, Mooney and Laugesen 1994). In the process, the aim of using competition to increase efficiency and responsiveness has met with some success (Robinson and Le Grand 1994) but it is difficult to determine whether this should be attributed to the reforms *per se* or to other factors.

What is not in doubt is that the shift from an integrated system to one based on contracts has unsettled established relationships and resulted in an increased capacity to tackle problems in service delivery. Against this, transactions costs have increased and although action has been taken to tackle this trend, there remain concerns about the proportion of the NHS budget spent on administration. The evidence on the respective merits of population centred and patient focused purchasing continues to be contested and is confounded by the emergence of a number of hybrid approaches. As far as purchasing is concerned, the main lesson from the UK is that purchasing in a publicly funded health care system needs to combine elements of the population centred and patient focused approaches, although these need to be effectively co-ordinated if the risk of fragmentation is to be avoided.

References

Audit Commission (1995) *Briefing on GP Fundholding*. HMSO, London

Audit Commission (1996) *What the Doctor Ordered*. HMSO, London

Black, D, Birchall, A and Trimble, I, (1994) Non-fundholding in Nottingham: a vision of the future *British Medical Journal* 309, 930–932

Bloor, K and Maynard, A 1994. An Outsider's View of the NHS Reforms *British Medical Journal* 309, 352–353

Bottomley, V (1994) National health, local dynamic *The Independent* 22 August

Bottomley, V (1995) *The NHS: Continuity and Change* Department of Health, London

Bradlow, J and Coulter, A (1993) Effects of NHS reforms on prescribing rates in general practice *British Medical Journal* 307, 1186–1189.

Brindle, D (1995) Spending up £1bn on NHS Bureaucrats *The Guardian* 6 February, 3

Carruthers, I, Fillingham, D, Ham, CJ and James, JH (1995) *Purchasing in the NHS: The Story So Far* Health Services Management Centre, University of Birmingham, Birmingham

Coulter, A and Bradlow, J (1993) Effects of NHS reforms on general practitioners' referral patterns *British Medical Journal* 306, 433–437

Coulter, A (1995) General Practice Fundholding: Time for a Cool Appraisal, *British Journal of General Practice* 45, 119–120

Dixon, J, Dinwoodie, M, Hodson, D, *et al*. (1994) Distribution of NHS funds between fundholding and non fundholding practices *British Medical Journal* 309, 30–34

Dixon, J and Glennerster, H (1995) What do we know about fundholding in general practice? *British Medical Journal*, 311, 727–30

Dowell, JS, Snodden, D and Dunbar, JA (1995) Changes to Generic Formulary: How One Fundholding Practice Reduced Prescribing Costs *British Medical Journal* 310, 505–508

Enthoven, A (1985) *Reflections on the Management of the NHS* Nuffield Provincial Hospitals Trust, London

Glennerster, H, Matsaganis, M and Owens, P with Hancock, S (1994) *Implementing GP Fundholding* Open University Press, Buckingham

Glennerster, H, Matsaganis, M and Owens, P (1992) *A Foothold for Fundholding* King's Fund Institute, London

Graffy, J and Williams, J (1994) Purchasing for All: An Alternative to Fundholding *British Medical Journal* 308, 391–394

Ham, CJ (ed) (1997) *Health Care Reform: Learning from International Experience* Open University Press, Buckingham

Ham, CJ (1994) 'Where now for the NHS reforms?' *British Medical Journal* 309, 352

Ham, CJ and Willis, A (1994) Think Globally, Act Locally *Health Service Journal* 27–28

Ham, CJ, Robinson, R and Benzeval, M (1990) *Health Check* King's Fund Institute, London

Ham, CJ and Shapiro, J (1995a) The Future of Fundholding *British Medical Journal* 310, 1150–1151

Ham, CJ and Shapiro, J (1995b) *Integrating Purchasing* Health Services Management Centre, University of Birmingham, Birmingham

Ham, CJ, Honigsbaum, F and Thompson, D (1994) *Priority Setting for Health Gain* Department of Health, London

Ham, CJ and Brommels, M (1994) Health Care Reform in the Netherlands, Sweden and United Kingdom *Health Affairs* Winter

Howie, J, Heaney, D and Maxwell, M (1995a) *General Practice Fundholding: Shadow Project – An Evaluation* Department of General Practice, University of Edinburgh, Edinburgh

Howie, J, Heaney, D and Maxwell, M (1995b) Care of Patients with selected health problems in fundholding practices in Scotland in 1990 and 1992: needs, process and outcome *British Journal of General Practice* 45, 121–126

Howie, J, Heaney, D and Maxwell, M (1994) Evaluating Care of Patients Reporting Pain in Fundholding Practices *British Medical Journal* 309, 705–710

James, JH (1994) *Transforming the NHS: The View from Inside* Centre for the Analysis of Social Policy, University of Bath, Bath

Klein, RE and Redmayne, S (1992) *Patterns of Priorities* National Association of Health Authorities and Trusts, Birmingham

Klein, RE (1995) *The New Politics of the NHS* Longman, London

Labour Party (1995) *Renewing the NHS* Labour Party, London

Light, D (1994) *Strategic Challenges in Joint Commissioning* North West Thames Regional Health Authority, London

Mawhinney, B and Nichol, D (1993) *Purchasing for Health* NHS Management Executive, Leeds

Maxwell, M, Heaney, D, Howie, J and Noble, S (1993) General Practice Fundholding: Observations on Prescribing Patterns and Costs Using the Defined Daily Dose Method *British Medical Journal* 307, 1190–1194

Mays, N and Dixon, J (1996) *Purchaser Plurality in UK Health Care* King's Fund, London

Mohan, J (1995) *A National Health Service?* Macmillan, London

National Audit Office (1994) *General Practitioner Fundholding in England* HMSO, London

Newton, J, Fraser, M, Robinson, J and Wainwright, D (1993) Fundholding in the Northern Region: the first year *British Medical Journal* **306**, 375–378

NHS Executive (1994a) *The Operation of the Internal Market: Local Freedoms, National Responsibilities* NHS Executive, London

NHS Executive (1994b) *Developing NHS Purchasing and GP Fundholding* NHS Executive, London

NHS Management Executive (1992) *Local Voices* NHS Management Executive, London

NHS Executive (1995) *An Accountability Framework for GP Fundholding* NHS Executive, Leeds

Nicholl, J, Beeby, WR and Williams, BT (1989) Roles of the Private Sector in Elective Surgery in England and Wales 1986 *British Medical Journal*, **289**, 243–247

OECD (1992) *The Reform of Health Care: A Comparative Analysis of Seven OECD Countries*, OECD, Paris

OECD (1994) *OECD Economic Surveys: United Kingdom 1994* OECD, Paris

Public Accounts Committee (1995) *General Practitioner Fundholding in England* Twenty Seventh Report Session 1994–95 HMSO, London

Radical Statistics Health Group (1992) NHS Reforms: The First Six Months – proof of progress or a statistical smokescreen? *British Medical Journal* **304**, 705–709

Radical Statistics Health Group (1995) NHS 'indicators of success': What Do They Tell Us? *British Medical Journal* **310**, 1045–1050

Redmayne, S, Klein, RE and Day, P (1993) *Sharing Out Resources* National Association of Health Authorities and Trusts, Birmingham

Redmayne, S (1995) *Reshaping the NHS* National Association of Health Authorities and Trusts, Birmingham

Roberts, J (1990) Kenneth Clarke: hatchet man or remoulder? *British Medical Journal* **301**, 1383–1386

Robinson, R and Le Grand, J (eds) (1994) *Evaluating the NHS Reforms* King's Fund Institute, London

Salmond, G, Mooney, G and Laugesen, M (eds) (1994) Health Care Reform in New Zealand *Health Policy* Special Issue, 29

Saltman, R (1994) A Conceptual Overview of Recent Health Care Reforms *European Journal of Public Health* **4**, 287–293

Saltman, R and von Otter, C (1992) *Planned Markets and Public Competition* Open University Press, Buckingham

Secretary of State for Health *et al.* (1989) *Working for Patients*, HMSO, London

Secretary of State for Health (1992) *The Health of the Nation* HMSO, London

Shapiro, J (1994) *Shared Purchasing and Collaborative Commissioning within the NHS* National Association of Health Authorities and Trusts, Birmingham

Sheldon, T, Smith, P, Browitz, M, Martin, S and Carr-Hill, R (1994) Attempt at deriving a formula for setting general practitioner fundholding budgets *British Medical Journal* **309**, 1059–1064

Smith, J, Bamford, M, Ham, CJ, Scrivens, E and Shapiro, J (1997) *Beyond Fundholding: A Mosaic of Primary Care Led Commissioning and Provision in the West Midlands* Health Services Management Centre, University of Birmingham and Centre for Health Planning and Management, Keele University

2 A public health perspective

Rod Griffiths and Bernard Crump

Introduction

This chapter is written at a time of intense change in the NHS. The election on 1 May 1997 produced a landslide for the Labour Party and a sea change at the centre of the NHS. The announcement in the subsequent Queen's Speech (1997) that the internal market was to be abolished effectively called into question everything that had stood for the last five years and more. At the same time the new Government made it clear that they understood the disruption that can be caused by major organisational change. At the time of writing relatively little of the new Government's ideas have emerged in enough detail to make substantial comment. This chapter therefore attempts to learn lessons from the experience of the market reforms of recent years and to analyse some of the challenges facing the new Government as it attempts to put its declared programme into action.

What have we learned from the reforms?

Probably the most dramatic lesson from the experience of introducing the reforms of the 1990s is the discovery of the extent to which people will change their role and behaviour on cue. Prior to the reforms the NHS was a coherent management system with no more than the usual interpersonal tensions. Suddenly different groups of managers were divided into two camps as purchasers and providers and told to be in conflict with each other and almost without exception people who had previously worked together entered into conflict relationships. It remains to be seen whether the new Government can undo the process by creating a duty of partnership.

The second significant lesson must be that the system does respond to incentives, so it is important to get them right. Saying that we want quality but giving incentives to volume will produce volume whatever the strength of the rhetoric about quality. At the moment more Health Authorities and

Trusts are overspent than ever before. Again this is probably because of the wrong mix of rhetoric and incentives. Ministers in the past frequently said that money would follow patients. Clinicians interpreted that to mean that they could treat as many patients as they could and that someone would pay. At the same time purchasers' budgets were capped and Trusts' contracts had limits in them. There were no incentives to clinicians to comply with cash limits so we ended up with a system where the game was to try and move the risk to the other party. Purchasers tried to create contracts where the risk for overperformance was with the Trust and the Trust tried to get the risk to the purchaser. Only seldom did purchasers and Trust managers try to work together to get the best service they could for the money available. The financial pressure caused by these fault lines in the system has built up year on year. The current system has failed to manage the financial risks. It could be that this is made worse by the overall financial position being tighter than usual but it is still the case that a publicly funded system should be able to manage within the funds available. If it cannot then there is something wrong with it.

The current system can also claim some successes; for instance, it can claim to provide a way of getting resources to populations on a formula that can be adjusted to meet need. That formula is now more complex and better adjusted to need than ever before. There are still some suspicions that additional political fudges have been added, like the market forces factor which appears to favour London. Fundholding has demonstrated that it is possible to give GPs more say in care. The challenge remains that this only works for those GPs with the skill and the will to take it on while others have no guarantee of influence. Patients' choice is not built in any effective way at the individual level although CHCs remain potentially effective at the population level.

In part, the problem has been one of direction, ie the pressure has been for achievements of volume, but part of the problem comes from the wish of trusts to succeed. At the moment the only measure of success is income, so all trusts tend to try to get bigger, do more work and expand. On a finite NHS budget this is doomed to failure and the current cash crisis is in part driven by this. It is likely that money will always produce incentives to get more so we need to reward quality rather than volume and find a way to limit the possibilities for Trusts to grow out of control. An additional lesson that has attracted political attention is that by putting an emphasis on contracts a huge volume of paper (or electronic records) has been generated along with spurious activity tracking money and patients in the system. It is often hard to see the connection between that activity and better health care, although clarity about what we get for the money may be a necessary precursor to decisions which can make better care.

What does the system have to achieve?

The NHS is funded from Government revenues and apart from a very minor income here and there from fees or commercial activities it gets all its money from the Government. The NHS therefore has to be accountable to Parliament. The Secretary of State is allocated money in the budget and is permitted by various Acts of Parliament to spend it on improving the health of the population, which he is expected to achieve by investing in health services. At the same time other Government Departments may also carry out Acts which may improve health or put it at risk. The extent to which these different activities are co-ordinated for the common good is a matter for the Government to decide, but they are not in the direct control of the Secretary of State for Health.

The health system has to get its money from the Exchequer to the providers of health care. At the same time there are a number of other things that it is desirable for the system to achieve (Box 2.1).

Box 2.1 What should the organisation of the NHS achieve?

- *To ensure equity of health outcome across the population*
  So that wherever you live your chances of good health are as near as possible equal

- *To give incentives to quality*
  To ensure that money is more likely to go into treatments that work best and hence that we get more health for the money

- *To manage financial risk*
  To ensure that we do not spend more than we are allocated

- *To get decisions and care as close to the patient as possible*
  Both through involving GPs in care and creating opportunities for patient choice

- *To give incentives to work effectively with other key players*
  Social Services are very important but so are other arms of Government like transport, housing and employment which are not effectively included at the moment

- *To make efficient use of public money*
  Once we are spending the money in the right place and on the right things it is still important to minimise the cost so that we get the most health care for the money

---

To ensure equity of health outcome across the population

In one form or another this has been a stated aim of Governments for a very long time. The appointment regulations for consultants which date back to the late 1940s and early 1950s (SI 1948, 1950) were intended to make standards the same across the country. Enoch Powell's hospital plan (Ministry of Health 1962) aimed to make access to good care available across the country by creating a network of modern hospitals. These early attempts at equity were aimed at setting standards, but since then we have concentrated more on aiming at equity of resource allocation. Since David Owen and Barbara Castle introduced the Resource Allocation Working Party (DHSS 1976) we have seen more and more refined formulae being developed with the aim of measuring need and allocating money to meet it. Each attempt has met two fundamental problems, the first is how to define need and equity with the statistics that happen to be available and the second is to manage the pace of change of any proposed redistribution that appears to be necessary when the new formula emerges.

Throughout this period the service has probably been gradually moving towards a more equitable distribution of resources but that does not mean that places with high deprivation have automatically been gaining throughout this period. Birmingham, for instance, which has some of the largest deprived populations, has been a loser throughout the last decade and more, principally because at the beginning of the period it had a large stock of old hospitals that used to provide services to the rest of the region around it. The deprived population are not necessarily made healthy by having masses of older hospitals but once the population have got used to them they are hard to close.

The pace of change that can be tolerated is influenced by several factors. If the pace is too rapid then there are high costs associated with redundancies and other costs of downsizing in the losing districts while at the same time staff cannot be trained and recruited fast enough in the gainers so money accumulates or is spent on things that appear unimportant. At the same time, where institutions have to close or services have to change significantly there are political costs and risks which make change more difficult. Achieving equity almost always means that more attention will be focused on the losers but there will almost never be enough money in the system to make it possible to achieve equity only by levelling up.

The new Government is determined to achieve equity but it has not yet said what it means by it. Aiming at equity of health outcome could open the way to break out of the current dilemmas about resource allocation. It may be that new concepts such as health action zones may be a possible route. Perhaps by changing the rules that get in the way of closer collaboration and providing some pump priming money it might be possible to concentrate efforts on attacking the causes of unequal health rather than trying to achieve an equitable distribution of health services. At best this deals with problems at too late a stage, after a heart attack for instance, and may be able to achieve nothing at all, as is frequently the case with lung cancer.

To give incentives to quality

One of the more remarkable features of the last few years has been the acceptance of the clinical effectiveness agenda and the concomitant rise in pressure for evidence based medicine. Embracing this agenda is an acceptance of the embarrassing fact that standards of care and outcomes vary widely across the country. The previous Government, backed by pressure from the Treasury, pressed very hard for efficiency which was measured in crude terms as activity per pound. It did not matter what the activity was.

There is no doubt that doctors found this distasteful, particularly as examples began to emerge where the pressure for crude efficiency was making good care harder to do and rewarding poor care. The most obvious example would be that if a patient was discharged too soon and this led to a readmission this appeared as two admissions and appeared to be more efficient.

Pressure from the professions led to the acceptance of the clinical effectiveness agenda, though the Government never accepted head on that the two agendas might be in conflict and no attempt was made to find a way of creating a balanced set of incentives which reconciled the two pressures. The challenge for the new Government will be to find ways of encouraging the system to deliver the right thing at the right price. The proposed new framework for measuring outcomes is a step in the right direction. (*The New NHS* Cmd. 3807 1997.)

To manage financial risk

Since 1976 when cash limits were first introduced one of the tasks of any system of organisation of the NHS must be to manage financial risk. The NHS is a large system and so its overall behaviour can be predicted with a fair degree of statistical certainty, but the individual parts are smaller and thus vulnerable to chance variation. In addition, the competence of the various managers varies as does the size of the agenda facing them at any one time. It is all too common to find instances where managers take their eye off the financial ball because they are distracted by other priorities. One of the prerequisites of the system as a whole is that there must be checks and balances and monitoring mechanisms which ensure that financial control is maintained.

To get decisions and care as close to the patient as possible

One of the successes of the last set of reforms has been the way that fundholding has got GPs into the system in a way that was never achieved before. Unfortunately it has also been accompanied by some of the worst aspects of those changes; increased bureaucracy and transaction costs and occasionally petty wrangling to no benefit to patients. What is needed is a method of preserving the involvement of GPs and the sensitivity to individual patient needs that this brings, while at the same time reducing the transaction costs and bureaucracy associated with fundholding. The White Paper has opted for locality commissioning where costs are reduced by working in larger groups, but the involvement of individual GPs is preserved. Some work needs to be done to determine the ideal locality and to decide whether it should be based on GP lists or on geographical areas. In rural areas these often amount to the same thing but in inner-city areas with high deprivation and population mobility the two approaches may be quite different to handle. The added problem of the inner-cities is that rather more of the GP practices are single-handed and this makes it harder to get groups of GPs to work together.

To give incentives to work effectively with other key players

The current system gives virtually no incentives to collaboration. The same could be said of systems in other statutory agencies. This is clearly a significant defect. If it could be remedied it would considerably help work on the wider public health agenda. The new duty of partnership a new idea which may be very radical despite its apparent simplicity.

The new public health agenda

The new Government has set out a number of aims including reducing waiting lists and management costs but as this chapter is concerned with public health it will concentrate on the public health agenda that has been established. This is the first Government to appoint a Minister for Public Health. While this makes it obvious that public health will be seen as more important in the future there is bound to be a period of uncertainty while the priorities of the new Minister emerge. At the time of writing the most useful guide is the speech by Tessa Jowell on 7 July 1997 (Jowell 1997) to a conference launching the new health strategy.

The speech covered familiar ground for those steeped in the history of public health. The Minister made it clear that public health was at the heart of a range of new Government policies. She referred back to Beveridge's five giants that were the cause of ill health and made it clear that there were going to be policies to tackle each of them. **Want** would be tackled through the minimum wage; **idleness** through welfare to work; **squalor** through improved housing, utilising capital receipts from the sale of council housing and though policies to improve the environment; **ignorance** will be tackled through policies to improve education; and **disease** through rescuing the NHS, tackling tobacco, and the Food Standards Agency.

It was made clear that action will be needed at a number of levels, across Government, at the local level and by individuals themselves. A Green Paper will be published which will set out how these levels relate to each other and make clear the most important areas for action. This sort of perspective, namely that improvements in public health require action across a range of social structures, is not new. The Ottowa Charter stated that the fundamental requirements for good health were:

- peace;
- shelter;
- education;
- food;
- income;
- a stable eco-system;
- sustainable resources;
- social justice;
- equity.

It is clear that the present Government is committed to action in all of these areas. The Ottowa Charter ends with a pledge which clearly defines the direction that this Government has adopted (Box 2.2).

Box 2.2 The participants in this Conference pledge:

- to move into the arena of healthy public policy, and to advocate a clear political commitment to health and equity in all sectors;

- to counteract the pressures towards harmful products, resource depletion, unhealthy living conditions and environments, and bad nutrition; and to focus attention on public health issues such as pollution, occupational hazards, housing and settlements;

- to respond to the health gap within and between societies, and to tackle the inequities in health produced by the rules and practices of these societies;

- to acknowledge people as the main health resource; to support and enable them to keep themselves, their families and friends healthy through financial and other means, and to accept the community as the essential voice in matters of its health, living conditions and well-being;

- to reorient health services and their resources towards the promotion of health; and to share power with other sectors, other disciplines and, most importantly, with people themselves;

- to recognize health and its maintenance as a major social investment and challenge; and to address the overall ecological issue of our ways of living.

Deprivation

The new Government has given significant commitments to tackling the health effects of deprivation. A new enquiry has been set up led by Sir Donald Acheson to look at what can be done. The complexity of the task can be illustrated by the contrasting data on a number of common diseases. Skin cancer is more common in the better off while lung cancer is much more common in the poorer groups. However when we look at the effects of treatment we find that the survival gradient for melanoma is much flatter than the incidence gradient. In other words, although poorer people are much less likely to get melanoma when they do get it they are less likely to survive it. In the case of lung cancer the disadvantage is doubled, not only are the poor more likely to get the disease but they are even less likely to survive when they do get it. The reasons for these differences are still being investigated. In the West Midlands we have looked at both heart attacks and breast cancer. In each case the relationship holds that irrespective of incidence, the survival rates for those who get the disease are lower in the poorer sections of the community. When we look at survival in hospital there is no difference. It appears that most of the difference in survival between different social groups has already been created before they get to the hospital service. This may be because poorer people get worse primary care, because they look after themselves less well, are exposed to greater health hazards or get more severe forms of the disease. Whatever the cause it seems clear that the research and the remedy lies in the community and in primary care rather than in hospitals. Attacks on social inequality are more likely to be effective by targeting resources in that direction than simply pressing to have a resource allocation formula that allocates money fairly, because 90 per cent of the NHS money at the moment goes to hospitals. In hospitals it no doubt does good work but it does not impact on inequalities.

Making a substantial difference to the health effects of deprivation will really require a different society. Public health, in the Acheson definition, is involved in organising the efforts of society to achieve better health. This means that public health practitioners should be key players in taking forward this agenda. The fundamental problem is to decide what agency is responsible for delivering the change. At the political level this is now clear; there is a Minister for Public Health. The kind of measures that are necessary are very wide. They span policies on unemployment, wage differentials, the range of social security benefits, housing, the environment as well as health. Only the Prime Minister's office covers the whole span. There have been suggestions from time-to-time that public health and its Ministry should be directly answerable to the Prime Minister. However, the decision has been made that the Public Health Minister is in the Department of Health. The White Paper with a foreword from the Prime Minister confirms that the lead role will go to Health Authorities. New legislation and guidance must therefore determine how the Department of Health and Health Authorities are to exert influence over this range of policy areas and co-ordinate them in such a way as to produce change in health status in the deprived parts of the community.

Organising the efforts of society

Patterns of disease

Some diseases and some health hazards are more common than others and none are distributed entirely evenly across the country. Furthermore, the population structure varies considerably in different districts, whether it be the presence or absence of different ethnic groups or the clustering of the elderly in certain favoured retirement areas. This means that no one form of organisation is likely to suit every circumstance. Rare diseases can be sufficiently uncommon that local Health Authorities simply do not have enough experience of them to know how to plan services. On the other hand, common diseases can be planned for and treated at the lowest level in the system because everyone sees enough to be familiar with what is needed. In the past health services have been organised around hospitals because they consumed the most money and therefore appeared to require the most management attention. If the health service was to be organised in order to maximise health then it needs to be organised around the patterns of disease and what causes them. The Calman–Hine report on cancer services has shown how this is possible. Common cancers can be treated in most acute hospitals provided they are able to maintain enough surgeons and oncological support to deliver site specialisation while less common cancers require collaboration over a wider area. In every previous version of the organisation of the NHS there have been some services that have been planned and funded at the national level, others at regional level and others by consortia of districts while the common diseases which make up the vast majority have been funded and planned for at the local level. It is inevitable that some similar mechanism will be required in the new arrangements. It is already clear that attempting to do without a regional tier is causing some problems, some specialised services have been lost and others seriously weakened by attempting to pretend that these can be organised by groups of districts. The districts always have local pressures which will take first place when funds are tight and there will be no-one to champion the rarer problems. Almost by definition this will not lead to immediate problems because the diseases are uncommon and it takes time for anyone to notice a pattern of poor care. The absence of a purchasing tier at the region is entirely unnecessary. The White Paper has remedied this problem by making the Region office responsible for creating an effective mechanism.

Patterns of social organisation

Just as diseases have their patterns, so does society. There have been various attempts to find ideal arrangements for governing below the national level. In the end most efforts tend to come back to using natural communities as the base to work from with some attempt at overview through some form of intermediate tier. It is interesting to make international comparisons. There are obvious issues created by geography and history as well as patterns of transport etc. It is noticeable however that most Western countries are either made up of populations of less than 10 million or are divided into regions which are that sort of size. In the USA there are about 200 million people in 50 states, an average of 4 million per state, although some are as small as a million and one or two are over 20 million. Across Europe we also tend to see units of Government at about the 3–8 million mark. Within the UK the three smaller countries are all in this range and the 8 regions of the NHS are a similar size, comparable to the Scandinavian countries, the Czech Republic or French regions. At the more local level cities of much over a million as unitary Governments are rare, though they are often surrounded by wider conurbations which are often not entirely part of the same local Government. Units below 100,000 are also uncommon. In part this arises from the way things are, presumably driven by economic and social pressures. Another important factor is the simple cost of Government. If the unit is too small the cost of maintaining a Government machine is too great an overhead to be borne by the taxpayer and however much smaller units may crave an individual identity they cannot afford a Government machine. The new organisation of the NHS will reflect exactly these social constraints.

If better public health is the aim then some way has to be found of working within these natural constraints of social organisation and epidemiology. It is inevitable that there will be no one organisational model which will fit all diseases. Public health activities must operate across these natural boundaries. Collaboration and multisectoral working are the key. Co-terminosity of boundaries with the other major players makes collaboration much easier.

Collaboration

Collaboration with other partners is known to be an essential part of gaining greater health in the population but it does not happen by accident. Experience over the last few years in the West Midlands shows that there are a number of prerequisites for good collaboration to happen. When the reforms began there were 22 Health Authorities and 11 FHSAs in the region. There are now 13 authorities each of which combines the functions of DHAs and FHSAs. This has meant mergers and divisions. Every year since 1990 there has been a different number of Health Authorities in the region. Over the same period there have also been substantial changes in personnel and some significant ups and downs on the financial side. Against this turmoil it is possible to see quite clearly that collaboration with local authorities requires organisational, financial and personal stability. Those authorities that have been least affected by these changes have the best record of collaboration. Collaboration is least good and most fragile in the places where there has been the greatest change in boundaries, people and financial position. It does not matter which party is subject to the upheaval. If either is subject to substantial organisational change or has a significant financial problem then effective collaboration will cease. Even if all these prerequisites are in place there may still be problems, created by other factors such as political differences and individual competence but it would be as well in the future to remember the losses of potential collaborative work that are inevitable if there is substantial organisational change. Any potential gains from collaborative work will be lost for two or three years if there is substantial organisational change.

Likely direction of changes

The White Paper is fresh off the press and many issues remain to be developed but some clarity can be distinguished.

A population base

There will be a population based Health Authority which acts as the unit to which resource are allocated. The public health responsibilities of these bodies are emphasised. This level will also be responsible for ensuring the performance of primary care. At this stage it is not clear how large the population will be that is cared for by such authorities. There has been some speculation that authorities might be larger. It could be suggested that this would reduce costs but larger organisations are significantly more difficult to manage and are inevitably more remote from the population they serve. Even if their main function is to oversee primary care the sheer numbers involved in authorities of over a million population are daunting. A population of 2 million could be expected to have 1,000 or more GPs. It would be difficult for a managing authority to maintain much of a personal relationship with that many GPs.

Primary care

If primary care is to have a significant impact on the rest of the system it has to be better organised. What the public want is a service with a single point of entry that provides polite and friendly 24-hour access to lifelong care. They want it to take their needs into account and give them access to more specialised care if they need it. Ideally they would like it to conform to publicly declared standards so that they can tell when they have just cause to complain.

At the moment primary care does not deliver this across the whole of the NHS. There are notable examples where the Service conforms to this ideal and goes further in committing itself to evidence based medicine as well. Some Health Authorities have set out standards and gone public about trying to enforce them. The Director of Public Health for Birmingham has included a map showing all the substandard practices in the city in her 1997 annual report (BHA 1997) together with a commitment by the Authority that the worst will be remedied by next year. There is no reason why this sort of performance management should not be standard practice.

Primary care is often confused with general practice. As long as we remain dependant on large numbers of single-handed practices and small partnerships this myth will be preserved. Good primary care requires a team of people in a co-ordinated range of roles. This does not happen without some structure and management and that is virtually impossible from a single-handed lock-up surgery. The most obvious method of organisation is to run primary care from health centres from which a range of staff and facilities can be provided. Gradually this is becoming the preferred model but there are still many practices and community health staff who do not work from decent premises. An obvious approach is to cluster a group of practices and their associated community staff together in one management unit so that complementary services that can be provided from such premises are available but the patients of each of the practices can be guaranteed access to a full range of facilities and skills within the cluster. These kinds of arrangement also facilitate locality commissioning. Some of these groups may in future be Primary Care Trusts.

If primary care is to deliver the benefits that it is capable of then there has to be a real attempt to manage it better. The most fundamental change is to move on from fundholding to a position where all of the health service activity associated with a particular practice or locality is made visible to that practice. Only if they can see all the activity can they be expected to think about how it could be better. It is not necessary that every item of health care be bought and sold with its associated transaction costs. The important thing is that it is visible to those who are managing primary care and hence capable of influencing the events surrounding each patient's care.

If Health Authorities are to be expected to improve primary care they are bound to want to see a more coherent management system. Without that there will always be a temptation to want to organise it themselves or contract it out to someone who can. If the essential fabric of general practice is to be preserved and developed within a comprehensive primary care system then it is almost inevitable that the Government will have to espouse some new models of organisation that are not in the Red Book.

The recent legislation, passed just before the Election, gives the necessary powers to pilot new ways of operating. The Government is fortunate to have these measures already on the Statute Book which should allow them to make changes far more quickly than if they had to resort to primary legislation.

Hospitals

The development of NHS Trusts freed hospital management to get on with what it saw as its job. In the best cases this produced better quality of care and more efficient hospitals. In other places it has produced insularity, defensiveness and inadequate control of quality. The performance management regime for trusts was only concerned with money. There is virtually no formal mechanism through which quality of care is monitored. The Patients' Charter provides a framework for examining what might be called hotel quality but it does not measure quality of health care. The only influence at the moment is the approval process for training posts that is carried out by the Royal Colleges and the Post Graduate Dean. A further source of information is the reporting of untoward incidents to the Regional Office but none of these amounts to a systematic survey of medical quality. The new Government is serious about making clinical quality an important benchmark and the White Paper introduces the concept of Clinical Governance in order to back this up. Quality will become part of the formal duties of Trusts.

Partnership

One major feature of any new change is bound to be a move towards greater partnership. It remains to be seen whether simply announcing that partnership is the order of the day will be enough. It would be possible to create pressures to make it work by making both parties responsible for failures. At the moment there is everything to be gained from negotiating a contract that leaves the risk with the other party. Similarly, although the system at the moment is supposed to be based on clear accounting principles, trusts will often try to hide information from their purchasers. If both parties to a contract were to be made responsible for its failure then the situation might begin to change. What would be required is that in the event of a serious problem with a contract both parties would report to the Regional Office on the reason for the failure and explain what they were going to do about it. Again the implication would have to be that in the event of serious failure that was not rectified by appropriate joint action then both parties would find that their performance related pay was reduced or in the worst case both were fired. Without such sanctions it is difficult to see what the incentives might be that would ensure that partnership gets off the ground in an effective way.

Implications for public health

Although the new system emphasises the importance of public health there are dangers for the specialty. The focus for public health activity is probably most appropriate at the district and regional level. Public health practitioners must effectively act in four main areas; within the NHS, currently mostly called commissioning; with other statutory agencies, mostly local authorities; in and alongside primary care, mostly working with GPs; and finally, directly with the public and other non-statutory bodies through health promotion in its widest sense. Current resources and constraints are such that very few districts manage to be fully effective in more than two out of the four areas. The greater emphasis on public health from the new Government means that demand for activity in each of these areas could increase significantly.

If locality commissioning became a major part of the system it is likely to need public health advice on a significant scale. Already there are a number of examples of total purchasing projects buying public health skills by contributing to the cost of consultant posts or having posts seconded to them. If each locality were to ask for as much public health advice as was provided in the Bromsgrove Total Purchasing Project (a population of 40,000) then roughly double the number of public health doctors would be needed. This could be done by other public health professionals but the total resources would still amount to a huge increase. Similarly, if there was a significant demand, as there should be, for more work in health advocacy and greater collaboration with voluntary bodies and with industry, then again there would be a need for more personnel and they would need to be able to adapt to working in these areas. The same could be said for work with local authorities and within the NHS if there is a greater demand for work on quality and outcomes. There is no way that the specialty as currently organised can accommodate such an increase in manpower.

With so many different demands there would be a great temptation for public health staff to move into the most exciting of the available projects leaving less interesting areas and Health Authorities short of staff. If that happens at the same time as the public health agenda for Health Authorities is expanded then the specialty could come under severe strain with real risk of fragmentation of effort and the risk of failure in unexpected ways. The Government has already exempted Public Health from management cost targets in an effort to get adequate staffing into place.

Where could the manpower come from?

Over the last three years there has been continuing debate within the Faculty of Public Health Medicine and in other bodies with an interest in public health about how different interests should best work together. Several years ago a study (Somervaille and Griffiths 1995) showed that there was a considerable number of non-medical staff working in and associated with public health departments. These staff were well qualified, having a variety of master and doctorate qualifications. They worked as epidemiologists, statisticians, information officers, geographers and in other *ad hoc* posts. Some are quite senior, while the majority are in junior posts in which there is rapid turnover and poor long term career prospects.

In the past this workforce was poorly organised with little attempt being made to provide consistent training to any agreed standards. By contrast, there is a well established training programme for doctors in public health but it takes five years to create a fully qualified consultant. Over the last 10 years there has been a concerted effort to train more doctors but it has largely been frustrated by early retirements made possible by frequent organisational change and increasingly stringent management cost targets which have squeezed out public health posts which appear expensive in the short term. If a similar enhanced recruitment programme was to be launched now it would produce consultants in public health medicine in time for the next Government.

Two things can be done in the shorter term. First by releasing management cost targets it should be possible to unfreeze vacancies and guarantee that able trainees do not leave the specialty. Furthermore, some of the recently retired might be tempted into at least part-time work. The second major opportunity is to enhance the training and career prospects of the public health profession from a multi-disciplinary background, scientists who clearly wish to work in public health but cannot find jobs. It is essential that they should have access to a full range of career posts. In other countries the medical profession is less possessive about hanging on to the top jobs. It is quite clear that some of the senior jobs must be filled by doctors, both because there is a clinical component and because there is a public expectation. At the same time it is impossible to imagine that there could never be a non-medical scientist who could run a public health department. If we are to have the people available to be able to do justice to this Government's desire to see improvements in public health then there is no choice but to move as rapidly as possible to a truly multidisciplinary profession. This means that the MPH or other suitable qualification must be agreed upon as the common currency and a national scheme of accreditation created. This would allow the creation of additional posts with a clear method of securing standards in the same way that the standards of the medical posts are ensured through the MFPHM qualification and specialist registration with the GMC.

Leadership in public health

Whatever the structure and funding that underpins it, public health practice is about getting other people to do things which will benefit society in general or sections of it. The actions are almost always done by particular individuals while the benefits are usually felt by unnamed individuals who often do not realise what has been done for them. Persuading people to act in these circumstances requires that they become committed to altruism without the normal person to person reward that goes with such acts in everyday life. It is generally recognised that legislation is the most powerful way to bring about such public health activity because it is the accepted method by which society encourages action for the general good. Unfortunately, legislation can frequently do no more than provide authority and sometimes resources for public health actions. On a day-to-day level such things must compete for priority alongside all the other pressures on those who might act. Getting public health activity to the top of the agendas of all the various parties who might be able to do something useful requires leadership.

Leadership in public health has many of the attributes of leadership in other areas but it has some distinct characteristics as well. The most significant difference from that required in general management is that public health practitioners must frequently try to lead people over whom they have no direct control. Leadership across organisational boundaries is the fundamental art and skill required in order to create intersectoral activity.

Little attention has been paid in public health training either to define what the necessary skills might be, to train for them or to select people who appear likely to develop them. The emphasis in the last decade and a half has been to secure an adequate manpower base for the specialty and gradually to recognise the importance within public health of the range of skills that can be brought to bear. The debate within the Faculty of Public Health Medicine about whether or not to allow full membership by examination to non-medical members has been a sad reflection on just how inward looking doctors can be. It has done nothing to focus attention on what it takes to achieve action across a multisectoral agenda.

Some of the necessary skills are already well embedded in training. For instance it is clear that public health practitioners must be able to collect, evaluate and analyse data from many different sources and bring it together to produce pictures of health and the threats to it. The reinstitution of annual reports by the Acheson Committee in 1988 went a long way to create a platform from which public health messages can be projected. Many different styles and methods of writing and production have been used to get the messages from annual reports into the media and on to the agendas of key players in the community. There is no doubt that skills in this area will continue to be vital. However if these messages are to be effective they need to be backed up by managerial and political activity that secures action. Public health doctors seem to have been less good at these latter activities. They face a daunting task. Their salary is paid by the NHS and they are accountable on a day-to-day basis to Chief Executives and Chairmen in the NHS. In order to be able to act in a multisectoral way they must first do enough within the NHS to prove their value to the Chief Executive and other Directors. When they have earned that respect and secured adequate resources they then have to persuade those same people that some of these scarce resources that they have come to value within the organisation must be deployed outside it, to no immediate gain for the organisation. To Chief Executives who for the last five years have been focused on a very short-term and efficiency driven agenda such multisectoral work can appear to be a distraction. Public health practitioners are effectively told to pull for the organisation or shut up. The leadership and persuasion skills necessary in order to both secure a seat at the table and leave it vacant part of the time are considerable. It is not surprising that many have opted for getting their seat and then sticking to the priorities within the organisation in order to maintain their base. Multisectoral activity has suffered as a result.

The real challenge to the new Government is not only to find ways of permitting public health practitioners to work across all segments of the agenda but also to develop people with the leadership skills to be able to function as leaders in each of these very different areas. As this chapter is being written, the Chief Medical Officer is leading a new project to look at the capacity of the public health forces across the different levels of activity. It is to be hoped that this project will pay some attention not only where leaders might come from and how many we might need but also to the skills they will need and the ways in which they can be developed.

References

Great Britain, Ministry of Health, National Health Service (1962) *A hospital plan for England and Wales* Cmnd 1604 HMSO, London

Great Britain, Department of Health and Social Security (1976) *Sharing resources for health in England: report of the resource allocation working party,* HMSO, London

Jowell, T (1997) *Public Health Strategy. Speech by the Minister of Public Health Tessa Jowell 7 July 1997* Department of Health Press Release H97 157

Report of the Director of Public Health (1997) Birmingham Health Authority, Birmingham

The Queen's Speech opening Parliament (14 May 1997)

Somervaille, L and Griffiths, R (1995) *The training and career development needs of public health professionals* Institute of Public Health, University of Birmingham

Statutory Instruments SI 1948 No1416 and SI 1950 No.1259 and Appointment of Consultants, Senior Hospital Medical Officers and Senior Hospital Dental Officers, Advisory Appointment Committees HMC(50)75

The New NHS Cmd. 3807 DoH (1997)

3 Planning and internal markets

Penelope M Mullen

The White Paper *Working for Patients* (DoH 1989a) stated its objectives thus:

- *to give patients, wherever they live in the UK, better health care and greater choice of the services available; and*
- *greater satisfaction and rewards for those working in the NHS who successfully respond to local needs and preferences.*

Among the most fundamental of the proposals designed to meet these objectives were changes in the method of allocating resources to Health Authorities and the separation of the provision of health services from their funding, using what many have termed an 'internal market'. How did these proposals affect health care planning – planning to meet the needs of the population, to secure equity and equality and to maximise health? How will the Labour Government proposals change this?

Allocation of resources

Working for Patients proposed that Regions, and eventually Districts, would be funded on a weighted per capita basis (with an allowance to the Thames Regions for higher prices in London). The previous 'cross-boundary flow adjustment' was abolished, leaving Districts to 'pay directly for the services provided for their patients by hospitals in other Districts . . .' (DoH 1989a, para. 4.11).

The allocation of resources has been problematic since the establishment of the NHS. The geographical distribution of its inheritance, both in terms of capital stock and medical staff, was very uneven. Resource distribution during the early years of the NHS was based on previous funding with additions for specific developments, thus perpetuating and even exacerbating the inherited geographical inequalities. The 1962 Hospital Plan (MoH 1962) and the 1971 Formula (DHSS 1970) did attempt to reduce these inequalities at Regional level, but inequalities within Regions were at least as great as those between Regions (Cooper and Culyer 1970). Prior to 1974, however, planning health care and equalising resources below the Regional level was difficult. This was due largely to the absence in the hospital sector of a geographically-based planning and management tier below the level of the Region. The pre-1974 sub-Regional tier, Hospital Management Committees (HMCs), were responsible for running a hospital or a group of hospitals and rarely had specific responsibilities to ensure that the needs of a defined population were met.

New opportunities for sub-Regional planning came with the establishment in 1974 of Area Health Authorities (AHAs) 'with full planning and operational responsibilities . . . responsible for providing or arranging for the provision of comprehensive health services . . .' to a defined population (DHSS 1972, p.20). In 1976 the new NHS Planning System was introduced. At the same time, but quite independently, the report of the Resource Allocation Working Party 'The RAWP Report' (DHSS 1976) made proposals for improving geographical equity both between Regions and within Regions. Regional target financial allocations were to be based on population weighted by age, sex and Standardised Mortality Ratios (SMRs) (as a proxy for morbidity), and adjusted for 'cross-boundary flow' using average costs per case by specialty applied to patient flows recorded two or three years earlier. Actual allocations to Regions would gradually be adjusted over several years so that they moved towards the target allocations. The RAWP Report proposed that the '. . . same principles . . . should . . . be applied to allocations below Regional level' (DHSS 1976, p.37).

The RAWP Report and its implementation have been the centre of considerable discussion, analysis and controversy (Mays and Bevan 1987) which is outside our scope here. However, the cross-boundary flow adjustment had far-reaching implications for health care planning, in particular for equity and priorities, especially at the sub-Regional level. While over the years there had been a considerable amount of work on costing such flows, a more important question from the point of view of planning was the fact that the home (exporting) authority was compulsorily required to pay for such flows while having no control over them (Brazier 1986, 1987, Mullen 1986). It was difficult for an authority to pursue its priorities and plan to meet the needs of its population while some of its resources were being used to pay for outward flows not figuring in those priorities. Importing authorities, on the other hand, complained that the cross-boundary flow adjustment did not fully compensate for the actual workload since, by using average costs, it did not fully cover the costs of treating high-cost cases. Further, the adjustment was based on historical data and, in any case, influenced only target allocations and not actual allocations. In addition, various perverse incentives appeared to be built into the system which were not conducive to good planning (Bevan and Brazier 1987). Indeed, not long after the RAWP Report was published Mullen (1978, p.11) suggested that:

> One partial solution to the problem of accounting for intra-regional cross-boundary flows would be to allocate resources to authorities taking no account of

> *the cross-boundary flows and to leave them to take the responsibility of paying for their own residents treated elsewhere . . . there would be far more flexibility for the Area planners to arrange health care for their population.*

In view of the problems, many Regions modified or even abandoned the RAWP cross-boundary flow adjustment method for their sub-Regional allocations.

Despite concern expressed about the methodology employed in the *Working for Patients* proposals for the allocation of funding (Mays 1989) and about subsequent funding methodologies (Peacock and Smith 1995), from the point of view of health care planning, the principle of funding authorities basically on a weighted per capita basis, with no allowance for cross-boundary flow, is to be welcomed. But did the accompanying proposals in *Working for Patients* for the provision of services hinder or help Health Authorities in fulfilling their planning role?

Funding and the provision of services

Internal markets

As noted above, the *Working for Patients* proposals for securing and providing services involved an 'internal market'. The origin of this term is usually attributed to Enthoven (1985a, p.39), who explained his proposals thus:

> *Each District would receive a RAWP-based per capita revenue and capital allowance. Each DHA [District Health Authority] would continue to be responsible to provide and pay for comprehensive care for its own resident population, but not for other people without current compensation. It would be paid for emergency services to outsiders at a standard cost. It would be paid for non-emergency services to outsiders at negotiated prices. It would control referrals to providers outside the District and it would pay for them at negotiated prices. In effect, each DHA would be like a Health Maintenance Organization.*

He also stressed that:

> *The theory behind such a scheme – which can better be called 'market socialism' than 'privatisation' – is that the managers could then buy services from producers who offered the best value.* (Enthoven 1985b, p.22)

This concept of the 'internal market' was adopted by most contributors during the debate prior to the publication of *Working for Patients*. For instance, the King's Fund Institute (1988 p.19) described the 'internal market' as having *inter alia* the following features:

> *Each district would receive a needs based, per capita allocation. It would be paid for services to outsiders at negotiated prices. It would also control patient referrals to providers outside the district and would pay for them at negotiated prices.*

However, statements from ministers and interpretations in the press, in the months leading up to the publication of *Working for Patients*, appeared to describe a rather different concept of the internal market – a patient-led system. For instance:

> the 'internal market', under which GPs could send patients to the health districts with the shortest waiting lists, with the money for their treatment travelling with them. (Brown 1988)

Classification of 'internal markets'

There were then two very different proposals being described under the heading 'Internal Market', which Mullen (1990) characterised as:

Type I 'Internal Market' Systems

With Type I systems the Health Authority receives funding for its population; has a specific responsibility for the health/health care of that population; and, in various combinations, provides and/or purchases services from other providers, public or private, to meet the health needs of the population. In the least 'radical' forms, the home authorities remain the main providers of services, but the purchasing of services from other Health Authorities is increased. In the most 'radical' forms, the home Health Authority does not provide any services directly, but puts out contracts (with or without competitive tendering) for the entire range of provision. With the Type I 'Internal Market' it is implied, although not always made explicit, that residents of the home Health Authority may be treated only by 'approved' or 'contracted' providers.

Type II 'Internal Market' Systems

With Type II systems, the Health Authority receives funding for its population; may be a direct provider of services; but residents can seek treatment anywhere and their home authority is obliged to reimburse the provider. This reimbursement may be either at cost or according to some laid-down scale or negotiated scale of charges. Popularly when this type of 'Internal Market' is mentioned, it is in terms of 'patients being able to shop around to find the shortest waiting list, with their Health Authority being sent the bill'.

The National Association of Health Authorities described this second model as 'automatic and immediate cross-boundary flow reimbursement', which it stated 'carries the internal market concept to its full fruition, involving transferring the initiative from the planners and treasurers, to the market customers (ie patients) and their advisers (ie GPs) with money following the patient' (NAHA 1988, p.19).

Experience from other systems

Some indication of the potential operation of the different types of 'internal market' can be obtained from examining finance and delivery systems elsewhere. The Type II system has many characteristics in common with an insurance-based system, where the insurance company reimburses the provider for care supplied. The Type I system has been likened to a Health Maintenance Organisation (HMO), with the difference that the Health Authority is compulsorily responsible for all residents of a particular location, thus having no choice over membership.

Insurance-based systems

Under most insurance systems, hospitals and health care providers supply services to insured patients and are then reimbursed for the services by the insurer according either to retrospective full-cost reimbursement, or to prospective reimbursement.

With retrospective full-cost reimbursement schemes, the suppliers of health care receive payment in full from the insurer for all expenditure incurred. Suppliers thus have an incentive to maximise income by encouraging as much activity as possible. They have an incentive to maximise the number of patients treated, maximise the length of stay, maximise the number of surgical procedures performed and the number of diagnostic tests carried out. Such systems are inherently inflationary as they encourage escalation of costs and there is no evidence that they give any encouragement to the cost-effective use of different procedures since the health care suppliers know they will be reimbursed whatever the cost.

In an attempt to control escalating costs, the US Government and insurance companies turned to a prospective payment system – a form of prospective reimbursement. Under this system, health care providers are reimbursed at a predetermined price for each defined unit of workload, regardless of the actual cost involved in providing that unit. The 'unit of workload' can be a day in hospital, a diagnostic test or a particular procedure, but more recently has been in the form of a case. This was associated with the development of Diagnostic Related Groups (DRGs) – a method of 'classifying inpatients into a manageable number of groups (467), which are both clinically meaningful and homogeneous in resource use' (Culyer and Brazier 1988, p.16). Providers are then reimbursed at a set price per case treated, according to the DRG into which the case falls. Prospective payment systems have the advantage that health care suppliers are paid for the amount of work they do and are encouraged to control the cost per case. However, incentives remain for suppliers to treat as many cases as possible; to treat the lowest cost patients within any group; to shift the cost of treatment to other agencies; and to classify patients in the highest cost group possible – known as DRG creep. Thus, with a prospective payment system the funding agency still cannot control total expenditure unless it can control the number of cases. Some insurance companies have attempted to do this by requiring prior approval for treatment.

Health Maintenance Organisations

HMOs were established in the USA in an attempt to control the escalating costs of health care. Instead of health insurance which reimburses the suppliers of health care usually on an item-of-service basis, HMOs enrol customers for an annual fee and in return guarantee health care for that year. 'HMOs usually employ their own primary care physicians . . . and either run their own hospital services or buy in from other suppliers' (Culyer and Brazier 1988, p.20). Costs are contained and efficiency encouraged since, unlike fee-for-service systems, there is no incentive on the part of the HMO to 'oversupply' services. This is supported by evidence that hospital stays and admission rates are lower in HMOs than under fee-for-service systems (Petchey 1987, p.494). However, there have been arguments that the lower costs result from reducing the level of care and jeopardising outcomes, at least to some of the poorer members (Ware *et al.* 1986, p.1021). There is an incentive for the HMO to reduce utilisation of services using, to some extent, general practitioners as gatekeepers. In addition, because HMOs can effectively choose which customers to enrol, there is some suggestion of 'cream skimming', ie HMOs are choosing to enrol lower than average users of services and have an incentive to discriminate against potentially high users of services (Petchey 1987). It must be remembered that the acknowledged success of HMOs in reducing costs should be viewed against the insurance-based systems they replace. The lessons may not have the same applicability in the UK where health care costs are already much lower (Luft 1991).

The White Paper proposals

'Internal markets' and the White Paper

Which model of the 'internal market' was proposed in *Working for Patients* – Type I or Type II? It has been suggested that the rhetoric was Type II, while the proposals were Type I. While this may be an oversimplistic observation, it would appear to contain some element of the truth. But what does a more detailed examination of the proposals reveal?

Health Authorities (HAs)
The central proposals, ie that (District) HAs should receive an allocation based on their population and should be responsible for providing or acquiring health care services to meet the needs of that population, are fundamentally Type I. However, there are several proposals in *Working for Patients* which introduced elements of a Type II system.

The first was the provision, designed to overcome objections to the loss of GP freedom resultant on the Type I system, that 'DHAs will need to allow for referrals by GPs to hospitals with whom no contracts have been placed, keeping some funds in reserve for this purpose' (DoH 1989a, para.4.24).

The second Type II provision related to emergency services. *Working for Patients* gave the assurance that 'the costs of emergency services and those requiring immediate admission to hospital can be met for every patient who needs them, irrespective of whether the patient is resident in a District which has a contract with the hospital' (DoH 1989a, para.4.18).

Thus 'if emergency admission as an in-patient is required, the cost should be met by the District of residence. This will require the hospital to levy a charge . . .' (DoH 1989c, para.2.18).

In respect of both these Type II provisions, 'charges for patients receiving treatment outside their District *and* outside the scope of its contractual agreements . . . should be recovered direct from the District of residence or from the GP budget holder' (DoH 1989c, para.2.19).

A further element of Type II was introduced later in respect of tertiary referrals – referrals made by a medically qualified consultant to another medically qualified consultant. From April 1993 providers were no longer 'required to obtain prior authorisation from the appropriate purchasing authority or GP Fundholder before accepting tertiary referral patients', with purchasers being required to pay for treatments on the same basis as for emergency ECRs (DoH 1992c, para.1).

In addition to Extra-Contractual Referrals (ECRs), proposals for cost-per-case contracts could also have Type II elements (DoH 1989c). In the absence of controls over referrals by non-fundholding GPs, the provision that under such contracts 'payment would be on a case by case basis, without any prior commitment by either party to the volume of cases which might be so dealt with', would appear very similar to a prospective payment system.

General Practitioners as budget holders

General Practitioner Fundholders (GPFHs) are also working with an 'Internal Market' which is mainly Type I. Initially GPFHs had budgets to purchase drugs, outpatient treatment and tests and a limited range of in-patient services. However, subsequent revisions to the regulations increased the range of services covered by the budget of what was later termed 'standard' fundholding. In addition, pilot schemes for total purchasing (or total fundholding), 'where GPs . . . purchase all hospital and community health services for their patients', were introduced (DoH 1994, p.4). Although GPFHs are working with a Type I 'Internal Market' there are some differences from the situation faced by HAs in that GPFHs are able to choose the population that they serve and most are not responsible for the full range of services.

However, GP Fundholding does potentially contain some features of a Type II model. In order to control and make best use of their budget, GPFHs must have full knowledge of the cost and scope of the services they are purchasing. However, once the initial referral has been made by the GP the provider, the hospital consultant, makes the diagnosis and determines the treatment (DoH 1989d, para.3.3). Thus, as the BMA (1989, p.12) points out, 'these costs would be beyond the control of the general practitioners but could fall on the budget'. While there is no formal provision for GPs to refer their patients for an 'estimate' before deciding whether or not they wish to proceed and pay for treatment, some GPFHs are making referrals 'for opinion only'. However, ethical problems could arise with this and the potential exists for disagreement about the amount and length of treatment, especially for items such as repeat visits to outpatients.

Health care planning and the White Paper

Against this background, what are the planning roles of the different purchasers and providers?

Health Authorities

Working for Patients said little about planning but stressed that, having been freed from the obligation actually to provide services:

> ... *DHAs can then concentrate on ensuring that the health needs of the population for which they are responsible are met; that there are effective services for the prevention and control of disease and the promotion of health; that their population has access to a comprehensive range of high quality, value for money services: and one setting targets for and monitoring the performance of those management units for which they continue to have responsibility.* (DoH 1989a, para.2.11)

The HA planning role was set out more fully in the guide for Self-Governing Hospitals (NHS Trusts):

> *3.2 Each DHA will have a responsibility to identify the total health care needs of its population and plan how these should be met. It will draw up these plans in the light of national policies and local priorities and resources. It will execute these plans by planning a coordinated series of contracts with selected providers and will then monitor them. The process will necessarily be a dynamic one with DHAs updating their plans annually and modifying their pattern of contracts both to reflect changing needs and to respond to new services becoming available from current or alternative providers.* (DoH 1989e)

The briefing pack accompanying 'Working for Patients' (DoH 1989h, section D5) claimed that at 'Regional and District level planning will be able to respond more effectively to the health needs of the population rather than being tied to details of the operational delivery of services'. However, *Working for Patients* warned that 'Health authority funding will continue to be cash-limited' (DoH 1989a, para.3.8).

GP Fundholders

The planning role of GPFHs is not clear. As noted above, firstly for standard fundholding their budgets only cover a limited range of services and, secondly, unlike HAs, GPs can select which patients to take on and thus include in their budget. Therefore, while they will have a practice planning role and, in the case of consortia, a multi-practice planning role, they do not as GPFHs have a population-based planning role. However, the operation of such practices could affect planning by their District(s).

Suppliers/providers

The role of providers – NHS Trusts and private suppliers – is the delivery of 'contracted services within quality and quantity specification to one or a number of clients in return for agreed levels of income' (DoH 1989f, p.4). Thus, providers have no formal responsibility to plan to meet the needs of a particular population, but do, of course, need to conduct business planning to secure and fulfil contracts and to attract and treat ECRs.

Health care planning with 'internal markets' and the purchaser/provider split

As noted above, elements of both Type I and Type II 'internal markets' appeared in *Working for Patients*. What then are the implications for health care planning of the different types of 'internal market'?

Planning with a Type I 'internal market'

Planning role

Through the placing of contracts, the planning of directly provided services, and control over where its residents may be treated, Type I systems give the home authority the potential to ensure that its priorities are pursued and that the planned balance between health care groups is maintained. Thus with Type I systems, Health Authorities have considerable potential for health care planning to meet the needs of their populations.

Equality and equity

If Health Authorities have different priorities and each purchases the health care which they consider to be a priority, then Type I systems can mean that residents of different Health Authorities may find access to some forms of health care even more unequal than previously. Other inequalities may result. There is evidence from HMOs that higher income groups gain greater health benefits from the system than do lower income groups (Ware *et al.* 1986). However, another potential source of inequality, 'cream skimming', which arises with HMOs, is removed in the case of HAs but not GPFHs since, unlike HMOs, HAs are compulsorily responsible for all residents and thus cannot select only the lower risks. However, HAs could suffer the secondary effects of such selection if GPFHs select only the lower risks leaving the HA with the higher-cost patients within any category. HAs would face an additional challenge in redressing any inequalities which follow from such selection without compensatory funding.

Expenditure control

The very nature of Type I systems means that home authorities have considerable potential for controlling both total expenditure and relative expenditure on different health care groups and types of treatment.

Planning with a Type II 'internal market'

Planning role

With a Type II 'internal market', the home authority would find its health care planning role very restricted with little scope for ensuring that local needs and priorities were met. This arises because patients are permitted to go anywhere for treatment, leaving the home authority to pay for this treatment, whether or not that authority considers such treatment necessary for that particular patient, whether or not that type of treatment figures in local priorities, and whether or not there are more deserving cases within the authority.

With such a system there seems little to prevent providers behaving in the same manner as providers elsewhere where reimbursement systems are in operation. Providers would place no restraint on the services provided or number of cases treated since they would be certain of payment. The home authority, on the other hand, could find its funds being compulsorily diverted to services and cases it considered low priority.

Equality and equity

The Type II model could lead to inequity between health care groups since large amounts of a Health Authority's budget would be compulsorily diverted to those areas where patients are more mobile and where providers find it most profitable to supply services, ie mainly elective surgery. Other health care groups, especially the so-called priority groups, could lose out. On the other hand, Type II systems could avoid inequalities resulting from differing District priorities, since patients can override local priorities by going elsewhere for treatment. However, new inequalities could arise between those patients with the resources and knowledge to seek care outside their district and other patients without such resources and/or knowledge.

Overall expenditure control

It is virtually impossible to conceive a completely Type II system operating successfully with cash-limited Health Authorities. All experience of retrospective and prospective reimbursement systems points to the difficulties of controlling overall expenditure. Thus, in practice, if a pure Type II system were operating, Health Authorities would find very large parts of their budgets being compulsorily removed to pay for a much higher consumption of acute health care (mainly elective surgery), with a consequent diminution of money available for other services.

It can be argued that a fairly radical Type II 'internal market' had developed during the 1980s in the care of the elderly where much of the provision was private but much of the funding was public. However, it is debatable how far this model can be extended to the rest of the health service. First, care of the elderly is essentially 'elective'. Second, the pre-April 1993 pattern of provision grew up initially on the basis of 'full cost reimbursement' and subsequently on 'prospective payment' – in both cases financed from non-cash-limited public funds. How far would it have developed with cash-limited funds?

Implications in practice

Of course, *Working for Patients* did not advocate a pure Type II system. Indeed, what was advocated was largely Type I. However, the existence of Type II elements, ie both emergency and elective ECRs and later tertiary ECRs, gives potential incentives to providers which are very similar to those under insurance-based systems. Unrestricted, the provision for ECRs would mean that providers have every incentive to treat as many patients as possible, in as high a cost category as possible, for 'referrals by GPs to hospital with whom no contracts have been placed' (DoH 1989a, para.4.24). Health care providers who have no contractual relationship with the home authority will have a financial incentive to 'over-supply' services, in the knowledge that they must be reimbursed. The HA would find some of its carefully planned resources being diverted to pay for services which might not figure in those plans. Barr *et al.* (1989, pp.122–3) went so far as to suggest that 'if the receiving hospital is allowed to "dump" excess capacity by charging no more than short-term marginal cost it will, in effect, be "stealing" part of another District's budget'.

These provisions could clearly lead to the cost-inflationary dangers associated with Type II systems. This point is recognised in an early departure from the principle of GPs' freedom of referral, which states that '. . . an open-ended commitment on the part of HAs to meet all non-contractual referrals would be incompatible with both the disciplines which the new system is intended to inject and with control of budgets' (DoH 1989c, para.3.3). It is stressed that 'DHAs will need to develop sensitive procedures . . . but will have the right to refuse . . . if there is no satisfactory reason for a distant or expensive referral' (DoH 1989e, p.9).

The difficulties in attempting to implement what is basically a Type I system, while retaining choice for GPs and patients, were further demonstrated in a more comprehensive description of the proposed provisions for ECRs. Starting from the general principle '. . . that GPs should be free, when necessary, to refer non-emergency cases outside the contract', discussion of the new role of HAs leads to the conclusion that HAs cannot 'be put in the position of being a mere cypher and reflecting individual GPs' wishes regardless of their effect on other patient services'. Thus, 'a presumption of the right to make an extra-contractual referral cannot therefore be a guarantee that the DHA would in all cases agree to meet the cost'. Further, a duty is also placed on the provider in that 'when a hospital receives an extra-contractual referral, it will need to discuss with the patient's DHA the financial arrangements and other terms . . .' (DoH 1989f, paras.3.14–3.16).

In practice, elaborate control mechanisms have been established and funds for ECRs, both elective and emergency, have been very limited – an average of only 1.33 per cent of cash limits being allocated initially in the first year (NAHAT 1991). Most Districts have required that each elective

ECR is individually approved, using decision rules for approval of varying degrees of strictness. For instance, some Districts refused on principle to approve elective ECRs where treatment had already started and some refused unapproved tertiary referrals (Williamson 1991). Thus before any referral is accepted, the hospital must go through a series of checks to ensure that the patient is covered by a GPFH, by an HA contract or by HA approval for an ECR (Mullen 1993, p.64). This strict control of ECRs came under heavy criticism from the Parliamentary Health Committee (House of Commons 1991) and the DoH subsequently issued guidance which limited the grounds for refusing ECRs (DoH 1992b).

There are naturally fewer formal controls on emergency ECRs, but in many cases the dividing line between emergency and non-emergency is very narrow (Ghodse and Rawaf 1991, Forsythe 1991). There is thus considerable scope for interpretation over how much treatment can be considered automatically 'authorised' following emergency admission and at what point during treatment, if at all, approval must be sought from the patient's 'home' authority (DoH 1992b).

The effectiveness of health care planning will be strongly influenced by the strength of the Type II elements in the internal market. Careful plans could be disrupted if unplanned Type II elements consume a large part of the HA's resources. However, planning problems also arise with a Type I system. These concern mainly contracting, the gatekeeper role, the relationship between HAs and GPFHs and rationing.

Contracting

With Type I 'internal markets', some or all of the health care services for an authority's residents will be purchased on the basis of contracts. The letting and operation of such contracts can have a profound effect on health care planning. Various types of contract have been proposed, all of which contain their own perverse incentives. Two types – block contracts and cost-and-volume contracts – predominated in the implementation of *Working for Patients*. Cost-per-case contracts, as originally proposed, appeared less in evidence possibly because of their Type II nature described above. With population-based block contracts, ie contracts to provide a defined population with its full requirements for a specified range of services, providers have an incentive to treat as few patients as possible, to undersupply and to reduce the level of service to the minimum specified in the contract. With cost-and-volume contracts, which specify the number of cases to be treated, the provider has an incentive to select the cheaper cases within the categories specified and to minimise the level of service per patient. In all contracts there is an incentive to shift the costs on to other services outside that contract, for instance, from hospital care to community care.

Further problems arise from the creation of 'packages' of services or care, a corollary of contracting and tendering for services and, to some extent, the purchaser–provider split. Much of the original debate on the 'internal market' appears to relate to elective surgery, which lends itself to 'packages' of care. It is easy to grasp the concept of tendering for the oft-quoted '200 hip replacements' and, apart from dangers such as 'cream skimming', this appears relatively non-problematic. However, *Working for Patients* proposed putting the entire health service out to tender – in discrete parcels. How a meaningful contract could be agreed for, say, general medicine, other than on a population basis, is difficult to envisage. If the contract is made for, say, 100 pneumonia cases, or for 100 fractures (or 100 births!), what happens to the 101st case that comes along? Basically, the choice of contract raises the fundamental question of 'which party carries the risk?' With block contracts providers carry the risk of catering for unplanned increases in demand and in effect accept open-ended contracts at fixed prices. With cost-and-volume contracts, the risk is carried by purchasers who have to provide additional funds if demand exceeds planned levels. As a result, a Type I 'internal market' needs a mixture of types of contracts and, in practice, a range of often imaginative hybrid contracts have been developed.

Other problems may arise as a result of contracting. First, what is the position of a Health Authority which, having identified a need for a particular service, cannot find a provider? Second, individual health providers entered the 'internal market' with different historical endowments of facilities and were unlikely to be able to compete equally for contracts. Third, problems might arise from the interdependence of services. Is it really possible to 'contract-out' some specialties and still retain a comprehensive service? Fourth, annual contracting poses planning problems for providers. They need a far longer commitment to feel confident in developing new services.

The gatekeeper role

While the home authority can plan and contract for the services it identifies as being required to meet the needs of its population, it is not clear how it will be determined which individuals will receive those services. In other words, which party, the purchaser or the provider, determines which patients will be treated on the contract? If it is left to the provider there could be strong financial incentives to select the lower cost, least complicated cases, within the contracted category.

The Department of Health (1989f, p.16) proposed that 'as a minimum, the contracting parties should consider specifying: . . . the criteria for admission and discharge of in-patients and for day/out-patient referrals'. However, it is difficult to see how such criteria can be formulated to ensure that treatment is received by the individuals that the home authority would have chosen.

Lilford (1989, p.1191) saw the ability of the home authority to choose who receives treatment as a major benefit to be gained from the system, stating that 'some patients will still go without treatment, but commissioning agents will help patients with the greatest need or best prognosis. Therefore, instead of the budget running out, say, after nine months of the year, the commissioner will preselect for the greatest perceived need'. However, Lilford gave no indication as to how this preselection might work.

Some HMOs 'employ' GPs to act as gatekeepers, and currently in the NHS GPs act as the initial gatekeeper to secondary care, with consultants and other hospital doctors acting as the final gatekeeper. It is not clear, with funding split from the provision of services, whether this system will work in compliance with the plans of the home authority. GPs are neither employees nor agents of the home authority and have no contractual, and little moral, duty to act as the authority's gatekeepers. Indeed, since GPs will feel that their primary duty is to their own patients, there will be no incentive to attempt to limit their patients' share of the contracts. Some HAs have attempted to involve GPs in purchasing, but there is little evidence to indicate whether or not such involvement influences individual referral behaviour. Hospital doctors are the agents of the provider, not the purchasing authority, and again cannot be expected automatically to take on the gatekeeper role. Some HAs via their Directors of Public Health have addressed this problem by agreeing admission and treatment protocols with consultants working for their contracted providers.

GP Fundholding overcomes this problem, since the GPs act as gatekeepers to their own budgets. However, there is an incentive to undersupply if GPs are permitted to retain budgetary savings. Bevan (1984, 1989) avoids this problem by proposing a simulated HMO based on GPs choices. Under this 'simulated market' districts would receive a population-based allocation and would pass this allocation 'down to GPs in the form of notional budgets for hospital and community health services; GPs would exercise choice . . . but that choice would be made against the notional budget, where GPs stand neither to lose nor to gain financially from how their actual use of services compares with their budget' (Bevan 1989, p.65). Indeed, several projects using such notional budgets have been established as alternatives to total fundholding.

Coexistence of HAs and GPFHs
Although HAs and GPFHs both face a largely Type I internal market, their coexistence raises some planning issues. As noted above, whereas HAs are explicitly responsible for meeting the needs of defined geographical populations, GPFHs are concerned only with the needs of their registered patients. The ability of HAs to plan for their populations can be constrained if substantial proportions of their population-based allocations are diverted to GPFHs, who may not share the planning priorities of the HA. To help overcome this problem, some HAs have attempted to involve GPFHs in the planning process. Even with such collaboration, HAs have faced problems resulting from the different budget levels set for GPFHs. In the first year of operation these budgets were established largely on the basis of imputed expenditure of the practice in the previous year, resulting in very great differences in funding per registered patient (Day and Klein 1991). However, even when, assuming it proves possible, the question of budget setting has been resolved, the incentive for GPFHs to select lower risk patients (Scheffler 1989) could leave HAs responsible for the higher risk patients, without commensurate funding. Indeed, there

may prove to be some 'natural' GPFH selection against higher risk patients, since such practices are less likely to be found in inner cities (Drummond *et al.* 1990, Dyson 1992).

Rationing

An advantage of the Type I model is that it enables the HA to determine its priorities and plan to ensure that the needs of its population are met. However, the more explicit regime brought about by the purchaser–provider split has led to increased interest in, and some advocacy of, explicit rationing (Mullen 1995). Such explicit rationing, where HAs specify which treatments they will and, more importantly, will not fund, which must be compared with the alternative of rationing by clinical judgement and waiting lists, can appear very attractive. However, explicit exclusion of whole categories of treatment, conditions and patient groups appears to make no allowance for variation in severity within any condition group. Thus, while on average one treatment may have a lower cost–benefit ratio than another, this may not be true of cases at the margin. Further, if waiting is used as part of the rationing system, patients at least have a choice between waiting, with zero direct money price, and not waiting, by paying for private treatment. If some classes of treatment are completely excluded, those unable to opt for private treatment also lose the option of waiting. Finally, can a national health system coexist with the freedom for individual local Health Authorities to exclude treatments which other authorities include?

Some HAs are setting priorities by limiting the number of certain types of treatment they will purchase – by using protocols to attempt to ensure those treatments are received by the highest priority patients. However, some consider such 'soft' rationing insufficiently rigorous for the new NHS and argue that HAs must face up to the necessity of rationing by excluding whole classes of treatment (Klein and Redmayne 1992, Millar 1992).

Markets and planning

The 'market' proposals in *Working for Patients* have other implications for health care planning, irrespective of the relative strengths of the Type I and Type II models. Many of these relate to the characteristics of the health care services that can be obtained to meet the needs of the population identified by the planning authority – the HA.

Volume of services

Many of the benefits intended to flow from *Working for Patients* appeared to be predicated on the assumption of an increase in the total volume of services provided. This is made explicit in an executive letter which stated that the 'objective of increasing the efficiency of the NHS will only be realised if competition delivers more in the value of savings and/or quality improvements than it adds to transaction costs' (DoH 1989g, p.4).

Thus, it was hoped that greater efficiency would achieve a higher volume of services. There is evidence from the US that 'substantial savings are achievable through the transfer of services from low volume, high cost, low efficiency centres' (Petchey 1989, p.86). On the strength of this Petchey (p.87)concluded that 'there is the potential for some cost saving even if we are unable to begin to quantify it'. However, there are countervailing forces which might result in a lower volume of services.

First, there are increased transaction costs and more staff are required just to work the system. The commentary to the Bill to effect the proposals estimated a permanent increase of about 3000 staff, in addition to short-term increases in staff (HMSO 1989).

Second, there is a risk that higher prices charged by monopoly suppliers will result in HAs being able to purchase a lower volume of services than that provided at present. As Barr *et al.* (1989, pp.121–2) put it:

> We must expect the new independent hospitals to act like any profit-maximizing firm. They will attempt to differentiate their products. Having many expensive specialist facilities this will not be difficult. We would expect them to corner discrete specialist areas of care and charge monopoly rent for the cases they treat. There will be no effective competition.

To counter this danger one of the working papers stated that '. . . the Secretary of State will need reserve powers to prevent a self-governing hospital with anything near to a monopoly of service provision from exploiting its position, for example by charging unreasonably high prices for its services' (DoH 1989b, para.2.15). However, NHS Trusts have power to fix pay levels and few have suggested that this will result in a general fall in pay – indeed, a general increase in pay levels is anticipated in an attempt to attract scarce staff (Maynard 1989). Much of the scope for pay reduction has already been exploited in the competitive tendering for support services. Unless entirely compensated by increased efficiency, increased costs will result in increased prices and thus lower volumes.

Third, a possible source of reduced volumes lies in the dividing up of services for the purpose of contracting. Many services offered by health providers can be considered as joint products. Thus it is possible that, as a result of letting out contracts for individual services possibly to different suppliers, the aggregate cost of the individual contracts (each of which would have to be independently viable) will exceed the combined cost of the original integrated services. Alternatively, a lower volume of services would be secured for the same cost.

Fourth, drawing on US and other international experience, Light (1991a, 1991b, 1993) suggests that competition itself may lead to lower efficiency and increased costs.

However, despite these misgivings, there was evidence of increased activity levels in 1991–92, and the Department of Health's later imposition of 'efficiency gains' on purchasers and providers has led to continuing improvements in efficiency as measured by the Efficiency Index.

However, several commentators warn against attributing increased activity to the introduction of the internal market. Petchey (1993, p.699) notes that the early increased activity was accompanied by a rapid growth in NHS funding (4.1% in 1991–92) and Light (1993, p.285) observes that large increases in NHS efficiency had been achieved in the 1980s. Analysis, including analysis of longer-term trend data, by the Radical Statistics Health Group (1992, 1995) suggests that many of the claims of improvements resulting from the 1991 changes are not supported by the data. Further, the distorting effect of use of FCEs (finished consultant episode) as a unit of activity has been widely noted (Munro 1997, p.68) and the Efficiency Index itself has been the subject of some criticism (Paton 1996, p.183, Appleby and Little 1993).

Waiting for services

One of the stated aims of *Working for Patients* was the reduction in waiting time for treatment. Indeed, one criterion for the placing of contracts and for monitoring providers is the length of waiting lists and the delay in treatment. However, it is possible that the rationing function of waiting lists will simply be moved to an earlier stage in the treatment cycle. A provider, being judged on the length of waiting lists, will simply accept for treatment the number of cases provided for in the contract, quite properly refusing further cases unless reimbursed on a cost-per-case basis. Indeed, there is anecdotal evidence of this happening (Mullen 1994, p.136). Refused cases will not appear on the waiting list. Further, by controlling the rate of acceptances for treatment, it will be possible for the provider to guarantee immediate treatment.

Location of services

The proposals, both Type I and Type II, involve 'purchasing' services, possibly at a considerable distance. This could lead to problems for a HA in planning equitable, integrated and accessible services for its resident population. Studies have shown that a proportion of patients are willing to travel to receive elective surgery more speedily, but there is little evidence on this question in relation to other services. For instance Lister (1988, pp. 69–70) asks: 'what comfort would it be for elderly and severely ill patients to hear of "competitive" NHS hospitals with vacant beds in Liverpool or Devon?' Culyer *et al.* (1988, p.31) stressed that 'care will have to be exercised to ensure that very sick and elderly patients are not treated or cared for long distances away from their homes and families'. Brotherton and Harris (1988, pp.69–70) pointed to increased difficulties in arranging back-up services and in discharging patients into community health services, if their hospital services had been provided far from their home locations.

Type of services provided

It is noted above that the main planning focus for providers is business planning to enable them to secure and fulfil contracts. Except in those cases where contracts are population-based, which exist although not officially envisaged in the post-review NHS, providers have responsibility only for those patients they treat and have no responsibility for any particular population. As Troop and Zimmern (1989, p.4) express it:

> . . . *at the hospital or service end the objective is entirely different. Its aim is efficient and effective service provision. It is the 'provider' of services. Its unit of concern is not the population but the patient episode and a well run hospital will know exactly, for each category of patient, the cost of care and its outcome.*

In the past some clinicians have been criticised for being concerned only with the patients they actually see and not with the wider population. As a result, considerable effort has gone into attempting to relate individual clinical decisions and actions to wider health and resource issues. However, the introduction of proposals which structurally divorce the providers of services from wider population considerations, may be considered by some to be a retrograde step and, in practice, may affect the type of care delivered.

Locality planning

Prior to 1991 there were various developments in health care planning with the aim of better meeting the needs of particular populations. One such development was Locality Planning, which aimed to plan integrated services for a community at a more local level than the District. The fate of such planning within the post-review NHS has been mixed. There have been experiments in locality purchasing, with schemes ranging from local input into HA purchasing decisions, to total devolution of resources to locality teams for them to secure the services required. However, such schemes raise questions not only of the availability of the necessary expertise for contracting at a local level, but the more problematic question of how large a population is required to act as a 'risk-pool' for different services.

Philosophy of health and health care

The underlying philosophy of health and health care provision, inherent in any system, has a profound influence on the nature and achievements of health care planning. This is a major area which can only be touched on here.

The emphasis in *Working for Patients* on services to individual patients, and provisions such as 'Life-Style Consultations' in connection with the 1990 Contract for GPs, and the introduction of the Patient's Charter (DoH 1991), can be viewed as a reinforcement of the individualistic view of health. This view has come under criticism from some commentators (Navarro 1976, Doyal 1979) because, they claim, it leads to treating the causes of ill-health as being individual, requiring individually orientated therapeutic responses or prevention through individuals changing their own way of life. Thus, it is claimed, the economic and political environment is absolved from responsibility for disease and collective responses are rendered unnecessary. Whether *The Health of the Nation* will reinforce or counteract this individualist bias will depend on the manner of its implementation (DoH 1992a).

Another related factor is the move towards treating health care provision as a tradeable commodity. Navarro (1986 p.30) claims that 'capitalism attempts to replace services pure and simple with commodities that can be bought and sold on the private market' and rather more strongly, Waitzkin (1983 p.677) suggests that 'from the standpoint of potential profit, there is no reason that corporations should view medical products differently from other products. The commodification of health care and its associate technology is a necessary feature of the capitalist political-economic system'.

The NHS and the Labour Government

The Labour Party (1995, 1997) has signalled its intention to end the 'internal market' but to retain the purchaser–provider split in the form of a 'separation in the planning and delivery of healthcare' (Labour Party 1995, p.20). The Secretary of State (Dobson 1997) foreshadowed a future NHS including both Health Authorities and NHS Trusts, albeit fewer in number. Health Authorities will continue to be funded on a weighted capitation basis.

The Labour Party (1997) proposes to replace GP fundholding with GP commissioning. In Summer 1997 applications were invited for about 20 pilot 'GP Commissioning Group projects' (DoH 1997a), and early action on fundholding involved deferring approval of the next 'wave' of fundholders (DoH 1997c Annexe A) and removing associated inequities in funding (DoH 1997c, Annexe B) and waiting lists (DoH, 1997d). The White Paper *The new NHS* (DoH, 1997e), published in December 1997, proposes the establishment of '**Primary Care Groups** comprising all GPs in an area together with community nurses [which] will take responsibility for commissioning services for the local community' (para.3.18).

Even with the publication of *The new NHS*, it is difficult to analyse how Labour Government policies will impact on planning. Integration and cooperation to replace competition, and frequent mentions of planning, including strategic planning, permeate many of the policy statements. To overcome fragmentation, *The new NHS* states that 'all those charged with planning and providing health and social care services for patients will work to a jointly agreed local Health Improvement Programme' (DoH 1997e, para.2.11). But, even with the removal of a competitive 'internal market', the retention of an institutional divide between HAs and providers means that their different planning roles will remain. Further, it means that elements of Type 1 and Type II 'internal markets' may, depending on how providers are to be reimbursed, also remain. Experience shows that no method of reimbursement can be entirely unproblematic. *Renewing the NHS* (Labour Party 1995) discusses allocated budgets and *The new NHS* proposes longer-term healthcare agree-

ments. But on what basis providers will receive their funding is not
entirely clear. However, various indications, such as HAs having choice
where to place agreements (Labour Party 1995, p.21) and restoring 'the
right of GPs to refer their patients to an appropriate hospital of their
choice' (Labour Party 1997), plus the proposals for commissioning by
Primary Care Groups, suggest that the relatively unproblematic system of
funding by global budgets may not prove appropriate. The impact of the
Primary Care Groups and primary care involvement in 'strategic commissioning, (Dobson, 1997) will depend very much on their nature, for
instance whether they are locality or (multi-)practice based and their
degree of freedom to control their devolved budgets. With GP
Commissioning Group pilot projects 'expected to cover populations of at
least 50,000' (DoH 1997a, para. 9) – the minimum survival size for
HMOs, according to Scheffler (1989, p.951) – and Primary Care Groups
typically serving 100,000 patients (DoH, 1997e, para.5.16), might we see
an NHS consisting of hundreds of mini HMOs?

Strong advocacy of Public Health, signalled by the appointment of a
Minister for Public Health, coupled with proposals to tackle the 'root
causes of ill health' (DoH 1997b) which go far wider than individual life-
styles, signals a fundamental change in philosophy. However, the proposal for a 'national schedule for "reference costs" which will itemise the
cost of individual treatments across the NHS' (DoH 1997e, para.9.20),
not only might perpetuate some of the costing problems identified by
Dawson (1994), but might also contribute to the commodification of
health care.

Conclusions

With the implementation of the *Working for Patients* proposals, the planning roles of the various parts of the health services were changed considerably and became more differentiated. The planning role of providers
largely revolves around business planning to secure and fulfil contracts.
Population-based planning relating to identifying the needs of a population and ensuring these needs are met – generally to promote the health of
a defined population – is the province of Health Authorities. This distinction seems likely to remain under the Labour Government.

Funding on a weighted-capitation basis, without compensation for
cross-boundary flows, should assist HAs in their planning role.
However, how to determine equitable weighting has proved problematic.
Labour has signalled its intention to improve the weighting to reflect
needs more accurately, but their proposals for dealing with cross-
boundary flows are less clear.

The separation of funding from the provision of services – with or without a competitive 'internal market' – can prove problematic for planning.
Two distinct types of 'internal market' have been identified, both of which
have considerable implications for population-based planning, for the
pursuit of priorities, and for equity and equality whether between

geographical areas, social groups or health care groups. Both types of 'internal market' were present in *Working for Patients* and there is evidence of tension between the two types of provision. Even with the publication of the 1997 White Paper it is not possible to determine whether the proposals of the Labour Government will retain any elements of Type I or Type II 'internal markets'. The outcome for planning to meet needs, to secure equity and to maximise health, will depend very much on the detail of the proposals in *The new NHS* and on the relative strengths, in practice, of any elements of the two types of 'Internal Market' which remain.

References

Appleby, J and Little, V (1993) Health and Efficiency *Health Service Journal* **103**, 20–22

Barr, N, Glennerster, H and le Grand, J (1989) Working for patients? The right approach? *Social Policy and Administration* **23**, 117–127

Bevan, G (1984) Organising the finance of hospitals by simulated markets *Fiscal Studies* **5**, 44–62

Bevan, G (1989) Reforming UK health care: internal markets of emergent planning?' *Fiscal Studies* **10**, 53–71

Bevan, G and Brazier, J (1987) Financial incentives of subregional RAWP *British Medical Journal* **295**, 836–838

BMA (1989) *Special report of the council of the British Medical Association on the Government's White Paper 'Working for patients'*, SRM2, British Medical Association, London

Brazier, J (1986) Is cross-charging the solution to the problems of cross-boundary flows?, pp. 26–42 in *Reviewing RAWP*, Social Medicine and Health Services Research Unit, Guy's and St Thomas's Hospitals, London

Brazier, J (1987) Accounting for cross boundary flows *British Medical Journal* **295**, 898–900

Brotherton, P and Harris, R (1988) *Their Hands in Our Safe* Socialist Health Association, p. 7

Brown, C (1988) Internal market could lead to hospital closures *The Independent* 9 July 1988

Cooper, MH and Culyer, AJ (1970) An economic assessment of some aspects of the operation of the National Health Service, Appendix A, pp. 187–250 in *Health Services Financing*, British Medical Association, London

Culyer, AJ and Brazier, JE (1988) *Alternatives for organising the provision of health services in the UK*, IHSM Working Paper No. 4 on Alternative Delivery and Funding for Health Care

Culyer, AJ, Brazier, JE and O'Donnell, OO (1988) *Organising health service provision: drawing on experience*, IHSM Working Paper No. 5 on Alternative Delivery and Funding for Health Care

Dawson, D (1994) *Costs and prices in the internal market: markets vs the NHS management executive guidelines* Discussion Paper 115, Centre for Health Economics, University of York

Day, P and Klein, R (1991) 'Variations in budgets of fundholding practices' *British Medical Journal* 303, 168–170

DoH (1989a) *Working for patients*, White Paper on the NHS, Cm555, HMSO, London

DoH (1989b) *Self-governing hospitals* NHS Review Working Paper 1, HMSO, London

DoH (1989c) *Funding and contracts for hospital services* NHS Review Working Paper 2, HMSO, London

DoH (1989d) *Practice budgets for general medical practitioners* NHS Review Working Paper 3, HMSO, London

DoH (1989e) *Self-governing hospitals: An initial guide* HMSO, London

DoH (1989f) *Contracts for health services: operational principles* HMSO, London

DoH (1989g) *Implementing the white paper: discussion document on pricing and openness in contracts for health services* EL(89)MB/171, DoH, London

DoH (1989h) *NHS review: briefing pack for NHS managers* DoH, London

DoH (1991) *The patient's charter* DoH, London

DoH (1992a) *The health of the nation* Cmd 1896, HMSO, London

DoH (1992b) *Guidance on extra contractual referrals* issued under EL(92)60, DoH, London

DoH (1992c) *Tertiary referrals* EL(92)97, DoH, Leeds

DoH (1994) *Developing NHS purchasing and GP Fundholding* issued under EL(94)79, DoH, Leeds

DoH (1997a) *GP Commissioning Groups* EL(97)37, DoH, Leeds

DoH (1997b) *Public health strategy launched to tackle root cause of ill health* Press Release 97/157, DoH

DoH (1997c) *Changing the internal market* EL(97)33, DoH, Leeds

DoH (1997d) *Fairness and equity for hospital treatment* DoH Press Release 97/169

DoH (1997e) *The new NHS* White Paper Cmd 3807, HMSO, London

DHSS (1970) Circular 3/70 to Regional Hospital Board Chairmen, London

DHSS (1972) *Management arrangements for the reorganised National Health Service* HMSO, London

DHSS (1976) *Sharing resources for health in England: report of the resource allocation working party* HMSO, London

Dobson, F (1997) *Speech to the annual conference of the NHS Confederation on 25 June 1997* issued under DoH Press Release 97/145

Doyal, L (1979) *The political economy of health* Pluto Press, London

Drummond, MF, Crump, B, Hawkes, R and Marchment, M (1990) General practice fundholding *British Medical Journal* 301, 1288–1289

Dyson, R (1992) quoted by MacLachlan, R in 'Report of the first annual conference of the National Association of Fundholding Practices' *The Health Service Journal* 102, 15

Enthoven, AC (1985a) *Reflections on the Management of the National Health Service* NPHT

Enthoven, AC (1985b) National Health Service: some reforms that might be politically feasible, *The Economist* **295**, (7399), 19–22

Forsythe, M (1991) Extracontractual referrals: the story so far *British Medical Journal* **303**, 470–480

Ghodse, B and Rawaf, S (1991) Extracontractual referrals in the first three months of NHS reforms *British Medical Journal* **303**, 497–499

HMSO (1989) *National Health Service and Community Care Bill* 50/3, HMSO, London

House of Commons (1991) *Public expenditure on health services and personal social services* parliament, House of Commons Health Committee, 3rd Report, Vol.1, Report 614–1, 17 July 1991

King's Fund Institute (1988) *Health finance: assessing the options* Briefing Paper No. 4, London

Klein, R and Redmayne, S (1992) *Patterns of priorities: a study of the purchasing and rationing policies of the Health Authorities* NAHAT Research Paper No. 7, National Association of Health Authorities, Birmingham

Labour Party (1995) *Renewing the NHS: Labour's agenda for a healthier Britain* The Labour Party

Labour Party (1997) *Policy guide – health*, Labour Party WWW site

Light, DW (1991a) Perestroika for Britain's NHS *The Lancet* **337**, 778–779

Light, DW (1991b) Observations on the NHS reforms: an American perspective *British Medical Journal* **303**, 568–570

Light, DW (1993) Escaping the traps of postwar Western medicine, *European Journal of Public Health* **3**, 281–289

Lilford, R (1989) Looking to a Better Future, *The Health Service Journal* 28 September 1989, 1190–1191

Lister, J (ed.) (1988) *Cutting the Lifeline: The Fight for the NHS* Journeyman Press, London

Luft, HS (1991) Translating the US HMO experience to other health systems *Health Affairs* **10**, 172–186

Maynard, A (1989) *Whither the National Health Service*, NHS White Paper Occasional Paper 1, Centre for Health Economics, University of York

Mays, N (1989) NHS resource allocation after the 1989 White Paper: a critique of the research for the RAWP Review *Community Medicine* **11**, 173–186

Mays, N and Bevan, G (1987) *Resource Allocation in the Health Service* Occasional Papers on Social Administration No. 81, Bedford Square Press, London

Millar, B (1992) Irrational behaviour *The Health Service Journal* **102**, 14–15

MoH (1962) *A hospital plan for England and Wales* Cmd 1604, HMSO, London

Mullen, PM (1978) *RAWP and Resource Allocation in the NHS* Discussion Paper 13, Health Services Management Centre, University of Birmingham, Birmingham

Mullen, PM (1986) 'Funding of supra-authority Services' *Public Money* **6**, 55–58

Mullen, PM (1990) Which internal market? The NHS White Paper and internal markets *Financial Accountability and Management* **6**, 33–50

Mullen, PM (1993) The future of Waiting Lists *Journal of Management in Medicine* **7**, 60–70

Mullen, PM (1994) Waiting Lists in the post-Review NHS *Health Services Management Research* **7**, 131–145

Mullen, PM (1995) *Is health care rationing really necessary?* Discussion Paper 36, Health Services Management Centre, University of Birmingham, Birmingham

Munro, J (1997) Has the internal market been a success? Contradictions in competition in Iliffe, S and Munro, J (eds) *Healthy Choices: Future options for the NHS* Lawrence and Wishart, London, 53–74

NAHA (1988) *Funding the NHS: which way forward?* A NAHA Consultation Document, National Association of Health Authorities, Birmingham

NAHAT (1991) *Spring Financial Survey 1991* National Association of Health Authorities and Trusts, Birmingham

Navarro, V (1976) *Medicine under capitalism* Croom Helm, London

Navarro, V (1986) *Crisis, health, and medicine* Tavistock Publications, London

Paton, C (1996) *Health policy and management* Chapman & Hall, London

Peacock, S and Smith, P (1995) *The resource allocation consequences of the NHS needs formula* Discussion Paper 134, Centre for Health Economics, University of York

Petchey, R (1987) Health maintenance organisations: just what the doctor ordered? *Journal of Social Policy* **16**, 489–507

Petchey, R (1989) The politics of destablisation *Critical Social Policy* **9**, 82–97

Petchey, R (1993) NHS internal market 1991–2: towards a balance sheet *British Medical Journal* **306**, 699–701

Radical Statistics Health Group (1992) NHS reforms: the first six months – proof of progress or a statistical smokescreen *British Medical Journal* **304**, 705–709

Radical Statistics Health Group (1995) NHS 'indicators of success': what do they tell us? *British Medical Journal* **310**, 1045–1050

Scheffler, R (1989) Adverse selection: the Achilles heel of the NHS Reforms *The Lancet* **I**, 950–952

Troop, P and Zimmern, R (1989) A model for the Post-White paper NHS *NHS Management Bulletin* July 1989, 23, 4–5

Waitzkin, H (1983) A Marxist view of health and health care In Mechanic, D (ed.) *Handbook of Health, Health Care and the Health Professions* The Free Press, London 657–682

Ware, JE *et al.* (1986) Comparison of health outcomes at a health maintenance organisation with those of fee-for-service care *The Lancet* **i**, 1017–1022

Williamson, JD (1991) Dealing with extracontractual referrals *British Medical Journal* **303**, 499–504

4. The changing NHS and the finance function

Tony Cook

Like many other aspects of the National Health Service, the finance function has changed and is continuing to change over time. In recent years that pace of change has been particularly rapid. This chapter aims to review the changing finance function and to speculate on how it will further change in the light of the result of the 1997 General Election and the change of Government.

We need to take an historical perspective of the developing NHS finance function and in my view this history can be broken down into four phases:

Phase 1. From the creation of the NHS in 1948 up to the NHS reorganisation of 1974.

Phase 2. From the 1974 reorganisation up to the end of 1988.

Phase 3. From the publication of the *Working for Patients* White Paper (WFP) until April 1997.

Phase 4. Following the election of the Labour Government in May 1997.

It is important to note at the outset the distinction between *financial* accounting and *management* accounting. Financial accounting concerns the need to have systems in place which ensure that financial transactions (such as the payment of wages) are properly conducted and that appropriate records are maintained. Management accounting is concerned with ensuring that appropriate financial information is provided to the management of the organisation to ensure that they can manage it as well as possible and (in the public sector) deliver the greatest value for money (VFM).

Phase 1: the NHS prior to 1974

It is a little unfair to limit the finance function in the period from 1948 to 1974 to a single paragraph. However, for the purposes of this chapter we will do so. Hospital accounting at that time was largely a financial accounting function of ensuring financial probity, maintaining appropriate records, and producing summary year end accounts. Nevertheless there were pioneers amongst NHS Finance Officers (particularly Charles Montacute) who recognised the inevitability of the need to develop management accounting information (Montacute 1962).

Phase 2: the 1974 reorganisation through to end 1988

Arguably this was the most productive phase in the development of NHS accounting with a series of developments under both Labour and Conservative governments.

Essentially the 1974 reorganisation created a structure (in England) of 14 Regional Health Authorities beneath which were a number of Area Health Authorities (AHAs), some of which, in turn, were divided into Health Districts. Funding for the hospital and community health services was on a simple 'top-down' basis with separate allocations of funds for revenue expenditure (ie day-to-day running costs) and capital expenditure (ie building new hospitals). Funding for the Family Practitioner Services (ie the local GPs, dentists, opticians and pharmacists) was provided separately and administered through Family Practitioner Committees (which were coterminous with the AHAs).

Following a further reorganisation in 1982 the AHAs and Health Districts were replaced by District Health Authorities (DHAs).

At national level perhaps the most significant subject of debate was how resources were to be distributed around the system. This became known as RAWP, following the creation of the Resource Allocation Working Party.

However, most of the developments concern financial management at local level. Figure 4.1 (which comes from the 'Korner 6th Report' NHS/DHSS 1984) assists in considering these in some detail. Note the three levels of expenditure analysis described as 'subjective', 'departmental' and 'patient care'.

Prior to 1974, hospital accounts were generally maintained only on the traditional income and expenditure account basis which showed only a 'subjective' analysis of expenditure (ie salaries for doctors, salaries for nurses, expenditure on drugs etc). This corresponds to level 1 in Figure 4.1.

Following the 1974 NHS reorganisation we had the introduction of what is now referred to as the departmental system of budgeting (as in level 2 in Figure 4.1). While it has been refined and improved in several respects this departmental system of budgeting is still the main tool of financial management on the vast majority of NHS hospital sites. Moreover, as Maynard demonstrated (1984) it proved to be effective in enabling Health Authorities to live within their means. Cases where Health Authorities had overspent usually stemmed from a failure properly to install and operate such a system. In VFM terms, if the only

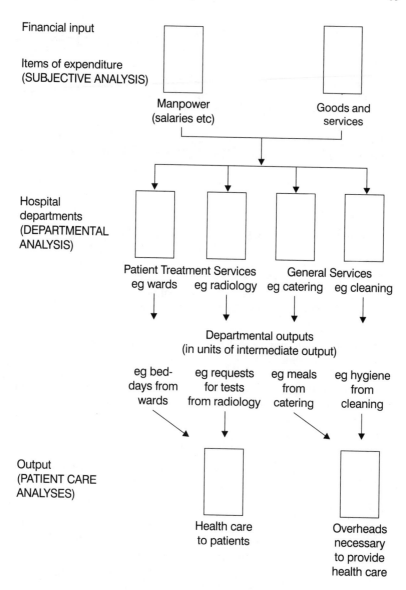

Fig 4.1 How money is used in a hospital day by day

financial objective is the achievement of 'economy' then the NHS was well served by the basic departmental system of budgeting.

However, we need to address the wider issues of VFM. If we accept the 'three Es' definition of VFM – economy, efficiency and effectiveness – then financial information systems need to be developed which will promote 'efficiency' and 'effectiveness' in addition to economy. It is in this wider context that the departmental system of budgeting becomes inadequate. In particular it is subject to three well documented limitations. They are:

1 It provides no analysis of expenditure by health care category – however defined. Thus, for example, if we wished to know how much we are spending on orthopedic surgery the departmental analysis of expenditure will not tell us. This is because part of that expenditure is incurred in the operating theatres, part in the wards, part in the X-ray department etc. However, the departmental system of budgeting contains no mechanism to identify those individual parts, nor any mechanism to bring them together to give a total for orthopedic surgery. This limitation is crucial, of course, to our ability to plan expenditure in health care terms.

2. Doctors – in discharging their clinical duties – make decisions which commit resources for which they are not the budget holders. Thus when a doctor asks for an X-ray or path lab test, or prescribes drugs, or decides that a patient should remain in hospital for a further two days, he is making a financial as well as a clinical decision. However, he is not presumed to be financially accountable for such decisions.

3 The corollary to point 2 is that it is budget holders – such as the chief pharmacist or chief pathologist – who are expected to manage their departments within a predetermined budget, although the level of activity in their departments is outside their control. The chief pharmacist, for example, has no control over the number of prescriptions that come into his department. However, he cannot refuse to dispense a prescription on the grounds that to do so would make him overspend against his budget.

Knowledge of these limitations is not new. The Royal Commission Report of 1978 (Royal Commission on the NHS 1978) identified them, and the next decade saw several initiatives to develop improved financial information and to overcome them.

All of these initiatives shared the common approach of adding an additional, clinical, analysis of hospital expenditure. We can, therefore, conceive of a simple three dimensional model (Figure 4.2).

Clearly as with the existing 'subjective' and 'departmental' analysis, so the clinical analysis of expenditure may be provided in greater or lesser degrees of detail. Conventional wisdom – as illustrated for example in Korner 6 – came to identify five possible levels of analysis for the clinical axis:

1 *to client group* (mental handicap, maternity, the elderly etc);

2 *to clinical specialty* (orthopedics, pediatrics, obstetrics etc);

3 *to consultant* (and his clinical team);

4 *by disease category* (hip replacements, appendectomies, strokes etc);

5 *to the individual patient.*

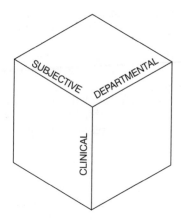

Figure 4.2 Three dimensional model

In fact attention was paid at different times and in different initiatives to developing financial information appropriate to each of the above levels of analysis.

For example, analyses of expenditure to *client group* were available at the national level since the mid-1970s. These have been calculated by a technique misleadingly known as 'programme budgeting'. This involves making very broad brush assumptions about how costs can be allocated to broadly defined client groups. Such figures are of limited value in that they contain no guide as to whether the resources have been spent efficiently or effectively. Likewise the title is misleading in that it is not a true budgeting system. Nevertheless, limited though their value was the NHS in England did not make consistent use of programme budget figures (unlike in Scotland where the Health Boards have produced historical and projected figures to assist health care planning).

From the 1987/88 financial year, Health Authorities were required to produce 'specialty costs'. These are, by definition, calculations of average costs per case at *specialty* level, prepared at the end of each financial year on historical bases. The technique had been existing for some years, and could provide information of use in identifying high levels of expenditure within a particular specialty within a District, (and now a Trust) and could be of value in assisting local planning.

If we can now move down the clinical axis to level 5 – that of the *individual patient* – there have been various trials in techniques of patient costing; designed by definition, to calculate the cost of treating each patient. Of particular interest here was the work of the Financial Information Project which had been in existence since 1979. There are arguments in favour of analysing costs down to the individual patient. However, it should be recognised that while it is possible to analyse costs retrospectively to the individual patient, it is not possible to plan prospectively to the individual patient. It is not possible for example to predict that Mr

Smith will have a heart attack or that Mrs Williams will fall over in the snow and break her leg. We cannot budget down to the level of the individual patient.

Thus all three of these techniques, programme budgeting, specialty costing and patient costing, are of some value but do not overcome all the limitations of departmental budgets.

Consequently the most significant developments concentrated upon what can be described as systems of 'clinical budgeting'. In the UK there have been three initiatives of note, and variants have concentrated on three levels – specialty, consultant and disease category – in our clinical analysis. These three initiatives are CASPE, 'Management Budgeting' and 'Resource Management'.

CASPE – an acronym for clinical and service planning evaluation – is a small research group based at the King's Fund College. It was also established in 1979 and developed systems of clinical budgeting – perhaps with varying degrees of success – at a small number of NHS hospitals. A key feature of the CASPE approach has been the emphasis on the planning rather than the control aspect of budgeting through PACTs (planning agreements with clinical teams). Discussions were held with consultants and agreements drawn up as to what would be the expected workload for the clinical team and what resources they may require to process that workload. The early CASPE trials were actually discrete information systems developed with little finance department involvement. In such cases the District Treasurer would have argued that financial control over the hospital remained with the traditional departmental budgets.

The development of 'management budgeting' was one of the recommendations of the Griffiths Report of 1983. In a supporting paper Blyth (1983) argued that the objective was to

> *develop management budgets involving clinicians at unit level with the emphasis on management rather than accountancy. The aim is to produce an unsophisticated system in which workload related budgets covering financial and manpower allocations and full overhead costs are closely related to workable service objectives, against which performance and progress can be compared.*

That is the key paragraph in a paper which logically argued the case for a better budgeting system and set out a number of principles on which it should be based. By and large those principles were soundly based although one could take issue with the question of 'full overhead costs'. This does not follow what is generally accepted as good industrial/commercial practice. The paragraph also contains a clue as to why management budgeting was perceived, by some, to be a failure in that it talks of an 'unsophisticated system'. It *is* possible to have a system which includes 'workload related budgets concerning financial and manpower allocations etc' but it is not going to be 'unsophisticated'. In that respect Blyth was unrealistically optimistic. Nevertheless, the overall principle is important. There is a need for workload related budgets covering financial and manpower allocations, related to workable service objectives, against which performance and progress can be compared.

In the light of Griffiths the DoH funded four 'demonstration districts'. These too had their successes and failures. They demonstrated that it is possible to construct systems of clinical budgeting in acute hospitals. However, they also threw up a number of problems. The need to have adequate supporting information systems in such key areas as patient administration, radiography, pharmacy and pathology is one of the technical problems. Even more important, however, are the organisational and behavioural issues: what are the correct managerial relationships between the medical, nursing and paramedical professions? Above all to what extent can clinicians be persuaded to accept that they are financially and managerially accountable for their decisions? And if they do, how should their organisational structure be incorporated into the managerial hierarchy of the hospital? Insofar as management budgeting was seen to be a failure it was because it was perceived to be too much of a finance-led exercise which did not adequately tackle the organisational and behavioural issues.

Hence we had the move, in 1986, to 'resource management' (the RMI). Health Notice (86)34 (DHSS 1986) initiated the change of title and the very real change of emphasis. It identified four lessons which had been learned from the management budgeting experience:

1 Doctors and nurses need to be centrally involved in management arrangements.

2 Doctors and nurses need to be centrally involved in specifying the information requirements of the new systems.

3 Effective financial management support is vital.

4 The pace at which management budgets are introduced will need to be carefully judged.

Six acute hospitals were identified to be pilot sites for the RMI. From a narrow accounting point of view the significant change was that they were to be geared to the introduction of patient 'case-mix planning and costing'. Such a system requires that patients suffering from similar diseases and requiring similar treatment regimes should be grouped together. The budgeting system then becomes capable of reflecting the complexity of cases handled, rather than the simple numbers of patients treated. In terms of our levels of analysis on the clinical axis we are now moving from level 3 (consultant), to level 4 (disease category). World-wide, there have been several approaches to case-mix accounting.

For example at Southmead – one of the original management budgeting demonstration districts – the approach was to ask each of the participating consultants to define the 10 or 12 case types which probably made up 80 to 90 per cent of their regular workload. For each of those case types a treatment pattern was identified and costs applied in order to build up a treatment cost for the typical patient. Such an approach is perfectly logical from a local management accounting point of view. However, it suffers from the drawback that each consultant is defining his own case type and will do it differently from another consultant in another hospital. It therefore makes comparison difficult.

Internationally the most widely used approach is based on the international disease classification developed at Yale University. Under this approach all acute patients can be allocated to one of 475 Diagnosis Related Groups (DRGs). Already this system has been extensively used in the USA where increasingly the Medicare and Medicaid systems are reimbursing hospitals on the basis of a price per DRG. In the UK all of the new resource management sites initially based their development of case-mix accounting on DRGs, although more recently they have been developing an improved British classification known as HRGs (Healthcare Resource Groups).

Yet another American approach is being developed at Johns Hopkins University. This recognises that even within the same disease category some patients are more severely ill than others and require correspondingly more extensive – and more expensive – treatments. This approach therefore introduces severity ratings whereby patients' illnesses are then classified into one of four categories of severity, within the same disease category.

It should be recognised that we are still in the early days of case-mix accounting. Moreover, difficulties arise simply because we are dealing with patients in a hospital rather than products in a factory. Inevitably therefore, even within one category, some patients are more severely ill than others, some have more complications, some respond to treatment better than others etc, etc. Crucially therefore the task is to identify groupings which make both medical sense – in that all patients in that group are clinically similar – and accounting sense – in that the treatment of all such patients will require similar resources. Although cumbersome, the expression 'resource homogeneous diagnosis related groups' well illustrates the problem. However, there is no reason to believe that it is incapable of solution. Probably it will require more categories of patients, coupled with some form of severity ratings. Nevertheless there are examples in the industrial/commercial world of organisations with several thousands of product variants. With modern data processing facilities the numbers of categories are not likely to be a problem.

Once we have definable categories of patients, each of which can have a defined treatment regime, it then becomes a fairly straightforward task to build up a defined treatment cost. Such an exercise involves setting standard costs for hospital units such as 'bed-days' and 'operating theatre hours' etc. This information can now readily be produced within existing clinical budgeting systems. In management accounting terms this is simply a standard product cost. Most industrial/commercial concerns will have such standard costs calculated for their ranges of products. They would regard them as essential information necessary to plan their activities, to prepare operating budgets and to assist in pricing their products.

All of the developments described above are concerned with the running costs, or 'revenue' expenditure in the NHS. Similar developments occurred in respect of capital expenditure. Before the reforms the NHS was much criticised because it did not have a comprehensive inventory of its fixed assets. It did not therefore have a commercial-type balance sheet which shows the value of those assets, nor did it take a 'depreciation' or 'leasing' charge for the use of those assets into its income and expenditure account.

However, as with revenue expenditure, recognition of these weaknesses is not new. They too were identified in the Royal Commission and, similarly, there has been a series of developments in the intervening decade. Three are particularly significant.

First, we have had the introduction in 1981 of a more formal and comprehensive Investment Appraisal Mechanism 'known as the Appraisal of Options Procedure (DHSS 1981). This was refined with the issue of the revised Capricode manual in 1986 (DHSS 1986). Second, we had the Ceri Davies Report of 1983 (DHSS 1983) advocating the need for Health Authorities to develop an estate management plan. Third, we had the 1985 report by the then Association of Health Service Treasurers on Managing Capital Assets in the NHS (AHST 1985), in the light of which work was commissioned at three DHAs on setting up comprehensive asset systems.

Now no-one could argue that all the problems of financial management – particularly as an aid to achieving the maximum VFM from limited resources – had been overcome by the end of 1988. Indeed the opposite is the case. Across the whole of the NHS there had barely been a scratching of the surface. However, all of the developments underway at the time – involving both capital and revenue expenditure – shared three particular characteristics: they were evolutionary, they were ongoing and they were incomplete.

They were evolutionary in that, although many of the 'trials' pilot studies' and 'demonstrations' had different origins, there was frequently a common thread linking one to another, and lessons learned from one have been applied in another. They were ongoing in that they were still at an early stage and the process of applying them right across the whole of the NHS would take several years – probably up to the end of the century. Finally they were incomplete in that even on the pilot sites, many issues had yet to be addressed. Four in particular could readily be identified:

1 In the case of the RMI there is a need to co-ordinate activities in the acute hospitals with activities in community units and in family practitioner services to ensure – overall – the best VFM.

2 There is a need to introduce more comprehensive variance analysis to explain differences between 'budgeted' and 'actual' expenditure.

3 There is a need to tie together developments in revenue accounting with developments in capital and asset accounting to ensure that the impact of capital is properly accounted for.

4 There is a need to develop flexible budgeting to ensure that actual expenditure is measured against a budget which has been flexed to take account of actual workload (recognising both volume and mix factors). Flexible budgeting is normal practice in the industrial/

commercial environment. In the context of acute hospitals in the NHS it is the logical next stage to follow case-mix accounting, and could have been introduced with some changes to the 'old' funding structures of the NHS. Several advantages can be identified, perhaps the most important of which is that it would remove the financial disincentive which existed for doctors, hospitals and Health Authorities to treat more patients.

Thus at the end of 1988, there was a full and ongoing agenda for financial management within the NHS. Clearly it would have considerable implications for the staffing and structure of finance departments.

However, that agenda did have the advantage that it could be developed on an evolutionary basis, and that further innovations could be incorporated without major upheaval.

Phase 3: the *Working for Patients* White Paper and the Conservative Government reforms

The *Working for Patients* White Paper of January 1989 (WFP) and the subsequent legislation (the NHS and Community Care Act 1990) created just that upheaval.

Despite the commitment that 'the NHS is, and will continue to be, open to all, regardless of income and financed mainly out of general taxation' its impact was revolutionary. The main feature of the proposed changes was the creation of an 'internal market' in which DHAs would purchase health care on behalf of their local population from hospitals and community units who would be the providers of health care. Of the five key aims of the changes listed in the White Paper, four were financial, namely:

1 To improve the information available to local managers, enabling them in turn to make their budgeting and monitoring more accurate, sensitive and timely.

2 To ensure that hospital consultants – whose decisions effectively commit sums of money – are involved in the management of hospitals; are given responsibility for the use of resources; and are encouraged to use those resources more effectively.

3 To contract out more functions which do not have to be undertaken by Health Authority staff and which could be provided more cost effectively by the private sector.

4 To ensure that drug prescribing costs are kept within reasonable limits.

Amongst the specific changes impacting on the finance function were:

1 The separation of responsibility for purchasing health care from that of providing health care. RHAs and DHAs were to have planning, commissioning and monitoring roles, while as many operational roles as possible are delegated to the hospitals.

2 Hospitals were able to apply for self governing status within the NHS as Hospital Trusts. They are not then funded directly but earn revenue from the services they provide.

3 NHS Hospital Trusts were to be run by a Board of Directors – including a Director of Finance – on 'business-like' lines. They would therefore be free to retain surpluses and build up reserves, or to manage temporary deficits.

4 NHS Trusts were to produce annual accounts similar in format to 'Companies Act' accounts. They therefore included a full balance sheet, income and expenditure account and cash flow statement. The liabilities side of the balance sheet includes:

  (a) Interest Bearing Debt (IBD), in respect of which interest payments must be made to the Treasury.

  (b) Public Dividend Capital (PDC) on which, in due course, dividends will be paid to the Treasury.

5 The assets of those hospitals becoming Trusts were to be vested in the Trust. Hence the Trust would manage its own capital programme and would be able to dispose of assets as it thinks appropriate and has borrowing powers, subject to an overall financing limit.

6 NHS Hospital Trusts could negotiate the pay and conditions of their own staff, and acquire their own supplies and services locally.

7 Contracts needed to be negotiated between purchasers and providers for hospital services. These contracts needed to specify the services to be supplied and prices could be in three forms:

  (a) 'block' contracts for certain essential 'core' services;

  (b) 'cost and volume' contracts specifying a price for a minimum level of service, with additional cases treated over that minimum to be supplied at agreed prices;

  (c) 'cost per case' contracts.

8 A new system of resource allocation was to replace RAWP enabling money required to treat patients to be able to cross administrative boundaries.

9 A system of 'capital charges' was introduced to reflect Health Authorities' use of existing capital assets and any new capital investment. The charges are set to cover the costs of interest and depreciation.

10 Family Health Services Authorities (successors to the Family Practitioner Committees) became accountable to RHAs and receive their funding from them.

11 Large GP practices were able to apply for their own practice budgets to enable them to purchase a defined range of services direct from hospitals. Such practices were known as GP Fundholders (GPFHs).

12 There was to be a closer monitoring of FHS drug expenditure. RHAs would distribute funds to FHSAs on a 'RAWP-like' weighted capitation formula. FHSAs will in turn monitor expenditure through 'Indicative Prescribing Amounts' for GP practices.

13 FHSAs, to continue the development towards actively managing – as opposed to purely administering – the FHS.

This was a formidable new agenda to be imposed – and implemented within a very short time scale – on top of the existing programme.

While the first of these changes came into effect on 1 April 1991, each anniversary of that date through to 1 April 1996 saw further changes. Moreover, on that latter date we saw the abolition of the Regional Health Authorities (being replaced by regional offices of the NHS Executive) and the (newly created) FHSAs being subsumed into the DHAs.

Collectively these 'reforms' created a new internal funding structure within the NHS, and a huge new agenda for the finance function.

The first point that needed to be considered was simply the mechanics of making it work. Existing finance departments were not designed to handle this funding structure. Consequently there needed to be a massive overhaul.

Moreover, initially the requirement was for largely financial accounting facilities to address such issues as:

- How do we collect the income which is due to us?

- How do we pay for clinical services which we are purchasing?

- How do we pay for the goods and services which we need?

- How do we pay the wages?

It was in fact a diversion of resources away from the priorities which existed at the end of 1988 which were to develop the management accounting skills of the NHS: particularly to promote the better use of resources through the RMI.

Thus despite the fact that the reforms required a substantial input of accounting resources, these were largely committed to the bureaucratic tasks of co-ordinating transactions between A and B.

Writing now in the summer of 1997, after the election of a Labour Government committed to the 'abolition of the internal market', it is perhaps appropriate to look back to the period of the Conservative Government's reforms and draw some conclusions. Space will not permit an exhaustive analysis but I believe it is appropriate to comment on four aspects of these 'reforms'. They are: information for pricing and costing, the impact of capital charges, capital expenditure and the Private Finance Initiative (the PFI was not a central component of the WFP but subsequently became a central plank of Conservative Government policy on the NHS); and the financial cost of the internal market.

Information for pricing and costing

A fragmented NHS, in which various organisations buy and sell clinical services from one another on a 'business-like' basis, requires information for pricing. The White Paper made the bland assumption that this would be provided by the Resource Management Initiative.

There were two major misconceptions here. First was the issue of the timetable for 'rolling out' the RMI to the 260 major acute units. WFP made the statement that the RMI would be 'extended and accelerated' with the aim of building up coverage to those units by the end of 1991/92. There was never any prospect of that happening and, of course, it did not happen.

A more serious misconception was that the RMI was designed to provide the appropriate information for pricing. This was never the intention of the RMI. In fact the case-mix accounting developments within the RMI were still in their infancy. The six pilot sites were concentrating on the use of DRGs (and their successors HRGs) which cover only adult acute in-patients. Outpatients (and other categories) were not covered. In addition there is much evidence that DRG/HRGs are not the appropriate classifications for pricing purposes even within adult acute inpatient cases. Certainly they did not correspond to the categories identified within WFPs, GP practice budgets.

In a comprehensive survey of NHS costing Ellwood (1992) concluded: *the role of the NHS accountant in ensuring the successful developments of the NHS internal market centres around his ability to deliver on costing and pricing contracts. Existing cost methods are far from adequate to ensure an efficient allocation of healthcare resources through the internal market.*

Inevitably, the truth of that statement was realised and 1993 saw the 'Costing for Contracting' initiative (DoH 1993). This contained guidance on an absorption costing approach to allocating costs to treatment categories and to producing prices (embodying the totally unrealistic principle that 'costs' equate to 'prices') for HRG categories. Costing for Contracting has developed since 1993 and for the 1997/98 contracting round all acute hospitals were required to produce HRG prices for all surgical specialties 'to inform the contracting prices'. In a follow-up survey Ellwood (1996) again concludes that:

cost methods have developed and, following detailed guidance from the NHSME, consistency has improved, but a lack of activity information remains. Price variations due to costing approaches rather than differing resource use still persist. The thorny problem of adequately defining the healthcare products for costing purposes remains to be resolved.

Moreover, the reality is that few hospitals have the internal budgetary control systems to enable them to monitor actual expenditure on a case-mix basis. In the absence of such systems, in the absence of more cost per case contracts, and in the absence of providers having the freedom to separate 'prices' from 'costs', there was never any prospect of the internal market actually behaving like a market. Instead it could be argued that it had become purely a very cumbersome system of resource allocation.

Capital charges

A feature of the reforms was the introduction of a system of capital charges. They had three objectives:

1 to increase awareness in health service managers of the cost of capital;

2 to create incentives to use capital efficiently;

3 to see NHS provision evaluated on a basis broadly comparable with the private sector.

Note, however, that funds for NHS capital investment continued (initially) to be provided by the Exchequer as a separate allocation within the overall programme. Capital charges therefore impacted on the distribution of revenue funds to Health Authorities (*sic*). Capital accounting is a difficult area and no one would seriously argue that previous NHS practice was satisfactory. Indeed the need for Health Authorities and Trusts to hold comprehensive asset registers was no more than basic accounting. There is no doubt that the introduction of capital charges has done something to increase awareness in health service managers of the cost of capital. However, there is a considerable diversity of practice in the treatment of capital charges at local level and by no means all Trusts follow the (somewhat doubtful) requirement to take capital charges down to the level of the individual budget holder. Thus it is not clear whether capital charges have 'created incentives to use capital efficiently'.

In addition, capital charges are to include a 'depreciation' and an 'interest' element. That of course is not comparable to the private sector where the return on capital element falls in the margin between calculated 'costs' and selling prices. In addition, assets are to be revalued (now) at intervals of five years. However, this too is not private sector practice. The private sector has, in fact, been struggling with the intricacies of inflation accounting for the last 25 years and has, by and large, abandoned the idea as being too difficult. Certainly there is no requirement in private hospitals to revalue their fixed assets every five years. Hence, far from seeing NHS provision evaluated on a basis broadly comparable with the private sector, the authors of WFP swung the balance in favour of private hospitals. Objective No. 3 is not achieved.

In fact, with regard to fixed assets, there are two important requirements to ensure that they are deployed efficiently. First, there is the need to get the original investment appraisal right. Here the NHS has made considerable progress in recent years since the introduction of the Appraisal of Options procedure. Second, there is the need to create a funding structure whereby managers are encouraged to treat as many patients as possible. If they can do that they will be using their resources (including fixed assets) efficiently. Flexed budgets coupled with case-mix accounting promises that.

Capital expenditure and the Private Finance Initiative

Although originally promised for the end of 1991 a new capital investment manual did not appear until 1994 (NHS Executive 1994). It was a review and rewrite of the procedures set in the context of the 'reformed NHS' which had an internal market of purchasers and providers.

Essentially the new manual was a (well written) restatement of the Appraisal of Options procedure but conducted by an NHS Trust and set in the context of its strategic business case. Some constructive criticisms can be made of this manual (HFMA 1996) but overall it was a welcome development.

Less welcome, however, was the Conservative Government's commitment to the Private Finance Initiative (PFI) originally outlined under HSG(95)15 (NHS Executive 1995) which made it clear that private finance must be 'significantly explored' before approval would be given to a major scheme. It is now clear that there are three valid criticisms of the PFI.

- In the long term it will be more expensive to the NHS. Private investors will be looking to a higher return on investment than the 6 per cent per annum required by the Treasury.

- The PFI process itself is cumbersome, bureaucratic, expensive and time consuming.

- PFI distorts the traditional funding structure of the NHS with its separate capital vote and revenue vote. Essentially it is committing revenue resources to pay for capital assets.

The financial cost of the internal market

It is quite impossible to put a precise financial cost on the internal market. However, it is significant. Already since the 1997 General Election a review of contracting by the Accounts Commission for Scotland (1997) shows the possible cost of managing the purchasing side of contracting as being up to 0.6 per cent of contract costs. Earlier surveys by the Healthcare Financial Management Association suggest that up to 2 per cent of HCHS revenue funding is committed to the purchasing function. If we assume that a similar amount is committed to the sales function, then up to 4 per cent of revenue resources are being applied simply to the mechanisms of operating the market. Currently that is £1 billion per annum. Perhaps £500 million is a reasonable 'ball-park guesstimate'.

Conclusions on phase 3

As we have seen, the 'reforms' introduced by the Conservative Government following WFP caused a huge and expensive upheaval to the NHS finance function. It has achieved moderate success in some areas but, arguably, it substantially delayed the development of the real management accounting information which occurred during phase 2. It was eight wasted years.

Phase 4: the NHS and the Labour Government

Here we are entering uncharted territory. Clearly the NHS will be different. What is unclear is how different. Writing in the summer of 1997 we have only a few straws in the wind that might serve to give us an indication of what is to come. Significant amongst these straws: are the speech of 3 December 1996 by Mr Chris Smith MP when Shadow Secretary of State for Health (Smith 1996); EL(97)33 of 22 May 1997 (NHS Executive 1997); and the speech of 25 June 1997 by Mr Frank Dobson MP, now Secretary of State for Health (Dobson 1997). Collectively, they promise us an NHS White Paper in the autumn of 1997 and a 'debate on commissioning models for the future'. This chapter is now written as a contribution to that debate.

Pending the White Paper we need to examine the Smith speech to glean any indication of the future structure of the NHS. From this we must presume:

- The purchaser–provider split remains (although the rhetoric will be changed to commissioners–provider).

- NHS trusts will remain in more or less their present forms (although there may be fewer of them).

- GP practices will continue in more or less their present forms (including GP Fundholders).

- GP Commissioning Groups will be created, each to serve a population of between 50,000 and 150,000. However, the precise structure, function, funding and membership of such groups is unclear.

- District Health Authorities will continue to retain a responsibility for the overall planning of health care. However, they are to contain between 5 and 15 GP Commissioning Groups. We must assume therefore that their average local population will be about one million. This in turn means halving the number of the present DHAs (which have only been in place in their present forms since April 1996).

- The 'internal market' is to be abolished.

Since the election it has also become clear that the Private Finance Initiative will continue to play a part (perhaps a reduced part) in NHS capital expenditure. The DoH has now gone through a process of 'paring down' the original list of 35 major schemes (outside of London) to 12. But they will go ahead. What will happen to the remainder remains unclear.

The dilemma now facing the Government is how to make it work. Crucial questions to be addressed include:

- How do we get the money to the NHS Trusts?

- How do we ensure that the objectives of the GP Commissioning Groups are achieved?

- How do we ensure that the objectives of the DHAs are achieved?

- How do we create incentives for the hospitals to treat as many patients as possible within the constraints of their facilities and subject, of course, to achieving clinical effectiveness?
- How are variations in workload to be funded?
- How are Extra Contractual Refunds (ie patients from outside the locality) to be funded?
- How is capital expenditure to be funded?

I believe that it is possible to resolve this dilemma and to answer the questions above satisfactorily. This can be achieved by a revision of the financing of the NHS in three ways:

- A revision of the overall funding structure of the NHS.
- A recognition that NHS Trusts are responsible for their own capital expenditure.
- The introduction at DHA level of local, flexible financial planning agreements.

Let us look at each of these in turn.

The overall funding structure of the NHS

Currently, Parliament 'votes' to the NHS separate allocations of funds for revenue expenditure and capital expenditure. In addition there is an element of 'funny money' revolving around the system. This originates as the interest and dividends paid by NHS Trusts to the Treasury (ostensibly as a charge for the use of their capital assets) and is then fed back into the system as part of the revenue allocations.

My view is that this link should be broken. NHS trusts should continue to be liable to pay interest to the Treasury on their IBD. However, the Treasury allocation to the NHS should be one allocation of funds and should cover revenue operating costs and an element (which needs to be calculated separately) for the use of the capital assets (of an appropriate standard) in delivering health care. There would cease to be a separate allocation of funds specifically for capital expenditure. In addition, there would be no requirement that the capital servicing element of revenue funds should equate to the sum of the present capital expenditure allocation plus interest and dividends received from NHS Trusts.

The abolition of the distinction between capital and revenue funding is not a new recommendation. It was made as long ago as 1985 in the then AHST report (AHST 1985). However, in my view it once again becomes relevant in the light of the blurring of that distinction which is occurring anyway in PFI schemes, and in the light of the need to define responsibility for capital expenditure.

NHS Trusts to be responsible for their own capital expenditure

The 1994 Capital Investment Manual was a valuable piece of work. It was essentially an updating of the Appraisal of Options procedure for capital expenditure, but in the context of the internal market. It was clearly based on the assumption that it was an NHS Trust that was responsible for initiating capital expenditure proposals. While this might not always be appropriate, I believe it to be a principle which should now be restated.

If an NHS Trust is receiving funding which includes a capital element, then the logic of the situation is that the Trust should be responsible for the financing of those facilities. This can be done in one of four ways:

- From internally generated funds (Trusts retain the 'depreciation' element of their capital charges).

- By borrowing the funds (either from the Government or commercially) to build their own facilities.

- By conventional leasing of facilities provided by a commercial company.

- By some form of PFI deal whereby a commercial company (or consortium of companies) designs, builds *and operates* facilities in return for payments from the Trust.

The issue of how they are funded is local to the Trust. It does not need to be a matter of national concern.

Local financial planning agreements

Within each new district of a million or so people it would appear that the Government is planning to create a new tripartite structure of:

- A District Health Authority which has an overall health care planning remit.

- A number of GP Commissioning Groups which will be concerned to see that the local providers deliver the health care they require.

- A number of NHS Trusts.

The problem is how to get the money to the NHS Trusts and to achieve the objectives of the DHA and the GP Commissioning Groups.

My view is that this can be achieved by means of local flexible financial planning agreements. To achieve this it would be necessary to set up a financial planning unit within each DHA. Such a unit would, however, need to work very closely with the GP Commissioning Groups and the local NHS Trusts. The objective would be to produce approved operating budgets for each of the Trusts based in a district. Such operating budgets would need, on the one hand, to incorporate the health care objectives of each of the local GP Commissioning Groups. On the other hand, they would need to conform to the overall funding constraints that are imposed on the DHA. The anticipated workload of patients from outside the District (ECRs in the current jargon) can be incorporated following discussions between each planning group and those of neighbouring districts. They would draw extensively on case-mix information (particularly HRGs) and would incorporate flexible budgets. (A memorandum on the use of flexible budgets appears as an Addendum to this chapter).

Conclusions

I believe it is possible to envisage a rational funding structure within the NHS which does abolish the internal market and which provides the incentives to deliver the greatest VFM from limited resources. I believe that the proposals outlined above provide the basis for this to be achieved. However, it will not be easy. Research is required into a number of obvious aspects including:

- Calculating the capital element of the combined revenue allocation.
- The continued development of case-mix accounting.
- A study of fixed, variable and semi-variable expenses in the NHS.
- Studies of expenditure programmes outside acute care.

Nevertheless, what the probable structure does offer is a return to the ongoing and evolutionary (and far from complete) nature of NHS financial management.

Addendum

Value for money, flexible budgets and NHS acute hospitals

There are many textbook definitions of a budget. The Chartered Institute of Management Accountants (CIMA) describes a budget as 'a quantitative statement for a defined period of time, which may include planned revenues, expenses, assets, liabilities and cash flows'. Putting it at its simplest, a budget is a financial plan.

CIMA then goes on to describe a flexible budget as one 'which by recognising different cost behaviour patterns, is designed to change as volume of activity changes'.

Flexible budgets are extensively used in private sector industry. Let us take a very simple example to illustrate their application. Assume that a company makes three products, 'A', 'B' and 'C', and has calculated product costs of £8.00, £10.00 and £12.00 each, respectively. In advance of the financial year the company will prepare its budget for the coming year. If the Sales Director believes he can sell 1,000 units of each product each week, this would give a weekly budget as shown in Table 4.1

Table 4.1

Product	Product cost £/unit	Sales volume	Budget £
A	8	1,000	8,000
B	10	1,000	10,000
C	12	1,000	12,000
Total		3,000	30,000

As part of the budget setting process this budget will have been approved by the Purchasing Director (who will agree that he can buy in the necessary raw materials at prices incorporated into these costs), the Personnel Director (who will agree that he can employ the labour needed at the wage rates incorporated into these costs), the Works Director and the Finance Director. So we have an agreed weekly budget.

What then happens, of course, is that the Sales Director goes out into the market place and comes back with an order book which inevitably differs from that budgeted. As an example, let us assume that it is Product 'A' – 800 units per week; Product 'B' – 1,100 units per week; and Product 'C' – 1,200 units per week. Note that the order book differs in total (3,100 units per week rather than 3,000) and also differs as to the mix of products required.

At this point the Works Director will say, 'Okay, I recognise that those are the products I must make in the factory and, of course, I will do so, but *don't expect me to do so within the original budget of £30,000 per week.*' The budget must be flexed as shown in Table 4.2.

Table 4.2

Product	Product cost £/unit	Sales volume	Budget £
A	8	800	6,400
B	10	1,100	11,000
C	12	1,200	14,400
Total		**3,100**	**31,800**

This revised, or flexed, budget becomes particularly significant at the next stage when we start comparing actual expenditure with that budgeted. If, in manufacturing the required production, the Works Manager incurs an actual expenditure of, say, £31,000 in a week it would be complete nonsense to say to him, 'You have overspent by £1,000 against the original budget of £30,000' when in fact he has achieved savings of £800 against the flexed budget. Yet that is exactly what has been happening in NHS acute hospitals for years – and continues to happen where there are 'block' contracts between District Health Authorities and NHS Trusts.

At this point we must introduce a further factor; the need to distinguish fixed costs from variable costs. CIMA defines a fixed cost as 'a cost which is incurred for an accounting period, and which, within certain output or turnover limits, tends to be unaffected by fluctuations in the levels of activity'. A variable cost, in turn, is one 'which varies with a measure of activity'.

This distinction is fundamental to management accounting. It recognises that in any organisation there are some costs (depreciation, heating, lighting, insurance, local authority rates, etc.) which are there (in the short term at least) regardless of the level of activity. On the other hand, there are some costs (raw materials and bought in components in a manufacturing environment) which vary upwards or downwards as the level of activity varies upwards or downwards. It is thus possible to draw a simple graph showing the relationship between costs on the one hand and the level of activity on the other (Figure 4.3).

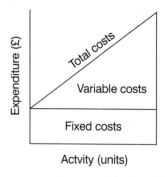

Figure 4.3 Relationship between level of activity and expenditure

In our simple example we assumed initially that all the costs were variable. If we now recast the budget on the assumption that there is a 50/50 split between fixed and variable costs, we have a revised original budget as shown in Table 4.3. Note that this still shows a total budget of £30,000 per week. It has simply been presented in a slightly different format.

Table 4.3

Product	Variable product cost £/unit	Sales volume	Budget £
A	4	1,000	4,000
B	5	1,000	5,000
C	6	1,000	6,000
Fixed costs			15,000
Total		**3,000**	**30,000**

However, the flexed budget is recalculated as in Table 4.4. Note that in calculating the flexed budget the variable costs have varied as the required numbers of each product have varied, but that the fixed costs have remained fixed.

Table 4.4

Product	Variable product cost £/unit	Sales volume	Budget £
A	4	800	3,200
B	5	1,100	5,500
C	6	1,200	7,200
Fixed costs			15,000
Total		**3,100**	**30,900**

We now have a much more meaningful total against which to compare the Works Director's actual expenditure of £31,000.

What then is the relevance of all this to the NHS in general and to acute hospitals in particular? On the one hand an acute hospital consists of certain fixed assets – land, buildings, operating theatres, scientific and X-ray equipment, etc – and it consists of a highly skilled workforce of doctors, nurses, professions allied to medicine and support staff. On the other hand the pursuit of Value for Money (VFM) requires that we make 'the best' use of limited resources. Usually VFM is defined in terms of the 'three Es' – economy, efficiency and effectiveness. Essentially it requires that limited resources are used to deliver a health service that is first and foremost 'effective' but also manages its resources 'efficiently' and 'economically'. Without then getting into any clinical arguments as to what is or is not 'effective' treatment, I would advocate that the pursuit of 'efficiency' requires that the management of an NHS acute hospital should be using their limited fixed assets and their limited manpower resources to treat as many patients as possible. However, this clearly has not always happened in our hospitals because of the effects of the rigid cash limits (and, currently, rigid block contracts) which can be seen to have placed too much emphasis on the 'economy' aspect of VFM.

How then can NHS acute hospital managers be given the latitude to treat as many patients as possible within the physical constraints of their facilities without costs running out of control? Flexible budgets hold the solution to this conundrum.

As in our private sector example above, hospital budgets must be prepared recognising the distinction between fixed costs and variable costs. And in the case of an acute hospital the bulk of the costs are fixed costs. All of the costs relating to the building are fixed, and traditionally all the staff costs have been regarded as fixed. Falling into the 'variable' category are the costs of drugs, dressings, X-ray supplies and some laundry and catering costs. Conventional wisdom has it that the fixed/variable split in an acute hospital is about 85/15. This is shown diagramatically to give an approximate picture in Figure 4.4.

This means that if hospital budgets can be prepared incorporating Healthcare Resource Groups (HRGs) which recognise the fixed/variable split, then the very real prospect arises of saying to hospital managers,

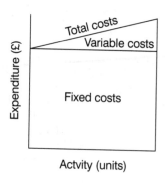

Figure 4.4 Relationship between level of activity and expenditure in acute hospitals

'there are your fixed assets, there is your cohort of doctors and nurses; now use them to treat as many patients as possible'. The HRGs would act as the equivalent of the product costs in our simple example above and provide the basis to 'flex' the budgets, recognising changes in the volume of activity and changes in case-mix. However, the fixed element of the budget remains fixed and the 'flexing' operates only on the variable costs. Thus the arithmetic remains in favour of retaining financial control. If we assume that the budget is prepared with an 80/20 fixed/variable cost split, then even if the hospital increases its volume of activity by 10 per cent over that originally budgeted, its flexed budget increases by only two per cent. At the same time it is using its physical resources to their fullest capacity, and this improvement in efficiency is clearly measured in that its average cost per case falls by 1.02/1.10, ie to 92.7 per cent of the original budget.

Conceptually it is very simple but, of course, there are problem areas to be overcome. I believe that four such problems can be identified.

1 Even after several years the development of case-mix accounting is still, in reality, at an early stage. The leading hospitals have accumulated a considerable amount of case-mix information and are beginning to develop systems of internal budgetary control incorporating HRGs. Others are only just beginning and lack the strength needed in their accounting departments and hospital information systems. However, work should continue. One criticism of the current internal market is not that the NHS is employing too many accountants, but rather that it is employing them in doing the wrong things. The 'reforms' following *Working for Patients* have required a huge input of resources on the purely financial accounting tasks of conducting transactions between DHAs, GP Fundholders and NHS Trusts. This in turn has meant that the development of real management accounting information has been neglected.

2 Even with a comprehensive system of case-mix accounting, not all the work of an acute hospital fits neatly into HRG categories. There will

probably always be some workload that falls outside such categories and must be accounted for separately. However, I do not feel that this invalidates the whole approach.

3 In the real world, not all costs fit neatly into the black and white 'fixed' and 'variable' categories. The reality is that there are shades of grey. Unfortunately, in the context of an NHS acute hospital, the biggest single item of expenditure – nursing salaries, which may make up as much as 40 per cent of the total costs – falls into the 'semi-variable' category where an increase in workload means an increase in expenditure, but not on a straight line basis. In reality the fixed/variable split itself varies, of course, between different specialties and between different case-mix categories within specialties. Some work has been done on defining the degree of 'variability' of semi-variable costs but that, too, is at an early stage.

4 Finally, the internal structure has never been created within the NHS which has made it possible to incorporate flexible budgets into the financial regime of acute hospitals. I believe that within the expected triangular proposal for enlarged DHAs, GP Commissioning Groups and local NHS Trusts, it would be possible. I would envisage a situation whereby it is the responsibility of the District Health Authority to negotiate financial plans for NHS Trusts within a District which incorporate flexible budgets. I recommend that this should be done – initially on a trial basis in a number of pilot districts.

References

Accounts Commission for Scotland (1997) *Bulletin 1. Expanding on Contracting* Accounts Commission for Scotland, Edinburgh

AHST (1985) *Managing Capital Assets in the NHS* AHST/CIPFA

Blyth, J (1983) *Budgetary Control/Management Budgeting.* Unpublished.

DHSS (1981) *DHSS Health Notice (81) 30: Health Services Management. Health Building Procedures* DHSS, London

DHSS (1983) *Underused and Surplus Property in the NHS, Report of the Enquiry* HMSO, London

DHSS (1986a). *Capricode : Health Building Procedures* HMSO, London

DHSS (1986b) *DHSS Health Notice (86) 34: Resource Management (Management Budgeting) in Health Authorities* DHSS, London

Dobson, F (1997) *Speech to the Annual Conference of the NHS Confederation* DoH, London

Ellwood, S (1992) *Cost Methods for NHS Healthcare Contracts* CIMA, London

Ellwood, S (1996) *Cost-based pricing in the NHS Internal Market* CIMA, London

HFMA Occasional Papers (1996) *The Appraisal and Financing of Capital Expenditure in the NHS* HFMA/CIPFA, London

Maynard, A (1984) *Budgeting in Health Care Systems Effective Health Care 2*, 41–48.

Montacute, C (1962) *Costing and Efficiency in Hospitals: a critical survey of management of hospitals* Oxford University Press (for Nuffield Provincial Hospitals Trust), Oxford

NHS/DHSS (1984) *Steering Group on Health Services Information: Sixth Report to the Secretary of State* HMSO, London

NHS Management Executive (1993) Executive Letter (93) 26. *Costing for Contracting*, DoH, Leeds

NHS Executive (1994) *Capital Investment Manual* HMSO, London

NHS Executive (1995) *HSG (95) 15. Private Finance and Capital Investment Projects* DoH, Leeds

NHS Executive (1997) *Executive Letters (97) 33. Changing the Internal Market* DoH, London

Royal Commission on the NHS (1978) Research Paper No. 2, *Management of Financial Resources in the NHS* HMSO, London

Smith, C (1996) *A Health Service for a New Century* Labour Party, London

5 Assessing efficiency in the NHS: a case of unfulfilled potential?

Michael Drummond

Introduction

Increased efficiency was one of the major objectives of the White Paper *Working for Patients* (DoH 1989). The document proposed a number of efficiency promoting measures, including the establishment of an 'internal market' for health services with contracts between 'purchasers' and 'providers', a voluntary scheme for those general practices that wish to manage their own budget and indicative drugs budgets for all general practitioners.

Since the pursuit of increased efficiency is one of the major objectives of the proposals, this begs the question of how efficiency will be assessed. Chapter 3 in this volume (Mullen) points out that the functioning of the internal market in health care is not a simple matter. One cannot necessarily assume that the operation of market principles *per se* will automatically lead to efficiency. Indeed, there is considerable evidence from the literature (Evans 1985) that this is not the case, whether the patient is the direct consumer of services, or whether the doctor acts as an agent on the patient's behalf.

There has been relatively little formal assessment of the efficiency of alternative health care programmes or treatments in the UK (Ludbrook and Mooney 1983, Drummond and Hutton 1987, Coyle 1993). Authors point to a number of possible explanations, including the lack of appropriate evaluative skills, the lack of available data and the lack of appropriate incentives. Indeed, the only formal standing requirement for economic evaluation of alternative plans or programmes in the NHS in recent years has been option appraisal for schemes where one of the options is a capital scheme with an initial outlay of £10 million or more (DHSS 1981). In such cases, the Regional Health Authority needed to submit a formal evaluation of the costs and benefits of options with its approval in principle submission to the Department of Health (Akehurst 1989). With the development of independent NHS trusts, option appraisal has continued to form part of a broader business planning exercise.

In addition, the Department of Health has undertaken, or commissioned, evaluations of health technologies at the national level (Buxton *et al.* 1985) and has issued guidance on the economic evaluation of medical equipment (DHSS 1988). However, it has neither been thought desirable nor feasible to require formal evaluations of alternative programmes, treatments or technologies at the local level. Rather, the emphasis has been on encouraging decision makers in authorities, trusts and general practices to behave in an efficient manner, through a mixture of information and incentives.

This chapter examines the prospects and problems of assessing the efficiency of health care alternatives since the 1990 reforms. In particular, it considers the following issues:

1 what methods are available for assessing the efficiency of health care programmes and treatments;

2 in what ways did the reforms offer the potential for more assessment of efficiency;

3 what evidence there is that the reforms have encouraged assessment of efficiency and what the remaining problems are.

Finally, a few conclusions are drawn.

Methods for assessing the efficiency of health care programmes

The methods of economic evaluation have been well documented elsewhere, so will only briefly be described here (Drummond 1980, Warner and Luce 1982, Luce and Elixhauser 1990, Drummond *et al.* 1997a). There are several related techniques, all having the common feature that some combination of the costs (resources consumed) of health care programmes are compared with some combination of the consequences (eg, improvements in health obtained).

The particular techniques differ mainly in the extent to which they measure and value the consequences. Some techniques, such as cost analysis and cost minimization analysis, proceed on the basis that the alternatives under consideration have been shown to be equivalent in effectiveness. Others, such as cost-utility analysis and cost benefit analysis, measure consequences in quality-adjusted life-years and money terms respectively. The most widely used technique is cost-effectiveness analysis, where the costs are measured in money terms and the improvements in health assessed in the most convenient natural units, such as 'years of life gained' or 'disability days avoided'. (The various components of economic evaluation are outlined in Figure 5.1.)

There are two features of economic evaluation that merit particular emphasis in the light of the NHS reforms. First, assessment of efficiency explicitly requires consideration of both the resource use and the improvements in health obtained from the use of health care

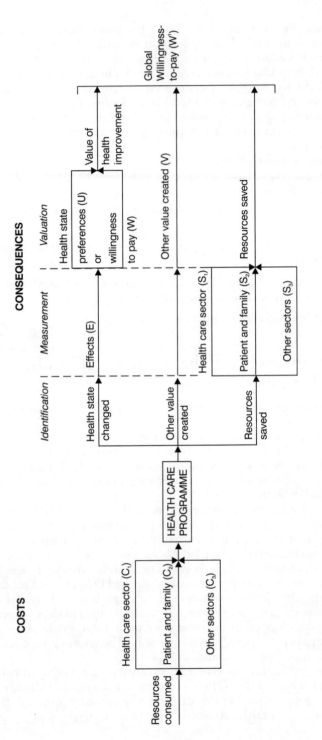

Figure 5.1   Components of economic evaluation (Source: Drummond *et al.* 1997a)

interventions. Therefore, improvements in efficiency need to be distinguished from cost-cutting measures, where no consideration is given to the reduction in the effectiveness of the programme when the resource commitment is reduced. Therefore, in the context of contracts for clinical services, or the establishment of community drugs formularies, the lowest cost option is not necessarily the most efficient.

Second, assessment of efficiency implies a wide consideration of the costs of health care programmes. For example, the consideration of cost is not restricted to the hospital, but includes also the costs in primary care and those borne by patients and their families. In the past, there has been a tendency in the NHS to shift costs from hospital to primary care budgets, through the earlier discharge of patients from hospital, or through restrictions in drug prescribing on hospital discharge. (Conversely, long waiting times for an outpatient attendance or for hospital admission also shift costs from secondary care to primary care. In the average district general hospital a significant proportion of medical admissions are emergencies.)

A key aspect of the reforms is that the Health Authority and Family Health Service Authority budgets are more interrelated. In addition, those general practices wishing to administer their own budgets under the GP Fundholding scheme have included in their fund a component to cover certain hospital-based treatments. However, this falls short of the health maintenance organisation (HMO) concept in the USA, where all the health care of enrollees is a charge on the HMO (Drummond and Maynard 1988). The total fundholding pilot schemes more closely resemble HMOs, but their future is in doubt given the new Labour Government's concerns about fundholding. Nevertheless, the reforms should, in principle, change the behaviour of key actors, such as general practitioners, in respect of the costs they consider relevant to their decisions.

Potential impact of the NHS reforms on the assessment of efficiency

It was mentioned earlier that, with the exception of option appraisal, the application of economic evaluation methods has been limited in the NHS to date. In 1987, Drummond and Hutton undertook a review of the economic appraisal of health technology (Drummond and Hutton 1987). They found that 50 economic appraisals had been published, covering a wide range of topics. This is still minute in relation to the number of health technologies used in the NHS, however.

Since 1987 the practice of economic evaluation in the UK has continued to expand with many more studies being published. In 1994 the Department of Health compiled a Register of Cost-Effectiveness Studies, with the assistance of researchers from the University of York (DoH 1994). This reviewed and classified 147 studies (from the UK and elsewhere) that contained cost-effectiveness data on around 500 health care interventions. The objective of the Register was to provide information to health care decision makers. More recently there have been a number of initiatives to ensure that the content and delivery of care in the NHS is based on high quality research, through the NHS Research and Development Strategy.

It is much more likely that the majority of assessments are currently undertaken either informally or indirectly. For example, the managers in most NHS trusts expect their clinical staff to be applying the most appropriate treatment technologies, either in their day-to-day practice, or in submitting bids for the development of clinical services. The extent to which this feeling is misplaced is unknown. Managers mainly comfort themselves in the knowledge that physical and financial resources for clinical work are in short supply in the NHS. This is therefore likely to encourage clinicians to search for more cost-effective procedures. However, it is known from the research into performance indicators that clinical teams with similar levels of resources produce different amounts of services (Yates and Davidge 1984). Also it is conceivable that NHS budgetary controls, while being effective in capping overall expenditure, may militate against the adoption of new, cost-effective, procedures if these necessitate financial outlays.

The discussion above has related mainly to the services under the management of Health Authorities. Even less is known about the assessment of efficiency in general practice. Prior to the reforms, general practitioners were largely free to employ the treatment technologies, mainly pharmaceuticals, that they saw fit, with no overall budgetary limitation. Similarly, there were no restrictions on referrals to secondary care, although long waiting times often acted as a limitation in practice.

Given the arrangements in primary and secondary care prior to the reforms, it is hardly surprising that there had been so little assessment of efficiency. There were no formal requirements and few incentives. As the reforms were implemented, the incentives changed quite considerably. The next sections of this chapter examine a number of the key proposals in relation to the impact they may potentially have on the assessment of efficiency.

The internal market in health care

For the first time, an element of competition has been injected into the provision of health care through the NHS. Health Authorities, through their role as purchasers, enter into contracts with a number of agencies, primarily NHS trusts, to secure health services on behalf of their population. The extent of choice available to the Health Authorities purchasers varies from one location to another, but most deal with a range of providers. The providers are not guaranteed a budget as in the past. Rather, they attract funds as a direct result of the contracts placed. In addition to the contracts placed by Health Authorities, others will come from those general practitioners who opt to manage their own budget.

However, although the extent of competition varies from place to place, all providers have had to think about their business plan. Namely, what markets are they seeking to serve and how are they going to serve them? Since the price at which services are marketed will also be a factor, one would expect that the business planning exercise will prompt an examination of the treatment technologies being employed and their relative cost-effectiveness. Some providers have already gone so far as to produce prospectuses outlining their services. Though these documents do not necessarily show evidence of cost-effectiveness thinking being employed in their production, they are one sign that market forces are having an impact.

Contracts for clinical services

The 1989 White Paper envisaged three broad classes of contract; block contracts, under which the GP or Health Authorities would pay the hospital an annual fee in return for access to a defined range of services; cost and volume contracts, under which hospitals would receive a sum in respect of a baseline level of activity, defined in terms of a given number of treatments or cases, and cost per case contracts, where payment would be made to the hospital on a case by case basis, without any prior commitment of either party to the volume of cases which might be so dealt with.

Although the precise management arrangements for each type of contract differ, the contracting procedure incorporates several key steps, many of which offer the opportunity for assessment of efficiency. In particular, someone, perhaps the Health Authorities or the individual GP, needs to decide whether contracts are to be let for particular services or not. Once this has been decided, a contract specification needs to be written outlining the services to be provided, the treatment technologies to be used, the volume of cases to be treated, the standards to be achieved (in clinical effectiveness and quality of care) and price. Finally, a monitoring system needs to be put in place to see that the work specified in the contract has been undertaken to the required standard within the agreed financial amount. Any deviations from the terms and conditions of the contract would thus have to be justified. These decision points are discussed in turn below.

Deciding whether or not to place a contract

In reality, the scope for choice here will depend on the nature of the clinical service concerned and the room for political manoeuvre. For example, the provision of emergency services locally may not be a matter of choice, although there are, no doubt, choices relating to the nature and extent of emergency cover, eg, number of accident and emergency units in a given geographical area and the extent of 24 hours a day, 7 days a week cover. For certain types of elective operation, there is likely to be much more scope for choice in whether or not to let contracts.

There is scope here for economic evaluation to inform priorities for health care. For example, Williams (1985) pointed out that coronary artery bypass grafting (CABG) for severe angina with left main disease gave much better value for money (£1,040 per Quality-Adjusted Life-

Year (QALY) gained in 1983–84 prices) than CABG for mild angina with
two vessel disease (£12,600 per QALY gained).

Prior to the reforms, priorities within open heart surgery were decided
solely by the clinicians concerned. The Health Authorities merely decided
the level at which it was prepared to fund its surgical unit. One would
expect that, all things being equal, clinical priorities would determine that
the most serious cases are operated upon first, with broader and broader
indications being accepted as funding becomes more widely available.
However, this was rarely expressed as explicit agreement between management and the clinical staff. Indeed, it is possible that clinicians would
treat cases which they find particularly interesting or challenging from a
clinical viewpoint, rather than those which offer the most returns (in
terms of health improvement) in relation to the cost. Many surgical waiting lists comprise large numbers of simple, low cost, procedures. For
example, an analysis of ophthalmology waiting lists has shown that the
vast majority of patients were waiting for cataract extraction (Drummond
and Yates 1991). However, crude calculations of the cost per QALY
gained from cataract extraction show this to be a high value for money
procedure (Drummond 1988). A similar situation exists in orthopaedics,
where hip replacement has been demonstrated to give good value for
money (Williams 1985).

Since the reforms, Health Authorities and GPs have been able to decide
which clinical needs should be met first through their ability to place contracts. In that respect, the reforms represented a major shift in decision
making about health care priorities. The extent to which Health
Authorities and GPs have exercised their new power is variable, although
the waiting list initiative (IACC 1989) demonstrated that the letting of
contracts with units, or the threat of taking the funds elsewhere, has led to
a change in behaviour of secondary care physicians.

Deciding upon the contract specification

Prior to the reforms, hospital physicians largely decided on the method of
treatment and (implicitly) the cost. While managers took some of the
decisions controlling resource allocation, such as the nature of the 'hotel'
facilities in hospitals, the major resource allocators were the doctors. They
decided when to admit the patient, the nature of the diagnostic work-up,
the treatment technologies to be employed and when to discharge.

With the advent of contracts, a specification for the care to be provided
needs to be drawn up, including the client group to be served, the treatment methods to be applied, the standards of care to be achieved and the
arrangements for monitoring.

Since a key feature of the contract is the stated price, this gives an excel-
lent opportunity for comparisons of options. For example, different treatment technologies may have different cost-effectiveness. Taking a simple
case, there may be evidence that day-care or short-stay surgery is just as
effective, but of lower cost, than traditional surgery (Russell *et al.* 1977,
Waller *et al.* 1978). Therefore, providers ought to be able to agree

contracts for these services at a lower price. Costs may also vary with volume. Although this has been relatively under-explored by economists (Labelle 1987), presumably those providers concentrating on certain clinical services may be able to agree large contracts at a lower implied unit price. An example of this would be the concerted efforts to clear the cataract backlog (Thomas *et al.* 1989).

Finally, there may be occasions where there is an explicit trade-off between higher costs and higher quality. This may be in terms of amenities in hospital wards, or in the actual clinical care provided. For example, some surgical implants may have a greater durability or offer greater freedom of movement to the patient than others. Here, part of the contracting process potentially forces the purchaser to make explicit decisions about the level of quality required. In essence, this requires assessment of whether the extra benefits exceed the higher costs. Providers may decide to offer a range of options at differing price.

Economic evaluation, with its explicit assessment of costs and health improvement, is again well placed to offer essential data to inform these choices. Prior to the reforms, they have been made implicitly by the providers, although general practitioners may have adjusted their referral patterns based on knowledge about their patients' preferences and clinical practice in given hospitals. Such 'consumer choice' exercised through the GP, has probably been most prominent in the field of maternity care to date.

Deciding upon contract monitoring arrangements
Although an important feature of the contracting procedure, this is one where economic evaluation currently has little to offer. Most evaluations of health technologies are performed *ex ante* and there are few examples of situations where researchers have investigated whether the preferred option, as indicated by their study, has performed well in practice.

However, it is clear that the monitoring of contracts is not a costless exercise, and it is known from more aggregate economic studies that the administrative costs of health care systems embodying a significant market element are much higher than those of the NHS (Maxwell, 1985). Therefore, there is a role for the economic evaluation of alternative monitoring arrangements; namely, does the increased cost of more comprehensive monitoring generate benefits in the closer adherence to contract specifications? It may be decided, for some forms of health care, that block contracts, or those with a more general specification, are all that is required.

Practice budgets for general medical practitioners

Following the reforms, practices serving at least 9,000 patients were able to manage their own budget under the GP Fundholding scheme. Under standard fundholding the budget covers various hospital services (such as a defined group of surgical inpatient and day-case treatment covering most elective procedures, outpatient services and diagnostic investigation of patients and specimens) and practice services and prescribing.

In general concept, GP Fundholding is similar to that of the Health Maintenance Organization (HMO) in the USA. While not nearly as extensive, it embodies several of the same incentives, such as to improve the range and quality of one's own services in order to attract more patients and to review carefully the appropriateness of utilising certain hospital services.

Whereas the White Paper working paper dealing with this topic points out that 'the scheme will be structured to ensure that GPs have no financial incentives to refuse to treat any category of patients', it is well known that, in the USA, HMOs reduced the number of hospital admissions dramatically. They also made much greater use of other health care professionals, such as nurse practitioners (Drummond and Maynard 1988). Whether or not these changes, whilst reducing costs, also brought about a reduction in the quality of care is open to debate (Ware *et al*. 1986).

Much of what was said above about contracts for clinical services also applies to GPs managing their own budgets. Potentially, they have an interest in knowing that the treatment technologies used in the secondary care sector are the most cost-effective available. Additionally, GPs should have an incentive to consider whether it is more cost-effective to refer patients to the hospital at all, or to handle the care themselves. An obvious issue would be the substitution of careful management by the GP ambulatory care, rather than requesting hospital admission. Also, some GPs undertake minor elective surgery. Potentially this could increase if it can be shown, in a cost minimisation analysis, to be equally effective but of lower cost.

Another major item of GP care is pharmaceutical consumption. This component of the practice fund is allocated in accordance with the principles outlined for indicative drugs budgets (discussed below). However, it has extra meaning for GPs operating the fundholding scheme because increased expenditure on drugs means that other items of expenditure, such as elective admission to hospital, are reduced.

For example, it has been shown that a drug (misoprostol), if used prophylactically, can reduce the incidence of non-steroidal anti-inflammatory drug (NSAID)-associated ulcers in those patients taking these drugs for their arthritis (Graham *et al*. 1988). Therefore, would it be cost-effective for the GP to prescribe the additional drug? This question could be answered by an economic evaluation of the prophylactic use of misoprostol (Knill-Jones *et al*. 1990). Similarly, it is known that prescribing long-term medication for elevated serum cholesterol reduces the number of fatal and non-fatal coronary heart disease events. An economic evaluation can investigate whether the benefits of prescribing the drug outweigh the costs (Pedersen *et al*. 1996, Pharoah and Hollingsworth 1996).

Indicative prescribing budgets for general medical practitioners

The working paper dealing with this topic as part of the reforms argued that:

it is generally recognised that some prescribing is wasteful or unnecessarily expensive. The objective of the new arrangements is to place downward pressure on expenditure on drugs in order to limit this waste and to release resources for other parts of the Health Service.

Despite this forthright tone, later parts of the document pointed out that 'the scheme will be structured in a way that patients will always get the drugs they need' and that 'it will ensure that budgets reflect the costs of patients needing a greater volume of drugs or more expensive drugs …' 'so that there will be no disincentive to practices to accept such patients or to begin to prescribe expensive medicine to such patients, if there is a clinical need to do so'.

The development of indicative prescribing budgets needs to be considered alongside two other initiatives; the feedback of information on prescribing behaviour to GPs through PACT (prescribing analyses and cost) and the development of community formularies. Therefore, whereas prescribing budgets are inevitably set in the aggregate, taking into account local social and epidemiological factors, both PACT and formularies are much more likely to lead the GP to consider why a particular drug, and not an alternative including no drug, should be given in a particular instance.

Both PACT and formularies give information to GPs on drug costs. This is to be welcomed. However, there are dangers in drawing up formularies in too simplistic a way. First, it is possible that a too narrow definition of comparative costs would be used. This should not only consider the costs of the drugs but the other medical care that is required. For example, a slightly cheaper drug may require a more expensive route of administration, demand more frequent patient monitoring, or lead to more side effects.

Second, it is possible that costs in the longer term may be ignored. This is particularly true of drugs that are used prophylactically, such as lipid lowering agents. These may require additional costs now, but the costs of coronary heart disease occurring in the future may be reduced. Although in an economic evaluation, costs occurring in the future have less weight, since they are discounted to present values. See Drummond *et al.* (1997a) for more discussion.

Third, it is possible that differences in the effectiveness of drugs will be ignored in the quest for cost-cutting. It was mentioned earlier that one must distinguish between economic efficiency and cost-cutting. Therefore, it is conceivable that a higher cost drug would be worthwhile, compared to the alternative, if it had much higher effectiveness. Nevertheless, some branded products may offer only marginal advantages over much cheaper generics.

Each local Health Authority or commission has one or more prescribing advisers, who may be a doctor with training in primary care or a pharmacist, and who monitors local prescribing. As professionals, they see the promotion of good clinical practice as their first duty, but as officers of the authority they are also aware of the limited budgets for health care and of the need to promote the cost-effective use of medicines. They are

responsible for the setting of prescribing 'budgets' for general practitioners, and for encouraging compliance with these budgets. The budgets in
reality are open-ended, and the advisers have no real sanctions to discour-
age overspending. They visit most GPs at least once a year, but those overspending (or underspending, which may be a marker of poor practice and
undertreatment) more often. The advisers are under considerable pressure
within their Health Authority to contain prescribing costs in the current
year, and might have difficulty in justifying a short-term increase, even if
this would lead to greater savings in the long-term in hospital budgets.

It can be seen, therefore, that the choice of drug is not a simple matter.
Certainly, greater efficiency would not be achieved by the use of the
cheapest available product in each case. Thus, there is a clear role for economic evaluation in investigating the relative cost-effectiveness of prescribing options, given the initiatives that have been taken since the
reforms.

Evidence on the use of economic evaluation

It was argued above that the NHS reforms have increased the potential for
the assessment of efficiency. However, is there any evidence that this
potential has been realised in practice and what are the recurring problems?

In general, very little is known about the use of economic evaluation in
the NHS, but these issues have been partly addressed by a survey recently
conducted by Drummond *et al.* (1997b). They surveyed, by mail ques-
tionnaire, three groups whom one might expect to use economic evaluations in the NHS. These were: (a) the prescribing advisers, who advise
GPs; (b) hospital directors of pharmacy, who play a key role in hospital
formulary committees and; (c) directors of public health, who usually
take the lead in purchasing by health commissions. Another relevant
group would be GP Fundholders. However, these were not surveyed for
fear of having only a low response rate.

The full details of the survey methodology and the main findings are
reported elsewhere (Drummond *et al.* 1997b). Overall, it showed that the
use of formal economic evaluations was rather limited. Respondents identified a number of barriers to the use of economic evaluation (Table 5.1),
which comprised a mixture of concerns about the validity of the studies
and the practical constraints, even in the reformed NHS, of moving
resources from one budget to another, or freeing resources in order to
adopt a new, cost-effective technology.

Of course, it is worth reaffirming that many decision makers may be
undertaking informal assessments of efficiency, particularly in situations
where formal economic evaluations are not available. The prescribing
advisers were asked about their sources of information on costs and outcomes (Table 5.2). A substantial minority admitted to using personal
opinion or the opinions of others, as well as giving the rational response
(of always consulting the literature).

Table 5.1 Barriers to use of economic evaluation
(All respondents)

	An important obstacle %	Most important obstacle %
Cannot move resources from secondary to primary care	64.8	17.5
Studies open to bias because of large number of assumptions	55.6	12.6
Budgets are so tight we cannot free resources to adopt therapy	50.4	8.3
DH not interested in CE, only cost containment	48.9	8.1
Industry funded studies not credible	58.7	7.6
Studies need to be interpreted by a trusted source	30.3	6.1
Savings in studies are anticipated, not real	42.8	5.6
Don't understand studies	7.5	4.0
Can't take a long-term view, budget this year important	30.0	3.4
DH funded studies not credible	9.0	0.7

Source: Drummond *et al.* (1997b)

Table 5.2 Sources of information on costs and outcomes used by
decision makers
(Medical and Pharmaceutical Advisers)

How would you assess whether a more expensive medicine is worth the extra cost?	%
Clinical articles in peer reviewed journals	96.1
Formal economic evaluations	77.5
Opinions of other advisers	48.9
Opinions of other colleagues	41.0
Personal opinion	35.4
Other	9.0

Source: Drummond *et al.* (1997b)

Conclusions: looking to the future

Despite the potential for assessing efficiency offered by the 1990 reforms, the use of economic evaluation is rather limited in practice, a case of unfulfilled potential. Therefore, does economic evaluation have a future, particularly in the light of possible further changes in the NHS?

First, it is possible that the informal use of economic evaluation, through application of the way of thinking embodied in these studies, is more substantial since the reforms. However, this is difficult to measure and would have to be taken as an act of faith.

Second, initiatives have been taken to overcome some of the barriers to the use of economic evaluation identified by NHS decision makers. For example, issues surrounding the quality of published studies have been addressed by the development of methodological guidelines in the UK (DH/ABPI 1994, BMJ Economic Evaluation Working Party 1996) and elsewhere (Gold *et al.* 1996). Also, issues related to the accessibility to studies may be partly addressed by the considerable investment in health technology assessment as part of the NHS Research and Development Programme and the development of databases of economic evaluations (NHSCRD 1997, OHE/IFPMA 1997).

Other barriers to the use of economic evaluation, such as the difficulties in freeing resources to adopt new, cost-effective technologies, may be harder to overcome. In the future it is likely that there will be a movement towards longer term 'contracts', or agreements between purchasers and providers. This begs the question of who would have the incentive, or capability, to undertake or use economic evaluations. In large block contracts it is not normal to specify, at least in a very detailed manner, the treatment technologies to be used. Therefore, it might be necessary to rely on other approaches, such as the development of clinical practice guidelines, to encourage cost-effective care. However, if this objective is to be achieved it is critical that 'evidence-based medicine' includes consideration of economic factors.

Finally, although the NHS will continue to be primary care led, the future of GP Fundholding is in some doubt, with the development of local GP Commissioning Groups being the favoured option. At first sight this suggests that some of the direct incentives for GPs to consider cost-effectiveness will be removed. However, the extent to which GP Fundholders have sought out cost-effective options is not clear. Perhaps the new commissioning groups, working in liaison with the Health Authority, may have more opportunity to implement treatment guidelines and local formularies. In turn this may encourage more assessment of the efficiency of treatment options.

Therefore, the future for the assessment of efficiency in the NHS is uncertain, although not totally pessimistic. It is likely that it will be applied in some situations and not others, as is the case at present. However, there is a continuing need to improve the quality of studies and the incentives to use cost-effectiveness evidence in health care decision making.

Acknowledgements

The Centre for Health Economics recieves a programme grant from the Department of Health for study of the economics of the NHS. However, all the views expressed are my own. I am grateful to Vanessa Windass for secretarial assistance.

References

Akehurst, RL (1989) What clinicians can contribute to 'option appraisal'. In Akehurst, RL and Drummond, MF (eds) *Clinicians as the managers of health care resources* National Health Service Training Authority, Bristol

BMJ Economic Evaluation Working Party (1996) Guidelines for authors and peer reviewers of economic submissions to the BMJ. *British Medical Journal* **313**, 275–283

Buxton, MJ, Acheson, R, Caine, N, Gibson, S and O'Brien, B *et al.* (1985) *Costs and benefits of the heart transplant programme at Harefield and Papworth Hospitals* HMSO, London

Coyle, D (1993) Increasing the impact of economic evaluations on health-care decision making. *Discussion Paper 108* Centre for Health Economics, University of York, York

Department of Health (1989) *Working for Patients* Department of Health, London

Department of Health (1994) *The DH Register of cost-effectiveness studies* Department of Health, London

Department of Health/Association of British Pharmaceutical Industries (1994) *Guidelines for the economic evaluation of pharmaceuticals* Department of Health, London

Department of Health and Social Security (1981) *Health Services Management. Health building projects* HN (81) 30. DHSS, London

Department of Health and Social Security (1988) *Option appraisal of medical and scientific equipment* HMSO, London

Drummond, MF (1980) *Principles of economic appraisal in health care* Oxford Medical Publications, Oxford

Drummond, MF (1988) Economic aspects of cataract *Ophthalmology* **95**, 1147–1153.

Drummond, MF and Hutton, J (1987) Economic appraisal of health technology in the United Kingdom. In Drummond, MF (ed.) *Economic appraisal of health technology in the European Community.* Oxford University Press, Oxford

Drummond, MF and Maynard, AK (1988) Efficiency in the NHS: lessons from abroad *Health Policy* **9**, 83–96

Drummond, MF, O'Brien, BJ, Stoddart, GL and Torrance, GW (1997a) *Methods for the economic evaluation of health care programmes: Second Edition* Oxford University Press, Oxford

Drummond, MF, Cooke, J and Walley, T (1997b) Economic evaluation under managed competition: evidence from the UK *Social Science and Medicine* **45**, 583–595

Drummond, MF and Yates, JM (1991) Clearing the cataract backlog in a not-so-developing country *Eye* **5**, 481–486

Evans, RG (1985) *Strained mercy; the economics of the Canadian health care system* Butterworths, New York

Gold, MR, Siegel, JE, Russell, LB and Weinstein, MC (eds.) (1996) *Cost-effectiveness in health and medicine.* Oxford University Press, New York

Graham, DY, Agrawa, NW and Roth, SH (1988) Prevention of NSAID–induced gastric ulcer with misoprostol: multicentre, double-blind placebo-controlled trial *Lancet* **11**, 1277–1280.

Inter-authority Comparisons and Consultancy (IACC) (1989) *Examining some of England's longest waiting lists: half year report* IACC, Health Services Management Centre, Birmingham

Knill-Jones, R, Drummond, MF, Kohli, H and Davies, LM (1990) Economic evaluation of gastric ulcer prophylaxis in patients receiving non-steroidal anti-inflammatory drugs *Postgraduate Medical Journal* **66**, 639–646

Labelle, RJ (1987) Planning for the provision and utilization of new health care technologies. In Feeny, D, Guyatt, G and Tugwell, P (eds) *Health care technology: effectiveness, efficiency and public policy* Institute for Research on Public Policy, Halifax (NS)

Luce, BR and Elixhauser, A (1990) *Standards for socioeconomic evaluation of health care products and services* Springer-Verlag, Berlin

Ludbrook, A and Mooney, GH (1983) *Economic appraisal in the NHS* Northern Health Economics, Aberdeen

Maxwell, R (1985) *Health and wealth* Lexington, DC Heath & Co, Lexington Brook

NHS Centre for Reviews and Dissemination (1997) *NHS Economic Evaluation Database* NHSCRD, York

Office of Health Economics/IFPMA Database Inc. (1997) *Health Economic Evaluation Database* OHE, London

Pedersen, TR, Kjekshus, J, Berg, K *et al.* (1996) Cholesterol lowering and the use of health care resources *Circulation* **93**, 1796–1802

Pharoah, PDP and Hollingsworth, W (1996) Cost-effectiveness of lowering cholesterol concentration with statins in patients with and without pre-existing coronary heart disease: life table method applied to Health Authority population *British Medical Journal* **312**, 1443–1448

Russell, IT, Devlin, HB, Fell, M *et al.* (1977) Day-care surgery for hernias and haemorrhoids: a clinical, social and economic evaluation *Lancet* **i**, 844–847

Thomas, HF, Darvell, RHJ and Hicks, C (1989) 'Operation cataract': a means of reducing waiting lists for cataract operations *British Medical Journal* **299**, 961–963

Waller, J, Adler, M, Creese, A and Thorne, S (1978) *Early discharge from hospital for patients with hernia or varicose veins* HMSO, London

Ware, J, Rogers, WH, Davis, AR, Goldberg, GA, Brook, RH, Keeler, EB, Sherbourne, CD, Camp, P and Newhouse, JP (1986) Comparison of health outcomes of a health maintenance organization with those of fee-for-service *Lancet* i, 1017–1022

Warner, KE and Luce, BR (1982) *Cost-benefit and cost-effectiveness in health care: principles, practice and potential,* Health Administration Press, Ann Arbor, Michigan

Williams, AH (1985) Economics of coronary artery bypass grafting *British Medical Journal* **291**, 326–329

Yates, JM and Davidge, M (1984) Can you measure performance? *British Medical Journal* **288**, 77–83

6 Managing information and information technology in the NHS

Fred Barwell

One of the biggest obstacles to successful management of the NHS, and also to any analysis of its current well being, is the significant lack of any valid information as to what the NHS does, how much it costs and where the money is spent.
Dr Jeremy Rogers (September 1996): UK Professional Forum of CompuServe

Information and evidence

Throughout all the hospitals, surgeries, clinics and laboratories of the NHS enormous amounts of data are endlessly being accessed, assessed and acted upon. The scale of Health Service activity is both vast and varied. Almost all of the working time of an 'army' of medical records staff, clerical officers and medical secretaries is spent pursuing, gathering and transferring NHS data. As Teasdale (1992) has pointed out, even a relatively 'small' health district could have a resident population in the region of 300,000 and have a purchasing budget around £70 million. Annually, this converts to approximately 50,000 in-patient admissions, 200,000 out-patient attendances, 500,000 community contacts and well over 1 million primary care contracts.

Not surprisingly, it has been estimated that approximately a quarter of all expenditure on hospitals relates to information and information services. In addition, the added requirements of establishing and monitoring all service contracts means that computerisation is the only possible way of handling this volume of information. This level of information-related activity places the NHS in the midst of what many commentators like to call an information 'revolution'. Many believe that IT will transform the collection, storage and utilisation of information to the extent that: 'the emerging electronic world offers enormous benefits to organisations of all types' (NHS Executive – Information Management Group). The view of the IMG is that the potential benefits of information technology to the NHS can be realised through a systematic and well-planned approach which supports the aims of:

- Improving the delivery of seamless and integrated health care;
- Increasing the efficiency in the management and development of health services;
- Enabling treatment and care to be responsive to the needs and wishes of patients.

Unfortunately, not all of the investment in installing resource management and hospital information systems has been targeted appropriately, and there have been some costly and well-publicised implementation failures, most visibly in the collapse of the computer systems controlling London ambulances and in the Wessex and West Midlands RHA procurement failures. In 200 UK hospitals, over a five-year period, the capital costs have amounted to £625 million (Dean 1993) and to this must be added the additional, and not insignificant, costs such as staff training, and system maintenance and development.

All too often, the real costs and benefits of various information systems have not been rigorously evaluated, and when evaluation has occurred, the outcomes have not always been as favourable as had been expected. For example, the recently published evaluation of the East Anglian Hospital Information Support Systems (HISS) consortium projects (carried out by management consultants for the NHS Executive's HISS central team) revealed serious problems in each of the four trusts which comprised the consortium. These included late system implementations, failure of systems to work properly, and a failure to deliver the expected benefits. It was reported that the West Suffolk Hospital Trust had expected savings of £70,000 in cash release but this had not been realised. Perhaps, more alarming is the reported finding that staff do not consider HISS to be a useful tool since they consider it provides neither improvements in patient care nor benefits to clinical staff.

Despite the general lack of hard evaluative evidence, there is a strong belief that information is itself a valuable resource which has the potential for improving the effectiveness of an organisation by facilitating cost savings, enhancing quality of decision-making, promoting motivation and playing a vital role in shaping organisational change. Smith (1990) has argued that since information is a resource then the use of information within the NHS should be subject to the same criteria of cost-effectiveness as other more conventional resources. He has suggested that the five key questions for the NHS are:

1 What is the cost of the information?

2 How much information should be sought?

3 What specific information should be recorded?

4 By what means should the information be disseminated?

5 How is the information to be used?

Straightforward questions such as these can be useful in linking information requirements to critical success factors for both individual managers and professional staff, who all use informational indicators to ascertain whether or not things are progressing successfully. These indicators represent the core information needs since they are linked to the activities and decisions which must be undertaken in the course of performing their job duties. There is a very real opportunity for the NHS to become a culture where actions and decisions are firmly tethered to the use of reliable and valid information and evidence. The value of using information in this way is recognised across all levels of the NHS and this perception continues to fuel demand for what many believe to be the only firm foundation for rational decision-making.

This chapter briefly describes the development of information systems in the NHS and examines the ways in which the burgeoning demands for information in the NHS may be supported by computers and other forms of information technology. Of course, in itself simply presenting data does not facilitate the speed or enhance the quality of management decision-making and the importance of understanding information as a process as well as a product is discussed.

Realising an information culture

The NHS has had a long tradition of using large information systems. Before 1976, NHS information systems consisted of the administrative collection of data through the use of voluminous paper-based manual returns to the Department of Health. These documents detailed costs and process variables such as length of stay. The introduction of mainframe computers in the late 1970s enabled Health Authorities to collect and analyse more complex data than had been previously possible and this new computing capability generated the data that has formed the basis of the specialised field of 'health service statistics'.

Although it has always been theoretically acknowledged that organisational excellence and information provision went hand-in-hand, many of these early computer systems could not deliver any organisational improvements. This was because they were not compatible and central monitoring of information remained a difficult, if not practically impossible, task. More recently, as the NHS has become increasingly complex, there has been a parallel growth in the demand for data and information. Fortunately, the combined recent effects of rapid technological developments and falling costs in flexible and adaptive microcomputer systems now presents the NHS with a very real opportunity to make the transition to a responsive and effective information culture.

As well as these technological developments, this cultural shift had been primed by two earlier initiatives. First, the series of Körner Reports (DHSS 1982) had identified the need for minimum data sets which resulted in the establishment of a national data collection system. This remains to this day as the basis for national performance indicators. Unfortunately, since these minimum data sets reflected input and process measures and generally ignored outputs and outcomes they have been widely criticised. The second explicit attempt to influence information policy was the Griffiths Reports (DHSS 1983) which had advocated a management budgeting approach and in doing so highlighted the pressing need for NHS information systems to provide outcome, quality or cost information which managers could actually use.

Of course, it has become a truism in the NHS to state that it is not NHS managers but clinical care staff who most strongly influence resource consumption, and consequently it is imperative to ensure that clinical decisions incorporate those issues concerned with the effectiveness of using resources. For many years, it has been recognised that the active involvement of clinicians in the management process is an essential prerequisite to successful resource management, although this itself is dependent upon good quality information based upon the systematic tracking of the resources used by individual patients during their entire stay in hospital.

The Resource Management (RM) initiative

The advantages of linking clinical activity data to resource utilisation data at both the individual patient and at the case-mix level is not a novel idea in the NHS and, over a decade ago, the RM initiative was launched by the Finance Division of the DHSS (1986). The primary purpose of the RM initiative was to expand the decision-making roles of those staff who are in the positions to directly commit resources to patient care. The RM initiative had evolved from the earlier 'management budgeting' initiative suggested by the Griffiths Report (1983). The new finance systems which the Griffiths report had facilitated were intended to facilitate the joint discussion of financial information between managers and doctors, but by 1985 it was becoming evident that doctors were not happy with the financial reports they had been receiving and many considered them neither readable not accurate.

The RM initiative was based on two substantive key themes (Buxton *et al.* 1989). The first was securing the direct involvement of professional staff (doctors, and, to a lesser extent, nurses) in the process of hospital management (often using the clinical directorate model). The second was the creation of an information system that was both accessible and relevant for all users. The Case Mix Management System (CMMS) was at the centre of this information initiative and was designed to allow both clinicians and managers to identify the types of patients treated together with the treatments provided and the resources used. To provide this information practically, it was necessary that CMMS were used to collect and analyse test and treatment costs for all patients. This necessitated that information from a wide variety of other systems (both computer and manually based) must be available to the CMMS from other feeder systems. These systems include the Patient Administration System (PAS), Nursing Information System, Radiology, Pharmacy, Theatres, and Physiotherapy and so on.

In 1987 and 1988 six experimental sites were originally chosen to pilot the RM initiative and by 1989 the intention was to roll out the approach across the whole of the NHS. However, despite a great deal of enthusiasm from many NHS managers, a rather negative evaluation report from Brunel University (Robinson 1991) concluded that it was impossible to either assess the efficacy of RMI or to isolate any measurable improvements in patient care. Many managers felt that the discouraging tone of this conclusion struck the wrong note, since they considered that the RMI had achieved a great deal in encouraging clinical involvement not only in service planning but also in resource management itself.

The managers' disappointment with the adverse evaluation was understandable since it had been nearly a decade previously that the Griffiths Report (1983) had recommended that NHS units involve clinicians more closely in the management process. Until the advent of the Resource Management Initiative in 1986 there were very few NHS units with clinical managers or clinical directors who held any budgetary responsibility. Another positive outcome was that the RMI had highlighted that resource tracking needs sophisticated computer systems and this recognition created a climate which was receptive to subsequent major developments in the information arena.

The roll-out of RMI from its original six pilot sites roughly coincided with the start of the internal market and as contracting developed within the NHS, other initiatives have been grafted onto the original RMI rootstock. All of these 'grafts' are themselves highly data-intensive and include enterprises such as Total Quality Management (TQM), the Patient's Charter, and medical and clinical audit.

Although the RM initiative has not been demonstrably successful, it is clear that ensuring that the information needed to manage the resources supplied for the care of patients is available and acted upon appropriately means that the legacy of the RM initiative continues to remain an important influence on management thinking. For a more thorough description of the nature and impact of the RM initiative, the reader is referred to the chapter by Spurgeon (1990) in an earlier edition of this volume.

Hospital Information Support Systems (HISS)

There are four basic kinds of information in hospitals – usually described as activity, financial, manpower and clinical information. Historically, different departments have dealt with these different types of data. For example, information personnel typically only deal with activity data (such things as number of in-patients, day-cases admitted, patient flow through departments etc). The Patient Administration System (PAS) supports the effective use of beds and support services, by recording patient, ward and clinicians' details. This provides key management information about the hospital's workload. The outpatient module records planned appointments and attendances and is essentially an appointment system for scheduling clinics. Clinical data are largely held in case notes although there is a small amount kept on Patient Administration Systems.

Good information is crucial to both the quality of decision making and to effective management in the NHS. Indeed the cost-effectiveness of any hospital largely depends on the quality of information available to managers. As Ambage (1995) has pointed out, all information must be credible, timely, complete and accurate, but for effective management it must also be suitable for both clinicians and non-clinicians, easily retrieved, relevant and malleable. Unfortunately, in many hospitals, the information services are not properly integrated and this often leads to problems with patient records and the contracting process.

Typically, the PAS system may be many years old, the contracting system is often PC based and not linked to the PAS, and the medical secretaries hold individual consultants' waiting lists on stand-alone word processors. Other data sources include manual systems such as nursing diaries, A&E logs, theatre books etc and various computers at trust and district levels. At the hospital department level there are numerous specialised sources of data including radiology, pathology, theatres etc. Manual data collection is typically non-standardised and rarely audited.

The HISS programme was started shortly after the start of the RMI with the intention of testing the feasibility of bringing together separate operational information systems into a single integrated system. HISS uses a common Master Patient Index (MPI) as its focal point, since this holds both the personal and administrative details of all patients treated in the hospital. The wholesale replacement of existing systems (the so-called 'big bang' approach) was tried out at a few hospitals sites as a means of supplying computerised information support facilities for most hospital functions including:

- Business Systems (eg Finance, Manpower, Estates and Supplies)

- Management Systems (eg Case-Mix, Contract Monitoring, EIS and Clinical Audit)

- Activity and Clinical Systems (eg Medical Records, PAS, Order Entry, Results Reporting, and Prescribing)

- Departmental Systems (eg A&E, Theatres, Pathology, Maternity, Radiology, Pharmacy, Oncology, Renal, and Endoscopy)

- Nurse Systems (eg Care Planning and Workload Rostering)

- External Systems (eg GPs)

The benefit of this type of comprehensive integrated system is that patient data does not need to be repeatedly entered into the system which can be updated by drawing information from the hospital's feeder operational functions. Using a common data source, a key advantage of HISS is that it can provide information to all levels of the organisation including managers, clinicians and other staff. Since HISS are designed to record not only costs for tests and items of care but also allow comparisons between expected and actual care profiles, they have the potential for enhancing the costs and quality of service provision.

Only a few trusts currently have a fully functioning HISS although many have started the process of integrating their operational information systems. Often the first priority is to replace old over-stretched Patient Administrative Systems in order to facilitate not only the integration of other computer systems (eg radiology, immunology etc) but also to enable the integration of a wide range of patient administration and clinical functions such as the following:

- **Patient administration**

  Master patient index

  Tracking of case notes

  Outpatient scheduling and management

  Admissions, transfers and discharges

  Waiting lists

  Bed management

  Contracting

  Patient identification and registration in A&E

- **Clinical activities**

  Ordering investigations, X rays and other services

  Improved information for theatres

  Improved information for maternity

  Results reporting to the wards

  Improved communication with GPs

A substantial volume of information processing is still undertaken manually, which is both inefficient and wastes a great deal of staff time. The establishment of computerised departmental and support systems (eg pathology, radiology, pharmacy) linked to wards and clinics means that tests and results requests could easily be transferred. The planned installation of 'clinical workstations' linked to a comprehensive electronic patient record (which includes clinical notes, results of investigations, previous contact information etc) will support the planning, delivery and development of patient care.

The impact of the White Paper

The publication of the White Paper (DoH 1989) detailed the health implications of the then Conservative Government's view that the introduction of 'competition' into the NHS through the introduction of a quasi-market was thought to facilitate the efficient use of resources. This formation of an internal NHS market (initially introduced in April 1991) was based on the idea that every product or service has a cost to its provider and a price to its purchaser. Accordingly, there was a necessity for each link in the market chain to be controlled by a contract that specifies both the quality and the price of the goods or services to be provided.

This radical transformation from functional management to product line management meant that a hospital's or a department's income would now depend upon the quantity and quality of the work undertaken. Under this scheme, it was apparent that purchasers must demand relevant up-to-date and useful information so that they are able to assess the relative cost-benefits of their purchasing options. From the information perspective, the implications were clear. To compete within this internal market, service providers must provide the necessary information for purchasers to make cost-effective purchasing decisions.

Implementing these proposals has had an enormous impact on the NHS and has resulted in the establishment of self-governing hospitals, the introduction of practice budgets and the continuing development of medical audit. Despite the recent change of government in the UK, the impact and organisational momentum of the market model will continue to have major implications for the processing of information in the NHS. Although the new Labour Government is ideologically opposed to the health market philosophy, none of their proposed initiatives are expected to require that organisational performance will need to be any less tightly monitored and controlled than it was previously.

Another aspect of the NHS reforms which reinforced the necessity for better collection of operational data and the interpretation and presentation of information is the establishment of fundholding for general practitioners. The creation of GP Fund Holding practices (GPFH) meant that the income that clinical units receive depends upon the volume of referrals it can attract from GPs. To do this effectively, the GPFH clearly needs appropriate information about the costs and quality of services which are on offer so that they can purchase the best care for their patients. The providers (ie the clinical units and the specialist service departments – such as laboratories or diagnostic imaging departments) must provide this information to GPs so as to encourage referrals and requests for tests. In this way, the success of any provider rests on the provision of information about the costs and quality of patient care.

This radical change means that each GPFH becomes responsible for choosing how the funds allocated for registered patients are spent in purchasing required care. In influencing how GPs make their choices for patient care it is clear that quality of service measures are of vital importance. These quality indices can be of many types but all rest on obtaining reliable and valid information. They include the following:

- speed of service – time taken for laboratory results, clinic and discharge letters, and discharge summaries

- in-patient and outpatient waiting times

- quality of clinical expertise and provision of care advice and monitoring arrangements
- patient convenience – short journeys, clinic waiting times, provision of medication
- economy, such as avoiding repeating tests or ordering expensive tests which GP regards as unnecessary.

The national strategic vision

In 1992 the NHS Executive unveiled its IM&T strategy for the service. Since the internal market was already well underway, there was little option but to focus on how IT could underpin market operations. The strategic proposals were ambitious in both scope and time scale. Within seven years it was proposed that a multi-million pound investment was to deliver an integrated information technology infrastructure across the whole NHS. Essentially, the national strategic vision comprised five key principles:

- Systems should be person-based
- Management information should be derived from operational systems
- Systems should be integrated
- Information to be stored confidentially
- Information capable of being shared across NHS

These five key principles are intended to be supported by various kinds of initiatives including what are called 'enabling projects' (such as HISS and EPR – electronic patient records), 'maximising VFM' – value for money – (such as POISE and STEP), and human resource projects (such as training, education and development).

A central plank of the national strategy was the intention to support the development of integrated information systems in large hospitals since these units represent a crucial element in the provider market. Specifically, by the year 2000 it was envisaged that large (defined as units with more than 400 beds) acute hospitals should develop a range of integrated patient-based systems. These operational systems are 'patient-based' since they use the information modules of the PAS.

The emergence of self-governing hospital trusts with considerable independence in managing both their revenue and expenses has created the need for new information outputs. Before self-governance, hospital information systems could separate resource consumption from patient need since resource allocation was based on precedent and was not patient-centred. Indeed, it has often been observed that the traditional types of management information systems in hospitals have often been inadequate not only because of the funding mechanisms, but also because of organisational structure and the accepted role of management.

It has often been observed that the differences between the old system of administration of a fixed expense budget and the new demands of management of revenue and expense streams require fundamentally different types of information. The expansion of information is necessary to cover the following activities:

- Planning on the strategic, tactical and operational levels
- Understanding consultants' operational decisions which control both the Trusts revenue and expenses
- Contracting with other organisations
- Providing appropriate financial information to management board
- Determining appropriate staffing levels
- Optimally managing case and service mix

The explosion of the availability of information technology has the potential to ensure that information is collected and processed more cost-effectively than ever before with the following technological benefits for both clinicians and managers:

- Workstation support
- Data storage technologies
- Networking and communications
- Multimedia and telemedicine
- Decision support systems

The costs and benefits of IT in the NHS

One of the key advantages of computer-based systems is that they have the potential to be flexible enough to respond to the information needs of an individual manager. In simple terms, a flexible computer system is able to respond to the requests which are made and is also able to present reports at varying levels of specificity and complexity. The manager is able to extract information at a level of aggregation and in a structure which he or she had decided best suits the situation in hand. This individualisation of information can be considered as a process by which the manager attempts to make his informational input, decision-analysis and actioning strategies as optimal as possible.

Monitoring any aspect of the organisation necessitates that there are information systems in place to provide the required data easily, promptly and at the required intervals. A good information system should have a retrospective and a prospective role and should enhance both monitoring and decision-making. Information acts as a control mechanism when used retrospectively if managers are able to evaluate organisational performance using various types of performance indicator. On the other hand, when used prospectively, information can be used to aid decision-making. The budget is the most common mechanism where information is used prospectively to act as a guiding framework for future action.

Over the years a variety of information systems have sprung up and have been developed in the NHS but in a rather chaotic and piecemeal fashion. There are numerous systems currently in use in the administrative, financial and clinical arenas of the NHS but unfortunately they often have the fundamental problem of not being fully integrated. According to some estimates, managing information accounts for 15 per cent of hospitals' budgets and 25 per cent of doctors' and nurses' time (Audit Commission 1995). The NHS spends about £220 million per year on IT in hospitals for which there is very little evidence of benefit.

Cost-effectiveness analysis is a method for assessing and summarising the value of a medical technology, practice, or policy. Underlying the methodology is the assumption that the resources available to spend on health care are constrained, whether from the societal, organisational, practitioner, or patient point of view. Cost-effectiveness information is intended to inform decisions about health care investments within this finite budget.

Unfortunately, in spite of what many believe to be the 'obvious' usefulness of the computer, the valuation of the role of IT in health care is beset with problems. Few would disagree with benefits which focused on better care for patients, better targeted care for populations and better use of resources, although increasingly the quality of the evidence which supports these 'obvious' benefits of computers to health care is coming into question. Accurate costs and benefits are often difficult to assess in the real world, and with IT initiatives in particular, it is generally impossible to clearly demarcate the effects of the IT initiative independently of all the other changes which will have been precipitated. These difficulties in performing systematic evaluations has resulted in a dearth of systematic evidence which others can use in guiding their IT investment strategies.

Lock (1996) has highlighted the irony of the situation where the NHS is constantly exhorted to strive for greater evidence-based cost-effectiveness and, with scant support of evidence, £220 million is spent annually on information technology in hospitals. Furthermore, as Donaldson (1996) has pointed out, the output of this incompletely evaluated IT is often the data on costs, quality and outcome on which the objective appraisal of health services themselves should be based. Of course, the cost-effectiveness of many services has not yet been established and information on costs and outcomes is inadequate for many interventions. Sometimes the cost-effectiveness analyses have not been undertaken, or their quality is insufficient to provide conclusive evidence.

Finally, the variation in cost-effectiveness analysis methodologies themselves often makes it difficult to take cost-effectiveness results at face value. Although there is a constant exhortation to examine cost-effectiveness results, often the methodology and analysis which has been used is flawed. In particular, often the quality and representativeness of data on costs and effectiveness are questionable and the opportunity costs of alternative choices that decision-makers should consider are not properly explored.

New directions

In this concluding section three themes are briefly discussed which are considered to be critical to managing information in the future NHS. The first theme (the meaning of information) is concerned with the cognitive representation of information; what information means to people is crucial if there is to be a shift from a product to a process view of information. The second theme (shared decision-making) follows from the first and highlights the importance of building shared models of the decision spaces which both medics and managers must address. The third theme (the key role of the information-provider) highlights how information provision is not a neutral work activity but is fundamentally important in shaping how managers and medics conceptualise their decisions.

The meaning of information

Over 15 years ago, Dretske (1981) observed that there are many books which have the work 'information' in their title although it is rarely to be found in the index. From this observation, he concluded that it was much easier to talk about 'information' than to offer a decent definition. This problem remains to this day and, rather than attempting to erect a definitive definition here, some contemporary aspects of health care information will be subsequently discussed in order to highlight the key issues which lie at the heart of managing NHS information systems.

As Wyatt (1996) has observed, information is the commodity which we all use to make decisions. In the context of health care, information should comprise not only patient and resource data but must also include clinical and organisational knowledge.

However, the word 'information' tends to be used in two distinct ways: either to refer to 'bundles' of facts or to the communication and transmission of those facts. This double meaning has often resulted in a great deal of confusion about what is actually meant by 'information' in a health care organisation. It is essential to contrast the traditional notion of information as a product, with information as a process. Information is often regarded as material 'stuff' because it has been embodied in papers, books, reports etc. However, there is a process involved in information acquisition which refers to the fact that the 'information' which is received is not a function of 'pages' but of the mental processes of understanding and integrating this data into our personal knowledge structures.

The word information is derived from the Latin *'informare'* which means 'give form to' and in keeping with this, it has often been observed that data become information only when meaning is attached through human interpretation. Thus a set of bed-occupancy figures only becomes information when it can be interpreted as increasing or decreasing over time. From this perspective, information is data that has been processed into a form that is meaningful to the user and is of real or perceived value in current or prospective actions or decisions.

Since information must always have a purpose, otherwise it degrades into data, it is useful to identify the following key characteristics of information. Unlike data, information must precipitate one or more of the following changes (Barwell and Spurgeon 1993):

- **Inform** – Change the characteristics which are ascribed to organisational events or situations

- **Instruct** – Change the probability that certain activities will be undertaken

- **Motivate** – Change the value of certain processes or outcomes

More data, however up-to-date or speedily accessed, does not necessarily imply more information to the user. Data can only become information when it has been selected and processed to make it useful. The old adage 'data has a cost; information a value' means that when data is used to help solve a problem or make a decision or perform an activity more effectively, then the active conversion of data to information is taking place. The link between external information and internal knowledge is complex but there is a simple hierarchy that succinctly describes this structure.

- Data   (numbers, words)
- Information   (statements)
- Intelligence   (rules)
- Knowledge   (combination of the levels above)
- Wisdom   (combined knowledge bases)

Although it is undoubtedly the case that 'data is the raw material that is processed and refined to generation information' (Silver and Silver 1989), another more subtle conception is the one provided by Lewis (1994). In his words:

> Data are important to the organisation not because, as is often claimed, they can be processed into information but because they, or processed forms of them, may be perceived as and used as information.

This is an important distinction because it places the information user centre-stage and emphasises the individual's use of their own cognitive frameworks or mental models as 'filters' which recognise certain facts as meaningful and uses these to create an understanding about organisational reality. Experience has shown that trying to understand and accommodate to the perceived realities of organisations is the most important precursor to the good design of information systems.

The mental procedures and knowledge structures developed and used by health care staff are vital to characterise since these factors are at the heart of individual differences between managers. Unfortunately, this sort of tailoring of computer output to an individual's information needs is not always possible. Often, information systems are not designed to capitalise upon information need beyond the group level and in these circumstances reports for general consumption are produced.

There is a growing recognition of the ways in which information can serve to support the efficient running of an organisation not only at the operational level of day-to-day routine transactions but also at the level of supporting managers' decision-making strategies and even at the level of structuring strategic planning and policy-making. Of course, we must be careful with definitions here. It is still the case that most information systems are still data-processing systems despite the current preference for the former term.

Another important consideration is the distinction that can be drawn between information and strategic intelligence. From the standpoint of management, intelligence is that information which can be put to strategic use. Consequently, most of the strategic intelligence that an organisation needs is drawn from outside the organisation and is not served by internal information systems. As Wilson (1995) has pointed out, at the strategic level of the organisation, intelligence systems are much more likely to be useful than information systems.

Strategic intelligence requires the input of human minds to determine what the information means for the future of the organisation. At the executive level, most of the intelligence that an organisation needs are externally drawn and are typically concerned with aspects of the competitive environment (ie markets, market trends, competitors' actions, economic trends and legislation).

Shared decision-making

Achieving a shared perception of the nature and value of key information indicators is an objective which has the real potential of improving the quality and efficiency of patient care. Ensuring that medics and managers share the same basic information base, will encourage cooperative working practices. If this is to be achieved, then the nature of both medics' and managers' activities, tasks and information requirements must be understood in much greater detail than is usually the case at present.

However, even if a common information base can be established as a platform for joint decision-making, it is not easy to make health care decisions, particularly those with important consequences for patient care. Many health care decisions are not procedural and require different types of information to be integrated if competing options are to be evaluated in a systematic and rational way. In a real decision, all options usually have a mix of desirable and undesirable aspects and in a rational decision these need to be systematically weighted and compared.

As both NHS managers and medics find it essential to expand their traditional problem-space boundaries, then the issue of how decision-making can be improved becomes an increasingly important practical concern. One method for improving decision-making rests on attempts to improve the measurement of performance. Precise, sensitive and valid performance measurement is a necessary but not sufficient input to good decision-making. Effective decision-making output depends not only upon a good quality measurement input, but also upon sound information processing. This means that a variety of different sorts of information still need to be brought together in a sensible way before any judgements can be made with any level of confidence.

The key role of information providers

The efficient and effective production of information depends not only upon appropriate information technology for data capture and processing and delivering information, but also on the education and training for data recorders, information producers and information providers.

Most of the formal, and much of the informal, information which managers use is prepared and presented by people who have been called 'information providers'. These knowledge workers may or may not be managers themselves but they provide support managers in the following ways:

- They contribute expertise and effort in gathering, filtering, analysing and presenting information.

- They reduce information overload on the manager by not presenting the raw data; rather, they tend to use verbal and statistical summaries.

- The provide a common database for group decisions.

The role of the information provider is often critical in shaping the ultimate solution or organisational decision and often goes well beyond merely supplying data and interpreting information. The critical role of the information provider is expected to increase as the increasing demand for information within the NHS continues. For many years the impact of each 'reform' has brought with it calls for accurate, extensive, comprehensive and up-to-the-minute information. MacDougall and Brittain (1992) have listed some of these information needs:

- Scientific, clinical and health service information (eg reports, literature, computer databases, on-line searches)

- Patient-generated clinical data (eg disease patterns, treatment procedures, screening, clinical outcome, morbidity statistics)

- Information for patients, carers and the general public (eg waiting lists and times, leaflets, condition-specific information, complaints, advice)

The raft of management-led initiatives comprising clinical budgeting, resource management, and establishing clinical directorates (and local variants, eg the speciality manager model in which the unit general manager and clinicians agree activity targets prior to the provision of full general management support), have successfully focused attention on the new work ethos in the NHS. Some would argue that these initiatives have been less successful either in relieving managers of work pressure or, more importantly, of causing clear changes in the pattern of clinical activity.

Perhaps the pace of real change will accelerate only when managers and medics share a common understanding of the issues involved in providing good quality care. Better education and training aimed at giving medics and managers a broader view of both clinical and resource issues have a very important role to play in developing this shared perception.

References

Ambage, N (1995) *Trust information systems* In Sheaff, R and Peel, V (eds) *Managing health service information systems: an introduction* Open University Press, Milton Keynes

Audit Commission (1995) *Setting the records straight; a study of hospital medical records* Audit Commission, London

Barwell, F, and Spurgeon, P (1993) *Information for effective management decision-making in the NHS* Longman Group UK Ltd, Harlow

Buxton, M, Packwood, T and Keen, J (1989) *Resource management: process and progress* Brunel University, Uxbridge

Dean, M (1993) London perspective: unhealthy computer systems *Lancet* **341**, 1269–1270

Department of Health (1989) *Working for patients* HMSO, London

DHSS (1982) A report on the collection and use of information about hospital clinical activity in the NHS. Steering Group on Health Services Information: Chairman Mrs E Körner

DHSS (1983) NHS management inquiry. The Griffiths Report.

DHSS (1986) Health Notice (86) 34: Resource management (management budgeting) in Health Authorities.

Donaldson, LJ (1996) From black bag to black box: will computers improve the NHS? *British Medical Journal* **312**, 1371–1378

Dretske, FL (1981) *Knowledge and the flow of information* Blackwell, London

Griffiths, R (1983) *NHS management enquiry (the Griffiths Report)* DHSS, London

Lewis, PJ (1994) *Information systems development* Pitman Publishing, London

Lock, C (1996) What value do computers provide to NHS hospitals? *British Medical Journal* **312**, 1407–1410

MacDougall, J and Brittain, JM (1992) *Use of information in the NHS* Library and Information Research Report, Boston, York

Robinson, R (1991) Roll-call after roll-out *Health Services Journal* June 1991 18–19

Silver, GA and Silver, ML (1989) *Systems analysis and design* Addison-Wesley, Reading, MA

Smith, P (1990) Information systems and the white paper proposals In Culyer, AJ, Maynard, AK, and Posnett, JW (eds) *Competition in health care: reforming the NHS* Macmillan Press, London

Spurgeon, P (1990) Resource management: a fundamental change in managing health services Chapter 5 in P Spurgeon (ed) *The Changing Face of the NHS in the 1990s* Longman Group UK Ltd, Harlow

Teasdale, K (1992) *Managing changes in health care* Wolfe Publishing Ltd, London

Wilson, T (1995) *Mapping the information user: the wider perspective* Paper delivered at the INFOTECH '95 Conference, Kuala Lumpur, Malaysia, November, 1995

Wyatt, JC (1996) Advances in communication and information technology Chapter 14 In Peckham, M and Smith, R (eds) *Scientific Basis of Health Services* BMJ Publishing Group, London

7 Proving and improving the quality of national health services: past, present and future

John Øvretveit

Introduction

Meeting the health needs of patients has always been the aspiration of the NHS, or perhaps, more realistically, meeting the health needs of those most in need. Quality methods are systematic ways of improving a health service's ability to meet patient needs, and to prevent harming them. Yet the NHS has been slow to adopt quality methods from the commercial sector which, in theory, would transform what many still regard as a professional bureaucracy into a modern knowledge-based service industry. What has been the experience of the NHS with quality methods, and why have these methods not had the impact which they have had in other industries? Is it because the NHS is not like other industries and these methods are not suited to a people-intensive service whose product is care and cure? Is traditional profession-specific quality assurance all that is necessary, modernised perhaps with evidence-based medicine and outcome measurement? This chapter considers some answers to these questions in the course of giving a short history of quality in the NHS and looking at current trends and likely future developments.

In the last 10 years the number of different activities and methods used to assure quality in the NHS has grown considerably, mostly without co-ordination either at a national or local level. By 1996, 25 separate quality initiatives were listed by one commentator, ranging from accreditation to total quality management (Taylor 1996). Quality in the NHS is certainly a confusing subject. The purpose of this chapter is to help readers to understand the different approaches and some of the reasons for the variety. One of the losses to the NHS in recent years has been the loss of a collective memory and an understanding of NHS history. Much can be learned from the history of quality in the NHS which is of use in planning and pursuing other initiatives, especially about the need to involve professions for change to be successful, and about how best to create win-win strategies for change.

Why the variety and the confusion? Because quality is political: ownership and leadership of quality is directly related to the power and autonomy of professions, including management, in the NHS. Raise questions about the quality of a service and practitioners automatically assume that their work will be scrutinised, criticised and controlled, probably by people who do not understand it. The variety is not because, like much else, quality is not planned and coordinated in the NHS. The confusion will not be resolved by oversimplifying and rewriting history, but in practice, by different occupations and interest groups negotiating and agreeing how they will work together to improve the quality of care: usually this only happens in small multidisciplinary quality project teams.

But we are moving too fast into reflection and analysis. What happened, and how did we get to this point: a proliferation of approaches, with little evidence of the effectiveness of much which is done under the name of 'quality' in the NHS? Looking back, and from 58 degrees north, some of the history of quality in the NHS makes more sense than it did when I was involved in pre- and post-reform quality development work.

> *Businessmen have a keen sense of how well they are looking after their customers. Whether the NHS is meeting the needs of patients and the community, and can prove it is doing so, is open to question.*
>
> Roy Griffiths

A short history of quality in the NHS

Methods to ensure quality are as old as medicine. What is new is the attempt to use methods developed in industry to co-ordinate the variety of occupations and complex services which contribute to a patient's care. But what has not changed is that quality methods in health care serve a double purpose – to protect patients and occupations. The function of these methods in protecting and advancing professional interests has not been sufficiently understood. Neither has the close link between the ideologies of consumer quality, free markets and the reduction of the welfare state. The importance of these factors becomes clearer when we take a historical and a comparative perspective, which also helps us to see future possible trends.

In the past, many occupations have been able to persuade the public and authorities that practitioners not belonging to the trade are a danger to patients and that the trade association is able to ensure the quality of practice. But fundamental changes have occurred in recent years:

- A recognition that traditional and professional-specific quality assurance is insufficient in a complex multiprofessional service, and where the overall quality of a patient's care also depends on interservice collaboration;

- The availability of new quality methods which make it possible to understand and manage systems of care;

- Management have acquired more power in relation to professionals which has allowed them to take more responsibility for quality and this, in turn, further increased their power in relation to professionals.

In simple terms, we can summarise the history of quality methods in the NHS as being profession-driven in the early 1980s, followed by a provider-managerial phase in the early 1990s, leading into a purchaser-consumer phase in the late 1990s (Box 7.2). Generally, before the reforms in 1991 there was very little interest in quality and the two years of near chaos afterwards put many quality initiatives 'on hold'. But from 1993 onwards there was a steady growth of and sophistication to quality, a greater understanding of the more effective and profession-friendly continuous quality improvement methods, and a convergence between these methods and those of evidence-based medicine (Sackett *et al.* 1996).

Professional approaches to assuring quality

We are not convinced of the need for further supervision of a qualified doctor's standard of care.

The British Medical Association's submission to the 1977 Royal Commission on the NHS

Up to the mid 1980s most quality activities in the NHS were profession-specific. Traditionally, professions regulated quality with state support by setting training requirements, registering those qualifying and by disciplining practitioners, but only rarely, for poor practice. This approach fits with the ideas that the individual is the source of quality, that their peers and their associations are the best judge and jury of quality and that, once qualified, the quality of their work would be assured by the negative incentive of disciplinary action and by occasional post-qualification education. These ideas are also the basis for professional power.

But professional practice and health services have changed. Two changes occurred in the mid-1980s. First, professional associations experimented with more proactive approaches to quality and increased their use of applied research to develop professional practice (Shaw 1986). Medical audit became more widespread, using a variety of systematic methods to review medical care. National audits included the confidential enquiries into perioperative deaths (Buck *et al.* 1987, NCEPOD 1989) and into maternal deaths (DoH 1989a) – the latter investigations in fact starting in the 1930s.

Examples of local applied research projects at this time were the Ealing hospital's comparisons of surgical mortality and morbidity data which led to a 50 per cent reduction in infection rates over three years (Sellu 1986), and the Lothian surgical audit involving 30 surgeons (Gruer *et al.* 1986). The Royal College of General Practitioners started a quality initiative in 1983 (RCGP 1983) which has grown and changed over the years. The late 1980s saw a number of publications outlining methods for medical audit and reporting these and other projects (RCP 1989, RCS 1989, Shaw 1989, Frater and Spiby 1990, Marinker 1990, RCOG 1990).

The purposes of medical audit are many and include professional education and self-development, research into effectiveness, increasing the local effectiveness of medical care, proving medical quality to purchasers or the public, reducing and preventing poor medical quality and reducing the costs of medical care. There are three predominant models for audit: the first is an 'audit cycle' which defines standards and procedures, monitors care against standards, identifies divergences and makes corrections (Shaw 1989, Øvretveit 1992). The second is the 'research model' where audit is what would otherwise be called a research project. The third is the 'continuous quality improvement model' which focuses on processes of care and uses experimental techniques to run small-scale experiments (Berwick 1996). There is an interrelation between audit, research and education, but Black emphasises the importance of recognising the differences between them (Black 1992) (Box 7.1).

Medical audit often also uses the results of treatment- and service-evaluations: the 'evidence-based medicine' movement views medical audit as one means of encouraging clinicians to make greater use of effectiveness research by using this research as a basis for audit standards and guidelines (Sackett *et al.* 1996). Evaluations of medical and clinical audit (ie interprofessional audit) in the UK are reported in Kerrison *et al.* (1993), Walshe and Coles (1993) and Kogan and Redfern (1995).

In the 1980s, nurses and other professions also began to promote peer review, standard-setting and audit cycle approaches to assuring quality (set standards, measure quality, correct where necessary, and then review standards) (Pearson 1987, Øvretveit 1988). One of the earliest and well-known systems was the nursing-process-based 'Monitor', which sets questions for assessing the quality of a nursing assessment of a patient, the physical and non-physical care given, and how care is evaluated (Goldstone *et al.* 1983). In 1988, a national nurses' working group proposed methods for raising the standards of quality in nursing care (NN & MCC 1988), and at around the same time nurses in West Berkshire were developing what was to become known as 'Dissy' – the dynamic standard setting system (RCN 1990). This approach became quite widespread in the NHS in the early 1990s, in part because it was relatively simple and suited to a ward and community context, and allowed nurses to define locally appropriate standards. Approaches used by other NHS professions at the time are described in Ellis and Whittington (1993) and Kogan and Redfern (1995).

Management initiated quality programmes

A second change in the mid-1980s was general management, following from the Griffiths report (1983). One effect was that some top level nurse managers were given 'responsibility for quality' (organisation- or district-wide) as their partial, or sole responsibility. Some have proposed this as an explanation for the separate development of customer-service and medical quality approaches in the NHS in the 1980s. Another change was the emergence of clinical directors – usually medically qualified managers of hospital departments ('directorates') – who also had a responsibility for the quality of their directorate services. A third, more gradual, change was the strengthening of management, which led to managers taking a wider interest in quality than they had in their previously more circumscribed role as administrators.

Managers began to create and coordinate district- and organisation-wide quality assurance, and to initiate customer service programmes. A number of districts establish full-time quality assurance positions. Examples were South East Staffordshire, which ran a development programme for managers in quality assurance in 1987, Wirral, which established a district quality assurance team and strategy in 1988, and the Dorset programme. Another was the Enfield Quality Improvement Drives Scheme ('QUIDS'): Marks and Spencer sponsored prizes for proposals for quality improvements produced by multidisciplinary groups of staff. The groups defined the customers of a service, imagined they were customers, imagined improvements, and described how these could be made.

But there were other developments which were to shape the quality movement in the NHS in the 1990s, and make it more 'hard nosed' and less naive. The rise of consumerism was one such, but perhaps more important was the use of consumerism as a populist political strategy by the Government and as a justification for what some have termed an 'attack' on the professions and on the welfare state. Customer service quality was one theme which characterised quality in the NHS in the early 1990s, supported by the NHS reforms white paper *Working for Patients* (DoH 1989b). The most well known of the quality initiatives in the NHS then was the Trent personal service quality programme (started in 1985) which put service quality to patients at the centre.

In some respects, quality as patient satisfaction became for a time more important than quality as patient survival, alienating many clinicians just when their occupational interests and the NHS required them to take the newer methods more seriously. This aspect of quality is epitomised in the Patient's Charter (DoH 1992) which skilfully skirted professional quality issues to set standards for waiting times and service quality. Notwithstanding the criticisms, the Charter did have an impact, at least with mangers. By the mid-1990s managers were taking their comparative performance on these standards very seriously.

Box 7.1 Quality terms

Health service quality: meeting the health needs of those most in need, within higher level requirements and at the lowest cost.

Quality Assurance (QA): any systematic activity to ensure the quality of services – a general term for activities and systems for monitoring and improving quality. Sometimes defined more precisely. In the USA, 'QA' is used in a more limited sense to describe an approach to setting and enforcing standards through an accreditation process.

Audit: most medical and clinical audit is setting standards or guidelines, comparing practice with standards and changing practice if necessary. Audits can be carried out internally for self-review and improvement, or externally by inspectors. Peer audit can use already-existing standards, or practitioners can develop their own. Most quality assurance in the UK is professional, multiprofessional or organisational audit.

Organisational audit: an external inspection of aspects of a service, in comparison to established standards, and a review of an organisation's arrangements to control and assure the quality of its products or services. Audits use criteria (or 'standards') against which auditors judge elements of a service's planning, organisation, systems and performance.

Quality accreditation: a certification through an external evaluation of whether a practitioner, equipment or a service meets standards which are thought to contribute to quality processes and outcomes.

Quality system: a co-ordinated set of procedures, division of responsibilities, and processes for setting quality standards and procedures, identifying quality problems and resolving these problems. (BSI 5750 and ISO 9000 are standards for a quality system.)

Continuous Quality Improvement (CQI): an approach for ensuring that staff continue to improve work processes by using proven quality methods to discover and resolve the causes of quality problems in a systematic way.

Total quality management (TQM): a comprehensive strategy of organisational and attitude change for enabling staff to learn and use quality methods in order to reduce costs and meet the requirements of patients and other 'customers'. Quality is 'a method of management' – quality is determined by systems of care, and management are responsible for the performance of these systems.

Quality programme: a set of systematic activities intended to ensure the quality of one or more organisations' services and products, usually planned and organisation-wide.

Quality project: a time-limited task to solve a quality problem or improve quality, undertaken by a specially created team using quality methods in a structured way.

Another development in the late 1980s was an increasing awareness of organisational approaches to quality and a willingness and ability to try these methods. This both coincided with and contributed to the rise of managerialism in the NHS. A number of organisational quality assessment systems were developed and tried: two of the earliest were the small hospitals' accreditation programme (Shaw *et al.* 1988) which was offered nationally in 1993, and the BSI 5750 quality system standard (BSI 1987). (ISO 9000 is a similar international standard, with ISO 9004–2 for services added in 1991). BSI 5750 was first adapted and tested in four health services in 1987 (Rooney 1988). Her conclusions were confirmed by many others in the years to come: that this standard for a quality system was most easily applied to, and could benefit support services such as pharmacy, laboratories, medical engineering, catering, maintenance, and supplies purchasing. In later years a number of services achieved registration by BSI for meeting the standard's requirements for a functioning quality system, services such as laboratories, a district purchasing organisation (Mid Staffordshire in 1992), and a small GP practice.

Slightly later developments were the King's Fund organisational audit (tested during 1989–1992), which was to become a hospital accreditation system in 1995 (Brooks 1992, Scrivens 1995), and quality award frameworks such as the US Baldridge award adapted for health care (Øvretveit 1994d). Total quality management (TQM) also made an appearance in the late 1980s, but it took a few years before a few hospitals actually started significant TQM programmes. Perhaps the most successful and long running programmes were those started in 1990 at the St Helier Trust in Carlshalton and at Trafford, although the latter dropped 'management' from total quality and emphasised standard-setting and customer audit in the early years (Sewell 1994, NHS ME 1993).

That total quality management could be tried also signalled that quality was no longer the exclusive province of professionals, although management still kept a respectful distance from clinical matters. TQM gave an ideology and a justification for management to raise questions about and take a responsibility for quality issues beyond those raised by patient complaints: the central tenet of TQM is that most quality problems are not due to incompetent practitioners but to poorly designed and operated systems of care. But TQM was a double-edged sword. First, if managers were responsible for systems of care, quality problems were their responsibility and could not be delegated to the professions. Second, the philosophy emphasised worker empowerment and supporting those working the systems to use quality methods to understand and change these systems: managers had to follow through and make the changes proposed by quality improvement teams, and also risk empowering already empowered professionals. Managers and their staff did not have the time, the resources, and the nerve to do this, especially with the pace of events at the turn of the decade.

> *As the chief executive proclaimed the virtues of TQM against a background of the savings the Health Authority would have to achieve over the coming years, hardly anyone in the audience was in eye contact with him, bodies were turned forty five degrees away, eyes were everywhere but at the lectern, faces were grim, and the cynicism was palpable.*

Morgan and Murgatroyd (1994) p. 73.

The 'watershed' years 1989–1992

These 'organisational' quality approaches were both thrown off-track and assisted by the NHS reforms, which also had an impact on professional quality approaches. In 1990 the Department of Health financed a number of TQM 'projects' and an evaluation of TQM in the NHS. The evaluation found that only a few hospitals' quality programmes had been able to 'weather' the NHS reforms and many had not survived changes of management, mergers and other effects of the reforms (Joss and Kogan 1995). Yet two hospitals had been able to use TQM as an overarching framework to co-ordinate different internal quality activities, and to create a sense of common direction for staff during this period.

After the 'initial turbulence' of the reforms, which in fact turned out to be a way of life, both purchasing and provider managers began to pay more attention to quality. It would be wrong to suggest that competition was a driving force for quality: where competition did exist, it was in relation to costs and waiting times. Neither did quality figure much in decisions about mergers or hospital rationalisation: the question about the relation between volume and quality of specialty services is still unresolved, and none of the London specialty reviews in 1993 really considered quality.

Quality in contracts and contracting
Yet as purchasers began to get more information about costs and activity by specialty and then by patient groups, they recognised that the third corner of the 'value for money' triangle – quality – was unspecified and unknown. The Department of Health and other guidance on quality in contracts was largely ignored in many specifications by the seven health commissioners with whom I worked between 1991 and 1994 (DoH 1990, Øvretveit 1994a). However, during 1993 more contracts began to specify quality requirements, first in terms of waiting times, and then clinical quality indicators requiring specific audits and regular reports. The initial arrangement was that each purchasing authority 'had a responsibility' for the quality of hospitals within their geographical area, although questions were raised early-on as to what this meant in relation to private hospitals. This responsibility was carried out largely through specifications in contracts of required quality for all hospital services and then for each service or speciality, and by requiring routine reports.

One example is the quarterly reports which were produced by one orthopaedic hospital for all of its purchasers in 1993, which included: three-line notes on all written complaints over the last three months; drug and patient incidents; infection rates; cancelled operations; plaster and pressure sore rates; unplanned readmissions; outpatient waiting times (per consultant); and a routine patient satisfaction survey showing quarterly trends in such factors as 'Satisfaction with nurses listening and explaining', 'Satisfaction with doctor's concern'. Other purchasers used the specifications of the host purchaser when contracting from hospitals outside of their area. One research study found little had changed by 1996, and that the quality of clinical care was referred to in 75 per cent of the general and 43 per cent of the service specific specifications (Gray and Donaldson 1996).

Little of this was useful for inter-service comparisons, but it did show providers that quality was becoming an issue for purchasers. What GP purchasers lacked in terms of time to specify and monitor quality, they made up for in being able to make a better assessment of clinical quality and of individual patient satisfaction, and this too began to have an impact on hospitals and community trusts. However, in most cases the purchaser provider relationship which was required to encourage quality improvement still has to develop in ways which are common in other industries (Øvretveit 1994b). Later, purchasers' attention shifted from specifying details of quality in contracts to ensuring that providers had an appropriate quality system. When purchasers found that they did not have the expertise to judge whether the quality system was appropriate, they became more interested in schemes where external experts judged and approved the system, and in accreditation.

One result of the costs and difficulty of specifying and monitoring quality was thus a demand by purchasers for both public and private hospitals to have a recognised system for ensuring quality, or a credible certification that the hospital met certain standards of quality. This demand was resisted for a number of years by the King's Fund organisational audit group, who emphasised that a 'good' audit report was no guarantee of future quality. They also believed that changing to an accreditation approach would damage the open and developmental approach which had been valued by both 'peer-visitors' and the host hospitals. By 1995 the pressures became too great and organisational audit became an accreditation scheme.

This theme – of the tension between inspection and development – runs through the history of quality in the NHS, and is related to another theme: do providers, both individuals and institutions, make faster and more significant improvements to quality when performance feedback is confidential or when it is public? Both are related to the third theme of professional power and autonomy, and to a fourth: the link between quality and markets – it is no coincidence that private hospitals were heavily involved in the early development of organisational audit.

Deafening silences

It is of interest that, whilst purchasers sought methods to ensure the quality of services which they purchased for the public, few raised questions about the quality of purchasing as a service (Øvretveit 1994b). How was it to be defined, measured and assured? Sometimes the subjects which are not considered, and the reasons why they are neglected, teach us more about the NHS than those which become 'issues'. International comparisons highlight a number of silent subjects in the history of quality in the NHS (Øvretveit 1997), for example not recognising the link between quality and human rights, the continual and breathtaking lack of interest in the economics of quality and the cost of poor quality, relicensing of practitioners (eg every five years), and the lack of attention in the UK to educating patients to assess quality, to primary care team quality, to the role of community health councils, to inter-sectoral quality, and to quality in public health and in health promotion (Øvretveit 1996a).

One international development which had an impact on the NHS was methods for providing information to patients, purchasers and referrers about the quality of a service. For all the rhetoric about patient choice and consumerism, there was nothing in the first five years of the reforms which enabled patients to make informed choices about which doctor or hospital to go to. The publication in 1994 by the Scottish Office of mortality data from Scottish hospitals and other performance data did not do much to increase choice, but it was a landmark in the UK and in Europe. The problems of adjusting for case-mix, severity of illness and other patient and population characteristic which confounded many of the possible indicators were well known by the Scottish Office and to those in the NHS with whom they consulted. It is perhaps the consultation and the way in which the figures were released which was the most important lesson. There was lengthy discussion within the NHS, and a recognition that internal publication was not an option with the potential media interest which had already made use of the Birmingham research comparisons and the Royal College of Surgeons' confidential audit data. If the data were to be collected, they had to be made public: after long debate, the Scottish Office finally published the data with a 'Government health warning' that the figures were not of themselves measures of quality of care (Scottish Office 1994).

Those south of the border were more cautious, or perhaps secretive, and only later began to consider clinical comparisons as part of the hospital 'league tables' data release. The question still remains as to whether the benefits to patients and others justifies the cost of gathering and publishing comparative quality performance information which is not misleading. A little knowledge is a dangerous thing if it is inaccurate and in the hands of someone not aware of the limitations of that knowledge. Whilst new information technology will improve matters, the costs of systems for gathering, analysing and publishing information which allows valid and reliable comparisons is still too high for all but a few indicators (Øvretveit 1996b). The recent history of the NHS shows that obsession with performance on the easily-measurable distracts attention from the more difficult to measure, but often more important, especially in the realm of quality.

Post-1995

> *Following a critical report from the UK National Audit Office in December 1995 it was reported that, 'The Department of Health is still unable to assess the benefits of clinical audit five years after it was first set up in the health service, the NHS chief executive admitted last week . . . Some MPs expressed astonishment that the NHS executive has still not measured the outcome of the estimated 100,000 clinical audits carried out by Trusts, Health Authorities and GPs. A Labour MP demanded to know how the NHS could justify spending £279m to data on clinical audit in hospitals – equivalent to recruiting 1,500 doctors a year.'*
>
> *Health Services Journal 21 March 1996, p. 7*

Amongst the developments in the second half of the 1990s was a questioning of the value and cost-effectiveness of much of what was being done in the NHS under the name of quality. Earlier reports had proposed ways to improve the effectiveness of audit activities (Black and Thompson 1993, Kerrison *et al.* 1993, Walshe and Coles 1993). These, together with the change in emphasis to multiprofessional approaches (code words: 'clinical audit') gave a stimulus to and a refocused audit, which was assisted by the growth of the 'evidence based medicine' movement. The 'grand designs' of comprehensive total quality revolution had not been as successful as was hoped (Joss and Kogan 1995, Øvretveit 1994c), and it appeared that what was effective were local small-scale initiatives, which has always been the case in the NHS. More practitioners began to recognise that there was more to quality than setting standards and external audit: the newer continuous quality improvement methods for team-based process improvement were not only effective for clinical processes, but more clinician-friendly, building as they did on an applied scientific attitude. An increasing number of projects were reported using this method, notably at the first European Forum for Quality Improvement in London in 1996, and also in the quality practitioner's journal published by the Association for Quality in Health Care (Box 7.2).

Other developments included purchasers improving their specification and monitoring of quality, the testing of business process re-engineering, and a new NHS complaints system. Improvements to Trusts' complaints system were also influenced by an increase in litigation as Trusts became financially liable for negligence and by a range of 'risk management' methods from the USA. There was discussion of 'disease management' and of the use of methods to improve the quality of episodes of care crossing sectors, but only a few inter-organisational quality improvement projects were actually conducted before 1997. Increasingly sophisticated computer-based systems for measuring quality were developed, and a number of 'benchmarking' programmes were begun.

What has been the effect of these initiatives? It is difficult to say, because few have been evaluated and because of the difficulties of evaluating these interventions to organisations. Yet between 1990 and 1994, formal complaints to CHCs doubled from 37,050 to 87,184, those to GP service committees rose from 2,205 to 2,490, and to the health service commissioner from 990 to 1,782. Did quality drop, or were patients more willing to complain and found it easier to do so? Or was the NHS getting better at recording quality information and following the gurus' dictum of treating instances of poor quality as 'treasures to be cherished'?

Box 7.2 Some events in the history of quality assurance in the NHS

1969: Health Advisory Service established, following revelations about poor quality care in psychiatric and metal handicap hospitals (undertakes peer review visits). The National External Quality Assessment Scheme is set up to inspect NHS pathology laboratories

1979: Royal Commission recommends 'a planned programme of peer review of standards of care and treatment'

1983: Griffiths report leads to general management and raises the question of customer service in the NHS and the use of 'industrial quality assurance'. Royal College of General Practitioners starts a national quality initiative

1986: Formation of 'NHS Quality Assurance Interest Group' with conferences, which grew into the later 'Association for Quality in Healthcare'

1988: The first quality system is adapted for British health services (BSI 5750 Rooney 1988). The National Association of Health Authorities proposes an accreditation agency to bring together the many inspection bodies operating in the NHS. The King's Fund report on accreditation schemes leads to a pilot organisational audit approach in 1989

1989: '*Working for Patients*' White Paper proposes all practitioners take part in 'medical audit' (DoH (1989c, d)). '*Caring for People*' White Paper proposes quality assurance and inspection arrangements for community care. Department of Health sponsors a national total quality management programme. International Standards organisation and British Standards Institute publishes a draft standard for a service quality system. NHS Chief executive asks managers to develop a quality assurance programmes and allocates £7.5 million for quality initiatives (EL(89)/MB/114)

1990: Welsh Office launches a quality strategy for Wales, and recommends total quality management. Department of Health publishes guidance on contracting, including how to specify quality. An award exceeding £1 million is paid in compensation for medical negligence which led to brain damage for a baby at birth. Birmingham University starts the first UK masters degree in quality assurance in health care

1991: The Government proposes a Patient's Charter, defining standards of service which patients could expect for waiting and other subjects. Trusts become financially liable for medical negligence. New guidelines for medical audit (DoH 1991)

1992: The Audit Commission, a Government inspection agency, issues a consultation document on its future role in assessing quality (AC 1992)

1993: With better information about costs and volumes, purchasers become more concerned about quality in contracts. The Department of Health promotes clinical guidelines and quality assurance (EL (93) 116), and the dissemination of research evidence through the *Effective Healthcare Bulletin* (EL (93) 115). Researchers raise questions about the effectiveness of many audit activities. Department of Health changes the emphasis from professional to multiprofessional audit. The NHS Management Executive promotes TQM (NHS ME 1993)

1994: Scottish Office publishes death rates for patients for 30 hospitals and other outcome measures. First publication of NHS 'league tables', showing Trusts' comparative performance against 23 standards, including the proportion of patients in eight specialties admitted within 3 and 12 months

1995: Organisational audit becomes an accreditation scheme. Patient's Charter II issued, which distinguishes between 'rights' and 'expectations'. Department of Health starts pilot of surgical quality indicators for wound infection, readmission and death in hospital, with the aim of using these in an extended hospitals' 'league table'. Changes to medical disciplinary process, and health minister says that doctors risk being sacked if they do not report negligence on the part of colleagues

1996: *British Medical Journal* organises the first European conference on quality in health care in London, emphasising CQI methods. NHS complaints system is improved

1997: Conservative Government uses quality in part to justify proposals to privatise social services – regulation, provision and purchasing within one organisation is said to be incompatible with quality. Labour party considers possible legislation on patients' rights, and access to quality performance information.

Current issues and future trends

What are the current quality issues and future trends in the NHS? The first is a clash of paradigms: between the standards-inspection based approaches and the newer continuous quality improvement approaches. Whilst it is unfair to characterise the former as the 'police and punish' method, inspection approaches do tend to be based on assumptions that highlighting people's divergence from standards is itself enough to produce quality improvement. This approach is not effective if people do not believe in the standards, if they fear the consequences of being shown to be below standard, and if they do not have the skills or power to make changes. The latter and newer CQI approach is based on the idea that people are prisoners of the systems in which they work, and are condemned to produce poor quality unless they use proven methods to understand and change the systems. This approach can only work when there is already a climate of trust, and the skills and time to use the methods.

Both are necessary: the NHS must have standards, inspection and regulation of quality, and indeed this may be a necessary precondition for CQI methods. The Americans use both, however much they criticise the former. Yet there is a tension and incompatibility between these approaches which is increasingly recognised: one between the old church (we are all sinners and must try harder) and the new liberal theologians (if you recognise the greater scheme of things you are forgiven, if you act on this understanding).

A second and related issue is whether quality performance information should be made public, or only be disclosed to and used by clinicians and others internal to the service. That quality must be measured is not in dispute, although which are the best measures will always be contentious issue, and even more so as our IT capabilities increase. If the measures are generally agreed to be adequate – they will always be inaccurate and unscientific for the poor performers – and also allow comparisons, then would publicising these data produce faster and more significant quality improvements than only releasing the data internally? Perhaps the question has now become, what right does the NHS have to withhold from patients and others those data about quality which it already has? Payers and consumers in the US have answered this second question without considering the first. In the UK the irrepressible British press will no doubt answer this question and act in the public interest.

The future of quality in the NHS will be shaped by external factors and internal influences arising from the now established quality movement within the NHS. As well as the demand for information about quality from purchasers and the public, other external factors will be:

- Continual pressure on finance, which will force consideration of the costs of poor quality and of the expected return on investment in quality projects and programmes

- A pressure for greater accountability for the time and money spent on quality activities, a call for an evaluation of these different approaches, and closer management of quality activities

- New information technology, making data capture and analysis for quality improvement quicker, less expensive, and allowing comparisons, but also leading to a demand for new skills in quality measurement and interpretation

- Rising patient expectations, as people compare the quality of health services with other services as they become better able to judge and insist on better quality, together with the growth of power and sophistication of patients' associations

- More litigation and less willingness on the part of the public to give the NHS the benefit of the doubt

- New and more effective techniques from commercial services for improving quality

- From some quarters, a pressure to ensure quality for the poor, vulnerable and voiceless, in part articulated through a movement for patients' and citizens' rights

- More European requirements for basic standards of quality, for quality assurance, and for harmonisation of patient rights across Europe

- Increasing competition between NHS services and with the private sector

- Pressures to assess and report on the quality of different purchasing organisations, as public services

- Methods to ensure inter-organisational quality and continuity of care: increasing fragmentation of services and other changes will lead to assessing and improving the quality of episodes of care

Influences arising from within the 'quality movement' in the NHS will also shape future developments. These include:

- An emerging occupation of health quality specialists (eg audit co-ordinators), with their own interests and also increased capabilities to facilitate team projects and manage information

- A convergence between evidence based medicine, outcomes measurement/management, and continuous improvement approaches

- Doctors and medical managers will increasingly recognise the compatibility between CQI and a scientific approach, that the values are consonant with their own values and will begin to take a greater part in quality programmes which include this approach

- Accreditation schemes for different services will become an established part of the NHS

- A greater understanding of the more effective quality methods and of how to achieve change, leading to better selection and management of quality projects

- A more realistic approach to total quality management and greater sophistication in adapting the ideas to particular services.

Conclusions

Hindsight is a wonderful thing, especially from abroad. This short, selective and subjective account has made more sense of the evolution of quality methods and approaches in the NHS than there was at the time. Quality in the NHS is confusing and complex, but also very simple. The purpose of these methods are to help the NHS do what it is meant to do: to meet patients' needs in a humane and safe way with respect for the person, and to do so without waste and errors. When used by individual professions and for profession-specific quality improvement, these methods do not radically alter power relations, but this approach is no longer effective. With the increasing complexity of care and of service organisation, we cannot rely on professional quality regulation and improvement alone. The main problems have been and are getting professions to work together to improve quality and to work with management to change systems of care. And it is here that professional interests and politics cut across the common purpose of giving the best patient care. The different definitions and meanings of quality which cause the confusion are not accidental and serve to maintain professional boundaries and autonomy: language may be the professions' last defence.

There are some within the professions who see quality methods as a further onslaught by management to control and direct, or as a Trojan horse containing the soldiers of cost control. The history of these methods in the NHS certainly shows the potential of some to add more bureaucracy, and for management and others to intrude into the very core of professional discretion and relations with patients. Yet it also shows the potential for professions to use quality methods to uphold professional values and to reassert principles which have declined in importance in the business of health. If professions use these methods to understand the systems of care within which they work, and to test changes to these systems, this then can provide a new basis for cooperation with other professions and with management.

Some key points of the chapter

- In order to protect patients and better meet their needs, the NHS has supported the traditional profession-specific approaches to quality assurance, but has also sought to apply and adapt approaches from the commercial sector. This has sometimes led to confusion.

- Quality is political: whilst it may not be a conscious strategy, occupations' control and ownership of quality issues serves to defend and advance their interests, such as their 'rights' of self-regulation and autonomy and their ambitions to direct others. The political dimension to quality in part explains the 'confusion' about quality and the less than startling success of many quality initiatives.

- The main approaches to proving and improving quality in the NHS can be classified as traditional profession-specific (including professional regulation, education and audit), multiprofessional audit (using a variety of methods), risk management, complaints and customer satisfaction approaches, organisational audit and quality award assessments of the organisation's quality performance, contract management of quality, quality systems (eg ISO 9000), continuous quality improvement team projects, and total quality management.

- Notwithstanding the rise of evidence-based medicine and management, there is little evidence about which of the many quality methods and approaches are most cost-effective in different settings. Generally, small scale team projects, with trained and well-facilitated staff persistently using systematic methods seem to have achieved more than the larger customer service or other programmes.

- The history of quality in the NHS shows a movement in definition and focus from professional to managerial and patient-consumer approaches. This shift was both a consequence and cause of shifts in power in the NHS in the last two decades. This shift is epitomised by the Patient's Charter and by the change of emphasis in policy about audit: from supporting to requiring profession-specific audit, and then to encouraging multiprofessional audit and its integration with other quality activities, and then to emphasising the role of purchasers in requiring audit and quality information.

- The future will see rising patient expectations, supported by patients' rights, more public information about quality generated by lower cost information technology and increasing sophistication in quality measurement, an increased concern with the cost effectiveness of quality activities and with ensuring that they are well managed, more attention to inter-organisational quality, and an increasing use of clinician-friendly continuous quality improvement methods.

References

Audit Commission (1992) *Minding the quality: a consultation document on the role of the audit commission in quality assurance in health care* Audit Commission, London

Berwick, D (1996) Improving health care *British Medical Journal* **312**, 605–618

Black, N (1992) Research, audit and education *British Medical Journal*, **304**, 698–700

Black, N and Thompson, E (1993) Obstacles to medical audit: British doctors speak *Social Science and Medicine*, **36**, 849–856

Brooks, T (1992) Success through organisational audit *Health Services Management* **Nov/Dec**, 13–15

BSI (1987) *BS 5750 Quality Systems part 1: Specification for design/development, production installation and servicing* British Standards Institute, London

Buck, N, Devlin, B and Lunn, J (1987) *Report of a confidential enquiry into perioperative deaths* Nuffield Provincial Hospitals Trust/King's Fund, London

DoH (1989a) *Report on confidential enquiries into maternal deaths in England and Wales 1982–84* HMSO, London

DoH (1989b) *Working for Patients* HMSO, London

DoH (1989c) *Working Paper 6 – Medical Audit* HMSO, London

DoH (1989d) *Medical Audit in the Family Practitioner Services* HMSO, London

DoH (1990) *Funding and contracts for hospital services, Working Paper 2, Working for Patients* HMSO, London

DoH (1991) *Medical Audit in the Hospital and Community Health Services, HC(91)2 January* DoH, London

DoH (1992) *The Patient's Charter* HMSO, London

Ellis, R and Whittington, D (1993) *Quality Assurance in Health Care: A Handbook*, Edward Arnold, London

Frater, A and Spiby, J (1990) *Measured Progress – Medical Audit for Physicians* NW Thames Regional Health Authority, London

Goldstone, L, Ball, J and Collier, M (1983) *Monitor: an index of the quality of nursing care for acute medical and surgical wards* Newcastle upon Tyne Polytechnic Products, Newcastle

Gray, J and Donaldson, L (1996) Improving the quality of health care through contracting: a study of Health Authority practice *Quality in Health Care*, **5**, 201–205

Griffiths, R (1983) *NHS Management Inquiry* HMSO, London

Gruer, R, Gunn, A, Gordon, D and Ruckley, C (1986) Audit of surgical audit *Lancet*, i, 23–6

Health Services Journal, 1996, March, 7

Joss, R and Kogan, M (1995) *Advancing Quality*, Open University Press, Milton Keynes

Kerrison, S, Packwood, T and Buxton, M (1993) *Medical Audit: taking stock* King's Fund Centre, London

Kogan, M and Redfern, S (eds) (1995) *Making Use of Clinical Audit: A guide to practice in the health professions* Open University Press, Milton Keynes

Marinker, M (ed.) (1990) *Medical audit and general practice* BMJ Publications, London

Morgan, C and Murgatroyd, S (1994) *Total quality management in the public sector* Open University Press, Milton Keynes

NCEPOD (1987) *The report of a national confidential enquiry into perioperative deaths* King's Fund, London

NHS ME (1993) *The quality journey: a guide to total quality management in the NHS* NHS Management Executive, Leeds

NN & MCC (1988) *Quality assurance in nursing: report of a working group* National Nursing and Midwifery Consultative Committee, HMSO, London

Øvretveit, J (1988) *A Peer Review Process for Improving Service Quality* BIOSS, Brunel University

Øvretveit, J (1992) *Health Service Quality* Blackwell Scientific Press, Oxford

Øvretveit, J (1994a) *Purchasing for Health* Open University Press, Milton Keynes

Øvretveit, J (1994b) 'Quality in health services purchasing *Journal of the Association of Quality in Healthcare* **2**, 9–22

Øvretveit, J (1994c) All together now *Health Service Journal* **Dec**, 25–27

Øvretveit, J (1994d) A comparison of approaches to quality in the UK, USA and Sweden, and of the use of organisational audit frameworks *European Journal of Public Health* **4**, 46–54

Øvretveit, J (1996a) Quality in health promotion *Health Promotion International* **11**, 55–62

Øvretveit, J (1996b) Informed choice? Patient access to health service quality information *Health Policy* **36**, 75–93

Øvretveit, J (1997) Learning from quality improvement in Europe and beyond *Journal of the Joint Commission for Accreditation of Healthcare Organisations* **23**, 7–22

Pearson, A (ed) *Nursing Quality Measurement; Quality assurance methods for peer review* Wiley, London

Rooney, E (1988) A proposed quality system specification for the National Health service *Quality Assurance* **14**, 45–53

RCGP (1983) The quality initiative *Journal of the Royal College of General Practitioners* **33**, 523–524

RCN (1990) *Dynamic Standard Setting System*, Royal College of Nursing, London

RCOG (1990) *Interim guidelines on medical audit* Royal College of Obstetricians and Gynecologists, London

RCP (1989) *Medical Audit – A First report. What, Why and How?* Royal College of Physicians of London

RCS (1989) *Guidelines to Clinical Audit in Surgical Practice* Royal College of Surgeons of England, London

Sackett, D, Rosenberg, W, Gray, J, Haynes, R and Scott-Richardson, W (1996) Evidence-based medicine: what it is and what it isn't *British Medical Journal* **312**, 71–72

Scottish Office (1994) *Clinical outcome indicators* The Scottish Office, Edinburgh

Scrivens, E (1995) *Accreditation* Open University Press, Milton Keynes

Sellu, D (1986) Audit: Its effect on the performance of a surgical unit in a DGH *Hospitals and Health Services Review* **82**, 64–69

Sewell, N (1994) Total Quality Management: Making it Work in the NHS *Journal of the Association for Quality in Healthcare* **24**–29

Shaw, C (1986) *Quality assurance – what the colleges are doing* King's Fund, London

Shaw, C, Hurst and Stone (1988) *Towards good practice in small hospitals: some suggested guidelines* National Association of Health Authorities, Birmingham

Shaw, C (1989) *Medical Audit: A Hospital Handbook*, King's Fund Centre, London

Taylor, D (1996) Quality and professionalism in health care: a review of current initiatives in the NHS *BMJ* **312**, 626–629

Walshe, K and Coles, J (1993) *Evaluating audit: a review of initiatives* CASPE Research, London

8 Managed care: a route map for exploring health policy changes

Judith Smith

Introduction

What is managed care?

Introducing a major Department of Health funded review of the US literature relating to the performance of managed care, Robinson and Steiner reassuringly justify the standard British confusion when confronted with managed care:

> In the United States, the term 'managed care' is currently used to denote a bewildering variety of structures and strategies for improving the performance of the health care system ... the terminology surrounding managed care has been designed more for marketing than for research purposes and so labels are often used in conflicting and confusing ways.
>
> (Robinson and Steiner 1998)

So what is managed care? What is it about the concept that captivates and yet infuriates managers and clinicians in the NHS? Are there lessons from the US experience which can helpfully be applied to the UK as it adapts to the health policy of an incoming Labour Government at a time of tight control of the public purse?

Managed care has been defined as 'healthcare systems in which the responsibility for payment is linked more tightly to decision making about the provision of healthcare services than in traditional indemnity insurance plans' (Pollner 1995). This bringing together of the financial and the clinical, of management and care, is the essence of managed care. The fusion can occur at the macro level of the health care organisation as seen in the bringing together of the responsibilities for purchasing and provision in health maintenance organisations (HMOs), or at the micro level of the patient, as seen in managed care techniques such as care pathway guidelines and disease management protocols.

This distinction between managed care organisations and managed care techniques is drawn by Robinson and Steiner in their review of managed care (*op cit* 1998). Techniques such as utilisation review, physician incentives and disease management are concerned with functions of the provision of care. Organisations such as HMOs, social HMOs and preferred provider organisations (PPOs) are concerned with the structure of health care funding and provision.

At the macro, structural level, managed care is concerned with a realignment of the relationship between the three key actors in health care:

- Payers
- Commissioners
- Providers

It has as its key aim the desire to ensure that those third parties (managed care organisations and plans) who commission care on behalf of the payers (individuals, employers, taxpayers) are able to influence the level and quality of care given by providers (hospitals, primary care organisations, doctors). To achieve this aim, individuals in the US are enrolled into managed care plans or organisations, for which a capitation fee is charged to the individual, the employer or the government (on behalf of taxpayers). The managed care organisation then uses its pool of capitation fees to purchase all necessary health care required by its enrolled population in the time period covered by the enrolment fee. It does this by allocating resources to providers through contracts. Levels and standards of service are specified and these are typically supported by complex and far-reaching monitoring arrangements.

The incentive for the managed care organisation is to maintain the health of its enrolled population and to minimise expenditure on health treatment services. Therein lies the origin of the name of the most common and most talked about form of US managed care, the health maintenance organisation (HMO). Robinson and Steiner (*op. cit.* 1998) summarise the role of health maintenance organisations as follows:

> . . . *all HMOs offer care to defined populations, who accept restricted choice, they transfer risk to providers through capitation-based funding and combine financial and resource management.*

> (Robinson and Steiner 1998)

For 'all HMOs', you could quite reasonably substitute 'the NHS' in its post-1991 reform state. Health authorities, GP Fundholders, GP total purchasers and locality groups consider themselves responsible for the commissioning of health services for a defined population. The general public effectively accepts restricted choice of GP, consultant, hospital, date of elective admission and more. Contracts or service agreements are used by commissioners as tools for transferring risk to providers, drawing together funding and activity, and putting the onus on providers to control costs in a world of apparently rising demand.

Some commentators have gone as far as to suggest that the NHS is 'one of the first and most successful managed health care systems in the world' (Hatcher 1995). Others, such as Kirkman-Liff (1996) point out that there are elements of US managed care which can be 'grafted on' to the NHS, particularly in relation to the commissioning of care:

> *Health care systems in Europe are similar to gardens . . . The American health system is similar to a jungle . . . Managed care, integrated delivery systems, care maps, outcomes research, and community health information networks are just some plants that have recently evolved in the American jungle . . . Transplanting a jungle plant into a garden is an easy way to introduce a weed, and one never knows what parasites are attached to the roots of a foreign plant. . . . I am suggesting that Europeans look at purchasing in the US health system and take selective 'cuttings' of American ideas which can be grafted onto good European stock.*
>
> (Kirkman-Liff, 1996)

Managed care can thus be examined at whole system or purchaser organisation level, or at individual patient level. The NHS may be a managed care system, a total purchasing project or a primary care trust could be said to be a managed care organisation, and the use of contracts and protocols a managed care patient technique. Before examining in more detail the application of managed care to the NHS, it is helpful to explore the history and development of managed care.

History and development of managed care

Although usually regarded as an American import to Europe, managed care can be seen to have its roots in nineteenth century voluntary health insurance in many European countries (Abel-Smith 1995). These organisations sought the best buy from providers and did not shrink from stimulating price competition, just as with US HMOs of the 1990s. Abel-Smith identified those features of the early European social health insurance/sick fund schemes which can be seen to have predated their US managed care descendants:

- Charging the same premium for each member leading to a budget ceiling for expenditure.

- Using a combination of salaried and contracted doctors.

- Paying doctors on a capitation or fee-for-service basis.

- Purchasing drugs from the supplier offering the best discount.

- Having a list of drugs approved as covered under the scheme.

- Using hospitals with the most favourable prices.

- Closely monitoring doctors' prescribing and referral patterns.

In the European context, it was the arrival of compulsory insurance which eventually led to a shift of power from consumers to providers. Providers sought to escape price competition and lay regulation. Only in the 1980s was there a discernible move back towards funder control over insurers and hence over provider development and pricing (Abel-Smith 1995).

In America, the drive to develop managed care arose from widespread concern about cost inflation associated with traditional fee-for-service or indemnity insurance plans. In a fee-for-service system, individuals in the fee-for-service plan, or their employers, pay premiums for health care coverage. Doctors and other providers make a charge for health services to a third party intermediary, usually an insurance company (or the government if the patient is covered by Medicare or Medicaid). Despite some restrictions imposed on clinicians by insurers, and some third party control of fees, there are typically few incentives to doctors and providers to control costs. The incentive is to provide as much treatment as possible in order to maximise income and protect against legal liability.

Managed care is designed to address the fundamental perverse incentives of fee-for-service, without adversely affecting patients' health outcomes. Kirkman-Liff (1996) identifies three distinct stages in the development of US managed care:

1 Prepaid group practice

A model which started in the 1930s in Minnesota. Doctors work on a salaried basis as members of a group and collectively care for patients. There is a single medical record, doctors freely consult with each other about patients and revenues are shared. Early pioneers in group practice added the concept of pre-payment, which, as we have already seen, was developed in Europe during the nineteenth century. Thus patients enrolled as members of the group, paid a monthly fee, and received care as deemed necessary by the doctors.

Prepaid group practice developed in the western states and industrialists increasingly saw the potential to be gained from contracting directly with the groups of doctors to provide health services for their employees and their dependants. Schemes were rarely for-profit, had few user charges, and were often linked with the trade union movement. They faced significant opposition from fee-for-service doctors who perceived group practice as a threat.

2 Health Maintenance Organisations (HMOs)

In the early 1970s, prepaid group practice started to gain acceptance and President Nixon was known to regard it as a means of lowering health care costs. It was Paul Elwood, a White House policy advisor, who coined the term 'health maintenance organisation' for the development of managed care. Insurance companies were often supportive of initiatives to expand managed care, seeing it as a route to reduce rising health care costs for patients already enrolled in insurance plans. HMOs were to be made attractive to enrolees by incurring few or no co-payments by patients, despite the restriction on patient choice of doctor (a doctor from the prepaid group had to be used).

3 Managed care plans

In the 1980s, it became apparent that HMOs were gaining in popularity with those working class Americans now having access to a choice of insurance plans. As prepaid group practices and HMOs proliferated, so insurers, hospitals and doctors developed new corporate structures for the contractual relationships underpinning managed care. The individual or the employer could now contract with a 'managed care plan' as the 'health benefit intermediary', which would act as the insurer or purchaser of services on behalf of member enrolees. Managed care plans were typically for-profit and increasingly contracted with fee-for-service doctors as well as with groups or HMOs. Some plans were floated on the stock market and managed care was now 'big business'.

Federal and state governments started to use managed care within Medicare and Medicaid health insurance programmes, with some even introducing mandatory enrolment in managed care schemes for those falling within state health insurance coverage.

The integration of commissioning and provision

Both Kirkman-Liff (1996) and Robinson and Steiner (1998) point to the current important distinction within managed care as being the extent of integration of health benefit intermediary (commissioner) and service provider functions. Some models of managed care resemble the original prepaid group practices with the organisation taking responsibility for both the levying of fees and the provision of primary and preventive care for its enrolees. In this sense they can be said to be truly 'health maintaining', the focus being on trying to keep enrolees fit and well and avoid referrals to costly secondary and tertiary care. Other plans are returning to a more traditional insurance emphasis, with attempts to 'cream-skim' low risk patients combined with significant use of managed care techniques such as review of clinical decisions and prior authorisation of treatments.

Integration of commissioner and provider may also occur in relation to secondary care. Some HMOs own the provider hospitals used by patients or develop 'preferred provider' arrangements whereby patients are incentivised to use those hospitals or doctors with whom the HMO has reached a preferred provider deal. The range of organisational forms within US managed care is therefore wide and complex. Commissioning and provision may therefore be vertically integrated (HMO owns provider) or virtually integrated (HMO has preferred provider or other contractual relationships). This distinction between organisational and network/contractual integration is highlighted by Robinson and Cassalino (1996) and is gaining currency amongst UK commentators on changes to the NHS of the late 1990s (Ham 1996).

Verdicts on managed care

Whilst managed care is generally acknowledged to have offered a route for controlling costs and managing demand in US health care, views are polarised in relation to whether it is in itself a 'good thing'. Herzlinger (1997) argues that managed care has succeeded in slowing the escalation of health care costs because it denies care, squeezes payments to providers, and shortens hospital stays. She concludes that it has done for health care what downsizing has done for industry – not very much. Rayner (1996) echoes this warning about the deleterious effects on patient choice and clinician freedom: ... 'managed care is essentially about controlling (ie reducing) the cost of healthcare by minimising the freedom of doctors to make expensive referrals, and reducing the choices available to patients'.

We return to our original question. Are there lessons from the US experience of seeking to manage costs and care which can helpfully be applied to the UK as it adapts to the health policy of a new government at a time of tight control of the public purse?

The relevance of managed care to the NHS

Managed care tends to evoke strong and often negative reactions among managers and clinicians in the UK. It is frequently seen as a US import and NHS suspicion is fuelled by the apparently enthusiastic interest shown by pharmaceutical companies. May (1995) reinforced this point: 'Developed as a means of curbing the excesses of the US healthcare system, "managed care" is a conveniently fuzzy blanket term – but the concept is being heavily promoted by multinational companies as the latest cure-all for the NHS.' In reaching an understanding of the relevance of managed care to the UK, it is useful to return to Robinson and Steiner's (1998) distinction between managed care organisations and managed care techniques. There are both macro/organisational lessons to be learnt from managed care in the US and micro/patient management techniques which can be, and are being, applied in the NHS.

Macro/organisational lessons from managed care

The key principle underlying the NHS reforms of 1991 was the separation of the purchasing from the provision of care. A system of contracts was to be used for the definition of both quantity and quality of patient care delivered by hospitals and community services units. In the words of Lady Thatcher (1993) there was an intention to 'loosen the excessively rigid control of the hospital service from the centre and introduce greater diversity in the provision of health care'. Just as managed care is concerned with the relationship between payers, commissioners and providers of care, so the politicians leading the NHS review in 1988–89 sought to find a system which would realign incentives in such a way that efficiency and quality would be enhanced. They examined and rejected an HMO model of purchasing, a suggested network of 'local health funds'(LHFs). Thatcher described this proposed model as follows:

> *People would be free to decide to which LHF they subscribed. LHFs would offer comprehensive health care services for their subscribers – whether provided by the*

LHF itself, purchased from other LHFs, or purchased from independent suppliers. The advantage of this system – which was also claimed for the American HMOs – was that it had built-in incentives for efficiency and so for keeping down the costs which would otherwise escalate as they had done in some health insurance systems.

(Thatcher 1993)

The original aims of the 1991 NHS reforms were therefore consistent with those we identified earlier for US managed care, the bringing together of the financial and the clinical in a tighter decision-making process about care purchasing and provision. Hatcher (1995) identified four key features of managed care which were directly applicable to the NHS in the 1990s (see Box 8.1).

Box 8.1 Key features of managed care

- Limiting consumer choice to those approved by the funding agency.
- The gatekeeping role of the primary care physician.
- Selective contracting between purchasers and providers.
- A financial incentive system for physicians.

Source: Hatcher, 1995

These activities are themselves crucial to the drawing together of the financial and the clinical, the effective management of scarce resources in a health care system, in short, the management of care. In the UK, limited consumer choice in health care has long been broadly accepted by patients, primarily within the context of the primary care gatekeeping role of the GP. Hospital specialists are chosen by the GP on behalf of patients and this decision has been further circumscribed since 1991 by the nature of local contracts for secondary care negotiated by the health authority or the GP fundholder. In primary care, limited choice is also implicitly accepted, GPs placing geographical boundaries for their catchment population and patients reporting difficulties in changing GP for reasons other than a change of address.

However, it is in the area of selective contracting and physician incentives that the UK has seen a greater shift towards some of the organisational features commonly associated with managed care. The relationship between payers, commissioners and providers has evolved and matured. The original model of the separation of payers (health authorities and GP fundholders) and providers (NHS Trusts) has spawned differing approaches to commissioning health services (Shapiro *et al.* 1996) such as multifunds, GP commissioning groups, locality commissioning and total purchasing. This 'network' of commissioners (Figure 8.1) can be likened to a US network of managed care organisations where each 'HMO' takes responsibility for the health care needs of a defined or enrolled population, placing contracts with providers, using resources allocated by the payers – taxpayers via the Department of Health in the UK, subscribers to managed care plans in the US.

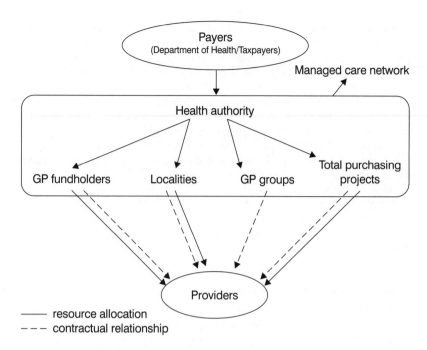

Figure 8.1   Multiple commissioners of care within a local 'managed care' network

Commentators have noted that it is these primary care commissioners who have tended to be able to exert a greater degree of selective contracting on service providers in leveraging service pattern and quality (Shaw and Richards 1997, Ham 1996). Whereas health authorities are rarely able to remove large contracts from local provider trusts in whose future survival the authority is likely to have an inevitable interest, fundholders and commissioning groups may not feel the same degree of loyalty. Resources may be withheld if quality standards are not met and there are examples of fundholder contracts being moved between providers as a means of stimulating service improvements (Audit Commission 1996).

In many of the new primary care organisations such as total purchasing schemes and the more radical locality commissioning projects, primary care commissioners display some of the organisational features associated with managed care, and with HMOs in particular (Smith *et al.* 1997). The commissioning and the provision of care are brought together in a single organisation. The primary care organisation has a capitated budget for its patient population and it provides as many services as it can in primary care, buying in the rest from hospitals, nursing homes, community trusts and other providers. Patients are accepting restricted choice of provider within the terms of 'enrolment' in a 'managed care plan'. Gatekeeping is a fundamental aspect of the organisation's functioning and selective contracting is used as the means of obtaining the best deals for the organisation and its patients. Physician incentives have been in operation; the GP has been able to make savings for ploughing back into the organisation or his/her practice, and they can develop an extended range of GP led services for which payments may be attracted.

Figure 8.1 depicts a local network of multiple commissioners within a single health authority. Fundholders, total purchasers, locality commissioning groups and GP commissioning groups may all hold delegated purchasing budgets for a defined patient population. Thus they become managed care organisations within a local managed care 'network', each organisation seeking to maintain the health of its population and placing contracts with providers to complement the services delivered within primary care.

What does this emergence of 'HMOs' in the NHS mean for the overall configuration of services? What are the strategic and operational implications for commissioners, providers and patients? The checklists in Box 8.2 illustrate some of the issues raised.

Box 8.2 Commissioners – a checklist

- How will standards for services be set?
- How will these standards be monitored?
- How will effectiveness of services developed by primary and secondary providers be assessed?
- How will strategy be co-ordinated across a health authority?
- How will the contestability of services be assured when purchasing and provision are combined in a single organisation?
- What will be the transaction costs of managing the network of small commissioners?
- Who will evaluate and compare the different models of purchasing and provision?

Providers – a checklist

- How will secondary care development and innovation be funded and co-ordinated?
- How will necessary reconfiguration of services be managed?
- What will be the transaction costs of relating to multiple purchasers?
- What support will there be for the short term costs of moving services from secondary to primary care?
- What will be the role of the community trust in a situation where primary care organisations increasingly seek to manage service provision?

Patients – a checklist

- Will information be made available about the benefits available from each primary care organisation?
- Will there be the possibility of moving between primary care organisations?
- Does diversity of primary care organisation enhance or compromise the equity of health care provision?

- What recourse will users have if they disagree with the care approaches and plans developed by primary care organisations?
- Will primary care organisations 'cream-skim' the healthier patients?
- Who will protect the interests of vulnerable patient groups?

Managed care therefore serves to highlight the relationship between the funding, commissioning and provision of care and throws into relief some of the risks and potential benefits to be gained within maturing commissioner–provider systems in health care. It is not, however, purely at the organisational level that managed care offers lessons for the NHS.

Micro/patient lessons from managed care

Managed care techniques in the US encompass a multitude of approaches to developing improved consistency and quality of patient care, including disease management, care pathways, physician incentives and penalties, physician profiling, and utilisation review (Robinson and Steiner 1998). Three approaches which are gaining particular currency in the NHS, often encouraged by the actions of primary care commissioners, are care pathways, disease management and utilisation review.

Care pathways

Care pathways can be defined as an example of a managed care programme which specifies a default template of care for a specific procedure or condition (Ellis, personal communication 1997). In an integrated care pathway (ICP), every element of care delivered by each member of the clinical team is explicitly described, all elements of the clinical process having been considered and evidence collected on best practice. The implementation of the pathway is supported by regular audit and analysis, including patient satisfaction surveys and results of ICP analysis are fed back to staff, and changes made to the ICP as necessary. In some settings, the use of care pathways has led to the abandonment of traditional nursing records and the use of a single record which is always available to the patient and their relatives.

The move towards establishing a 'gold standard' pattern of care for a clinical condition enables variances from 'plan' to be noted and analysed and may facilitate a greater degree of informed review of care delivery (Ellis 1997). It is generally accepted that ICPs should be developed and run by clinicians and that advantages are to be gained from supporting the implementation of ICPs with a parallel development of advanced nurse practitioners. In a micro-management technique such as ICPs, managed care is concerned with providing the best possible clinical care based on a careful evaluation of the evidence and supported by planned programmes of care, integrated across professional boundaries.

Disease management

Disease management is often viewed as a construct of the pharmaceutical industry, an approach to patient care whereby a pharmaceutical company determines the overall therapeutic regime for a patient, ensuring that the preferred product is one belonging to the company. In reality, disease management is a much broader concept, concerned with the micro-management of patient care. Pollner (1995) describes disease management as

> ... *[encompassing] not just the best way to use a particular drug in a given context but a total approach to managing particular disease entities which may or may not entail drug therapies at a given juncture ... Put simply, disease management means integrating pharmaceutical care with hospital and physician services.*
>
> (Pollner 1995)

This integration of health care entails focusing on the longitudinal experience of disease by a patient (as in care pathways), devising guidelines for diagnosis and treatment which go across the traditional organisational boundaries of providers. This co-ordination of care should lead to more coherent care for patients, a tool for auditing outcomes, a vehicle for patient education, and a greater degree of communication between professionals involved in a particular programme of care.

Utilisation review
Utilisation review is concerned with reducing unnecessary care by means of a scrutiny of past, current and planned services (Robinson and Steiner 1998). It is a technique which focuses on individual patients and is often viewed as relatively aggressive, challenging clinical practice and in turn the 'clinical freedom' of doctors. Utilisation review is increasingly being employed as a technique in UK total purchasing projects. Typically, a senior nurse is employed to review the care given to and planned for the total purchasing project's patients in hospital. The review nurse will go into the hospital on a daily basis, visit patients and discuss their care with hospital nurses and doctors. On occasions, the nurse will challenge decisions made by the hospital and seek to facilitate early discharge to the care of the primary care organisation, or make other changes to care being given by the hospital. While utilisation review is often criticised as being a costly means of addressing the management of care, others see it as a means of adding 'teeth' to contracts with providers and a way of challenging the previously unchallenged 'right' of hospital clinicians to determine the pattern of care received by patients.

The relevance of managed care thus operates at both a macro and a micro level. It enhances understanding of the relationships in health care markets and underpins attempts to develop greater consistency and accountability in the delivery of individual patient care.

Current developments and future implications

What then is the future for managed care? What are the recent developments in the US and what do these tell us of the likely direction of NHS commissioning and provider organisations? Does managed care enhance our understanding of the potential implications of the 1997 White Paper (Department of Health, 1997)?

In the US, substantial change is taking place within managed care organisations, as identified by Gabel (1997) in his list of the 10 key changes in the HMO industry in the 1990s (see Box 8.3).

Box 8.3

1 The rapid growth of for-profit HMOs

2 The rapid growth of network and individual practice association (IPA) models

3 The growth of mixed-model HMOs

4 Product diversification

5 Industry consolidation at the national and local levels

6 The decline of community-rating methods (weighted enrolment fees)

7 Altered payment arrangements with physicians

8 Increased patient cost-sharing

9 Declining hospital use

10 Increased use of clinical guidelines

Source: Gabel (1997)

Many of these changes strike a chord with changes currently taking place within the NHS. Declining hospital use is a goal for the majority of commissioners and lengths of stay for many procedures continue to fall. The use of clinical guidelines is being encouraged by commissioners keen to demonstrate clinical effectiveness. In relation to models of commissioning and provision, the UK equivalent of HMOs, significant change may be afoot.

A situation of mixed models of commissioning was allowed and indeed encouraged to develop under the Conservative administration. GP commissioning groups co-existed alongside multifunds, localities, total purchasing projects, GP fundholding and health authority purchasing. As seen in Figure 8.1, a network of commissioners often acted as the 'managed care network' for a population. A key issue for the NHS as it lived through the early days of a new Labour government was 'will this diversity of mixed models be allowed to continue?' Will a single group model such as the GP commissioning group be imposed in all areas of the NHS, or will different commissioning approaches be nurtured within local health authority managed networks?

The publication of the White Paper on replacing the NHS internal market (Department of Health, 1997) offers some clues in response to these questions. Primary care is placed at the heart of health commissioning, with some 90 per cent of health care resources to be commissioned by groups of primary care professionals. There is no proposal to impose a single model for this primary care led commissioning, but instead a 'stepped' process for stages of commissioning approach, ranging from a primary care group which advises a health authority through other intermediate stages to a free-standing primary care trust. This primary care trust will be accountable to the health authority for commissioning care and will, at level 4, have added responsibility for the provision of community services for their population. Thus we see the possibility of a truly integrated commissioning and provider organisations. The primary care trust will manage a unified budget for primary and community health services whilst also managing their staff and taking responsibility for commissioning hospital and other health services for their 'enrolled' list population. Perhaps we have witnessed the conception of the UK HMO.

Prior to the publication of the White Paper, commentators were beginning to detect a move away from diversity and competition towards a greater emphasis on collaboration and integration (Ham 1997, Shaw and Richards 1997). Discussion about the implementation of the Calman-Hine Report on Cancer Services and changes to medical staffing has increasingly led analysts to suggest that networks of care, or care programmes, are likely to be developed above and beyond traditional organisational boundaries (Ham *et al.* 1998). Commissioners in the form of primary care groups and trusts may become more like managed care plans, offering defined 'packages of care' to those enrolled with them, placing contracts for whole clinical services with a 'network provider'. Thus it can be seen that managed care again offers a framework and experience which informs and elucidates exploration of the UK health system.

Returning to Kirkman-Liff's analysis (1996), managed care offers some new plants for grafting onto specimens in the UK garden (utilisation review, care pathways, disease management). It also provides a route map for exploring the potential UK jungle of diverse models of health care commissioning which at times starts to resemble its US equivalent.

Conclusion

Managed care is a much used and abused term. A careful consideration of managed care in the US does, however, offer valuable insights into macro/organisational and micro/patient aspects of care delivered in the NHS. A new degree of clarity is possible when examining the interrelationships between the funders, commissioners and providers of care. While the US has reached managed care by means of a desire to control costs and manage providers, the UK appears to be 'grafting' the principles of managed care onto its attempts to understand the emerging commissioning process, as well as 'planting' some new managed techniques as a means of improving and focusing the provision of certain services.

Robinson and Steiner (1998) sum up the caution which is essential when examining managed care: '. . . These micro-management techniques in the USA . . . [should be viewed] as hypotheses for testing in the UK context rather than methods of proven effectiveness for direct application.' They also issue a timely warning about international health policy comparisons: 'On any health policy topic . . . evidence from abroad should be no more than a springboard for encouraging innovation at home and evaluating it in its own cultural context.'

References

Abel-Smith B (1995) *Health Reform: Old Wine in New Bottles Eurohealth, June 1995* LSE Health, London

Audit Commission (1996) *What the doctor ordered* HMSO, London

Department of Health and Welsh Office (1995) *A Policy Framework for Commissioning Cancer Services* Report of the Chief Medical Officers' Expert Advisory Group on Cancers, London

Ellis, B (1997) Managed Care: a hospital clinician's view *Journal of Managed Care* 1 Department of Health 1997 *The new NHS, modern, dependable* Cmd 3807, London

Gabel, J (1997) Ten Ways HMOs Have Changed During the 1990s Health Affairs **16**

Ham, C (1996) *Public, Private or Community: What next for the NHS?* Demos, London

Ham, C (1997) Big bang reform bows out. *Health Service Journal* **24 July 1997**, 20

Ham, C, Smith, JA and Temple, J (1998) *Hubs, Spokes and Policy Cycles: an analysis of the policy implications for the NHS of changes to medical staffing.* King's Fund, London

Hatcher, P (1995) Demystifying Managed Care *Health Services Management Centre Newsletter* 1, 1–2

Herzlinger, R (1997) *Market Driven Health Care: Who Wins, Who Loses in the Transformation of America's Largest Service Industry* Addison-Wesley, Wokingham

Kirkman-Liff, B (1996) *Commissioning Care: an American Perspective on UK Reforms* Health Services Management Unit, University of Manchester

May, A (1995) Over hyped and over here. *Health Service Journal* **9 March 1995**, 14

Pollner, F (1995) Management Matters *Odyssey* 1, Issue 3

Rayner, G (1996) Bureaucrats at your bedside *Health Matters*, **Issue 27**, 12–13

Robinson, J and Cassalino, L (1996) Vertical integration and organisational networks in healthcare *Health Affairs* **15**, 7–22

Robinson, R and Steiner, A (1998) *Managed Health Care: US Evidence and Lessons for the National Health Service* Open University Press, Buckingham

Shapiro, J, Smith, JA and Walsh, N (1996) *Approaches to Commissioning: the dynamics of diversity* NAHAT, Birmingham

Shaw, PA and Richards, JI 'Shifting The Boundaries: Partnerships in Total Healthcare' in Spiers, J (ed) (1997) Dilemmas in Modern Healthcare, Social Market Foundation, London

Smith, JA, Bamford, M, Ham, C, Scrivens, E and Shapiro, J (1997) *Beyond Fundholding: a mosaic of primary care led commissioning and provision in the West Midlands* HSMC, CHPM and West Midlands NHS Executive, Birmingham

Thatcher, M (1993) *The Downing Street Years* HarperCollins, London

9 Human Resource Management in the NHS – AD 2001

Hugh Flanagan

This chapter summarises a recent Delphi type survey on Human Resources (HR) in the NHS carried out by the author.

While in many ways there is less consistency of view about the structure, organisation and local detail of HR than previous similar surveys have indicated (Flanagan 1990, 1993), there are nevertheless a number of key issues or themes which keep re-occurring. These are encapsulated in the three key words of 'change', 'flexibility' and 'security'. Change, being the constant feature of the NHS work environment; flexibility, being the prime requirement in the management of human resources; and security, being the principal need of the NHS workforce.

The apparent diffusion of views about the detail of HR, how the function should be organised, and how it works in practice in different NHS Trusts is probably a reflection of the relative organisational fragmentation and the freedom of NHS Trusts over the last five or six years; though many people comment on the continuing degree of centralisation and central control in comparison to the Trust freedoms expected back in 1990.

The survey attempted to get people to step over some of the immediate and current debate around issues such as local pay and to take a medium to long term view by focusing on the year 2001. Though not that far ahead – think back four years – it still has a futuristic ring to it. The responses to the survey have been grouped into three sections which form the structure of the remainder of this chapter. First, a look at some of the emergent characteristics of the future NHS workforce, next, an exploration of the work environment in which this workforce will deliver health services, and finally looking at the overall HRM capability required by the NHS to manage and maintain the process of change.

What kind of workforce will be required to deliver health care in AD 2001?

There does appear to be a general consensus that the NHS workforce is and will increasingly be made up of three sets of staff, not dissimilar to

Handy's Shamrock model (Handy 1989) but with some slightly different features. The NHS Future Shamrock model (Figure 9.1) suggests that there will be three core groups of staff:

1　A core group of highly skilled and specialised staff built around the traditional professions of doctors, nurses and some of the professions supplementary to medicine/scientific professions groups.

2　A core group of clinical support workers to provide basic flexibility and which will be much more generic in the basis of their skills.

3　A management core group which will provide not only the basic management functions and administrative infrastructure, but will be the means through which non-core support services such a hotel services will be managed, along with a group of non-core clinical staff and a group of non-core management support services through a variety of agency/contract for service arrangements.

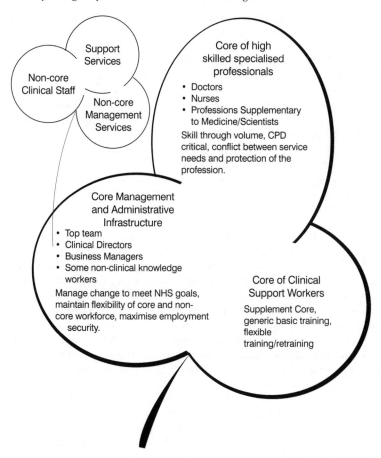

Figure 9.1　NHS future shamrock

There are a number of features surrounding the core clinical professions in the NHS on which there is some consensus, some of them paradoxical. First, that they will be required to undertake an increased volume of specialised work in order to build skills, as work in some areas becomes more complex and difficult, often due to the contribution of science and technology. At the same time, elements of work will also become more routine as they are developed and will be passed on to non-core clinical support workers. Second, because of the volume–skill factor there will in some respects be decreased flexibility between professions and between specialities within professions. At the same time certain technological developments, such as endoscopy and the provision of ward-based routine radiography services, will blur some of the demarcation lines between specialists both within and across professions, eg endoscopy between surgery and general medicine and the routine X rays taken on wards between nurses and radiographers.

At the same time there will be a continuing drive for flexible work patterns with flexible responses to changing service needs and for responses to the changes in services and facilities offered by science and technology. Core professionals will be required to work more flexibly to build up skills and to re-skill and be available across a greater variety of hours and shifts than previously. This will increasingly include senior medical staff. We will also see an increasing shift between work undertaken by doctors and that undertaken by nurse practitioners, particularly as their skill and training increases along with their confidence and their acceptability within the medical profession.

There is a strong view that service needs, costs and science and technology will be key drivers in forcing the NHS professions to act and train more flexibly. At the same time there is a view that the professional bodies may be faced with the dilemma of balancing the continuing employability through flexible skilling and reskilling of professional staff and protecting the borders of the profession.

Professional organisations must take account of the future employment prospects and therefore general employability of their members, but if they are too rigid in maintaining current boundaries based on current skill sets they may find other professions or support workers in professional/clinical areas step in to provide alternative means of meeting service needs. These paradoxical forces driving the current and future changes in the professions are not yet fully understood or fully worked out.

The increasing core of clinical support workers reflects the demand for more flexible support staff of a lower skill level than the core professionals who can adapt more readily to changes and developments. It seems increasingly likely that common core training may provide some of the inherent flexibility and that there will be less direct control of this area of training by professional bodies through increasing use of NVQs.

The core management role is also anticipated to become increasingly flexible, moving on to a 24-hour 365-day provision with generally increased flexibility in contracting arrangements, on call, weekend, night cover etc. Again, much of the driving force behind these changes will be the need to maximise the use of all health service facilities and services to meet the needs of the population and to increase the productivity and use of equipment and staff. Core management will centre around not only the top team/strategic direction and the provision of key management services, but will also include the business management of clinical and non-clinical services, possibly continuing to be based on a directorate type model. They will also manage the peripheral workforce, meet fluctuations in workload etc, and ensure the provision of non-clinical services. There will continue to be a need for high quality hotel services and these will increasingly be viewed as not part of the core of NHS business, along with some of the general management and support services required by the organisation: eg financial, pay services and some HR services such as recruitment and management of non core workforce.

The main purpose of the core management group will be to manage the process of change, maintain and increase flexibility in responding to needs and to maximise the long term employment security of the NHS workforce. The distinction between specific job security and general security of employment is increasingly being stressed.

A number of characteristics of workforce supply and demand were frequently identified. First, the overall numbers of staff servicing the NHS, by and large, remains constant. Clearly there have been some adjustments in terms of how people are employed; ie what form of contractual arrangements exist to provide the service and to engage the services of the staff required. The central argument is that, overall, the need of the NHS for a large number of highly skilled, semi-skilled and lower skilled staff does not radically change. There are redundancies in the NHS but, overall, they are not large-scale and more generally reflect changes in local patterns of employment and specific changes in methods of employment, eg contracting out. Mergers and reorganisations tend to affect the number of more senior staff required, but by and large have less impact on more junior staff and on professional staff.

There is a general view that restrictions in training input and resources of the last six or so years have led to a cut back in supply in some key professions, which has helped to fuel the growth in support staff (eg Health Care Assistants and NVQ based training and development for clinically oriented staff), both in order to increase flexibility and the speed with which gaps in the workforce can be plugged. Other features, such as the increasing attractiveness of working in the primary care arena as compared to secondary care, the rise of new professionals working in alternative therapies, and some decline in the use of bank staff in favour of external agency staff due to issues around accrual of employment rights, are all features that have been noted as significant, but which are not necessarily totally consistent across all NHS organisations. The centrality of the medicial and nursing profession remains, though many changes in the relative roles, remit and skills are noted.

Where there are major local changes, they are in job content and job structure linked to the organisation of work and services. Various forms of re-engineering and re-configuration of services in the organisation of work lead to new patterns of work and therefore new groupings of work-related tasks and new jobs which in turn often require new sets of skills. If there existed a higher level of flexibility in employment practices greater provision of (re)training, with increased ability and willingness on the part of the workforce to avail themselves of the re-training and re-deployment processes offered, then it should be possible to meet the underlying need for employment security in the NHS workforce. As a strategic aim this may have to be made much more explicit, in the sense that the current focus is still largely on job/grade/pay rate security.

There is a strong perception that staff are increasingly demanding an improved quality of life, which may in part be a reaction to the constant process of change and of itself is likely to contradict the need for increased flexibility. Most members of staff equate high quality of working life with stability and minimal change and, in particular, with predictability of income and work pattern. This is required in order to plan home and personal life. Perhaps some strategic rethinking, or clarification of existing thinking, around the need for flexibility both in employment practices and in work-force response, and the need to offer long term employment security to the workforce could provide the basic principles on which the framework of an NHS strategy for HRM could be built. This needs to be tackled if the capacity and readiness to change of the NHS workforce are to be enhanced.

The amount and frequency of change over the last 15 years could be said to have destabilised the NHS workforce to the extent that any form of change is now achievable, because there is minimal resistance. Staff and staff organisations find it difficult to get a firm footing in order to resist effectively. Staff feel insecure, even if the overall reality and evidence of employment prospects in the NHS belie this. Productivity is constantly increasing and there will continue to be cost pressures causing the search for different and better ways of providing services to continue. The effect will be to make staff feel less secure and probably less motivated if these overall workforce issues are not handled well. A negative effect could be for staff, through their trade union and professional organisations, to seek increasing collective protection in order to resist change.

On the whole, trade unions and professional bodies are probably feeling more confident and are now better organised than they were, and a protective response could have the effect of freezing the change process or at least bringing much more conflict into it. On the other hand, given that the NHS has overall become more used to change, this could be built on in a positive way laying the foundation for continuing long term change in the NHS. More effective management of change depends on enhanced communication of the need for change and the reasons for change, aimed at convincing the workforce that there is no sinister agenda and being open-handed enough to demonstrate the inherent truth of this approach. By underlining the inevitability of change and the reasons for it, by being more sensitive in management practices which facilitate change and ultimately by ensuring that HR policy is geared to trying to find ever better means of ensuring the long term employability of the NHS workforce, a strategic shift in the management of HR could be achieved. This is the central purpose of the core management infrastructure of the NHS.

Enabling frameworks for NHS workforce planning at national level, as with pay, seems to be a recurrent theme, possibly reflecting that on the whole NHS organisations have established a greater degree of local autonomy in the management of the workforce to reflect local needs and conditions. What is not clear is whether local variations in approach and emphasis always genuinely reflect local differences and needs, or whether in some cases they reflect inconsistency of skill, commitment and understanding by local managers. Examples are quoted of the differences in effectiveness and efficiency with which changes in the management of junior doctors' hours and the development and work of Training Consortia have been undertaken. Fundamentally there needs to be a clear national framework which will ensure adequate information and control of supply based on intelligent demand analysis. Clearly the professions and other staff organisations need to be involved in this process, but perhaps have less control over it.

Maintaining the employability of individuals in the NHS workforce needs to be a tripartite relationship incorporating the individual practitioners themselves, their employers (representing the needs of the work environment and the population served), and the regulating bodies that control the professions and their training. (Figure 9.2.)

What kind of environment will exist in 2001?

The term 'psychological contract' is often used to describe the set of expectations and assumptions, often implicit, which underpin and charac-

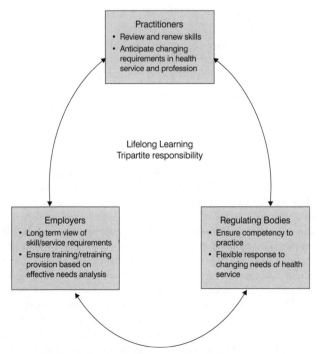

Figure 9.2 Maintaining individual employability

terise the employment relationship. The psychological contract that existed in the old NHS pre-1980 was pretty clear – 'the state as a good employer'. That which emerged during the 1980s and early 1990s also had particular characteristics but many uncertainties around the nature of employment in the NHS, (Fredman and Morris 1989). Staff are now probably becoming more demanding of management and mangers. They are less tolerant of poor management practice.

The National Audit report 'Finders Keepers' (Audit Commission 1997) indicated just how badly the NHS can treat staff and the impact of bad management practice in terms of reduced productivity and quality of service. An earlier NAO report drew attention to the wide variation in clinical productivity attributable to the effectiveness of people management (Audit Commission 1994). At the same time managers and management are less certain of their role and security of employment and as a group feel undervalued and unrecognised.

As the economy builds up and employment increases, a significant number of NHS staff may find options for employment elsewhere, even through second/third careers, which could add to the potential labour shortages created by earlier reductions in training.

There have been many local staff surveys in the NHS but there are certain common expectations on the part of staff which seem to emerge from these studies, eg:

- staff want the opportunity to use their skills;
- they want training and support in developing, maintaining and applying their skills;
- they want the support of management to manage the work environment and to help reduce the effect of various stressors resulting from rationing, funding and general change issues;
- there are some indications that staff are becoming less concerned about job security *per se* and are recognising the need to look at long term employment security.

These findings are echoed in other more general surveys (McHenry 1997).

Managers in the NHS are the key to managing the work environment effectively, but demotivated managers (Wall 1997) are less likely to be effective. Bad publicity and continual vilification in the press and regular bashing by politicians will not help build high morale and quality management practice in the NHS (Flanagan 1997). Staff are right to have a high expectation of management competence, but to ensure this we need to review and develop the nature of management and the managers in the service continually. We need to remove unnecessary management tasks both at local and national level by being clear about priorities, by looking at systems, by being serious about devolution and empowerment and we need to link this to a much more precise remit and clarity of job purpose for managers. The core of the manager's role should be based on enabling others to provide the services; in other words managing the environment of the NHS so that health and care services can be delivered by the right number of skilled professional staff, whether core or support, backed up by adequate support services. Real agreement on the purpose of the NHS, the priorities that can be met within the existing funding, and openness with the public about this would all help.

If managers are to manage the continuing changes in the NHS effectively they must be able to expect a reasonable degree of investment in their development. To ensure effective investment in management development there needs to be much more sophisticated and supportive appraisal and assessment processes for managers to avoid the natural tendencies of managers, as with clinical professionals, to work within their comfort zone (Parker 1995). Managers need to be more willing to change and to be much more flexible about when and where they work and how they manage. If we are expecting professional staff to think in terms of a 24-hour 365-day service to maximise utilisation of available resources, then managers have to think in those terms as well and reconfigure their own working arrangements to effect this.

Referring back to Figure 9.1, managers need to concentrate on managing the three core groups of the shamrock plus the three non-core. The key themes being flexibility, anticipation of changing needs and patterns of work and proactivity in managing the workforce and the work environment to avoid the trauma of sudden and reactive changes which could result in short term redundancies. There is obviously going to be a series of mergers within Health Authorities and Trusts over the coming few years. What is the best way of taking the pain out of these? Ensuring that top managers are given clear guidelines on their own position would enhance their leadership of the change process. Groups of chief executives and groups of directors and senior managers vying with each other for the jobs in the future organisation is unlikely to enhance their concern for maintaining quality of service during any change process and ensuring the employment security of professional and other staff in the organisations.

The theme of family friendly, flexible employment practices has been a fairly constant one over the last decade not only in the NHS but across many public and private sector organisations. Increased concern in terms of providing a healthy work environment is also linked to this and to the underlying theme of increasing and maintaining the quality of working life. Issues around term time working, annual hours, creches, paternity leave, career breaks, job design, ergonomics and the physical work environment, health facilities for staff and managing out unhealthy working practices have been the subject of a number of initiatives in the NHS and in other organisations.

The impact of Investors In People, Charter marks, Health at Work and similar initiatives, as a real investment in staff capability and security and long term quality of service provision, though often dismissed cynically, should not be underestimated. As always it is a question of how the acquisition of these 'badges' is approached, eg are staff involved, is there a real belief in and commitment by top management to the process, or are they just going through the checklist? Unfortunately, some of these processes also seem to carry unnecessarily bureaucratic external baggage. The problem in the NHS is that most of these activities are viewed as a cost rather than an investment in the workforce. There is a reluctance to be seen to be investing large sums of money in staff facilities, improving management practice and in the work environment, even though there is an increasing body of evidence which underlines the economic and business sense of making these types of long term investment in human capital provided they are all properly managed and remain clearly seen as a means to an end and not an end in themselves (Gratton 1997) . They require that the NHS operates within a long term timescale that is appropriate to people's development and maturation.

Employment contracts in recent years have seen an increasing variety of individual contracts and an increasing variety of contracting bodies, eg Statutory NHS Bodies, GP Practices, with and between groups of professionals etc. In many ways the employment contract is a more flexible and enabling document and is likely to become increasingly so, setting the parameters for managing and rewarding the work relationship. The differentiation between full time and part time employment is likely to become increasingly meaningless. Core professional knowledge workers are likely to be much more involved in negotiating their own individual contracts to suit their own circumstances. The issue of the work base is likely to become less fixed especially for the core staff who may work across a number of sites and centres of excellence providing a specialist service, possibly for more than one employer. Information technology will affect the nature of the working relationship in terms of where work is done. It will become increasingly important for the contract to define the terms surrounding fitness to practice on the part of the employee and defining the employer's commitment to maintaining long term employment security and the general employability of the staff member.

In terms of employee relations (ER) and the role of staff organisations, it seems to be generally felt that with some exceptions, Trust status has enhanced local employee relations and that local pay has in many cases also given a boost in the sense that local managers have taken more control of employee relations through more meaningful partnership with local representatives of staff organisations. A number of Trusts remark on the dichotomy between national and local perspectives on the part of trade union staff in their perspective on local ER. There are as many perspectives on ER and the impact of local pay as there are employing and staff side organisations. Not surprisingly, the staff side tend to have a less positive view of the impact of local pay (Thornley 1996). Research underlines the long-standing view that management get the ER they deserve and that their approach is largely value driven. Proactive managers managed local pay proactively and positively by often enhancing local ER (Corby and Higham 1996). A key finding emerging from many studies and documents on 'pay' is that it must be located in a broader Reward/HR strategy related to the NHS agenda and not as an isolated facet of HRM locally negotiated but centrally controlled (Black Country Personnel Consortium 1997).

What HRM capability will be required?

Given the future changes in the workforce and the work environment identified as emergent or required, the inevitable question is does the National Health Service have the HRM capability to deliver? When talking of the HRM capability of NHS management, it is line managers plus specialist HR departments that are being addressed.

Responses on HRM capability in the survey can be clustered around four basic issues:

1 The performance management/added value of HRM.

2 The HRM infrastructure and models of delivery.

3 Uncertainty about the nature of HRM, particularly the concept of strategic HRM.

4 The need for a strategic policy framework for HRM in the Health Service.

These are not discrete issues, and discussion of one weaves in and out of the others, but for the sake of discussion the responses have been grouped in this way.

There is currently a lot of concern about what whether HRM, and in particular specialist HRM departments, are 'delivering'. This has always been a concern not just in the NHS, because HRM inevitably has a large software component as well as 'technical' hardware. There are various discussions of what we mean by 'hard' and 'soft' HRM. But much of HRM is about the less tangible issues of process, behaviour, motivation, values, etc. The natural orientation of many managers, including HRM specialists, is to see and to conceive of HRM as a task-based activity, partly because some managers feel uncomfortable with process/software issues and partly because this gives a (spurious?) credibility to HRM in terms of contributing to 'the bottom line'.

Many of the concerns about delivery and about adding value led on to the need for 'bench marking' in HRM. Bench marking as an idea has been around for sometime and has probably been talked about and acted upon within HR departments over recent years, but it is currently receiving an additional amount of publicity in clinical as well as management services in the NHS. It is an internationally known method of judging effectiveness and is international in its application to HR (Hiltrop and Despres 1994). The only danger is a tendency to focus on function process and outcome measures which may not be related to stategic organisational goals.

Concerns about the effectiveness of HR centre on:

1 The effectiveness of senior HR staff, particularly directors.

2 Policies and practices.

3 The quality of line management expertise.

Effectiveness in management is often a subjective concept based on implicit criteria and mental models (Flanagan and Spurgeon 1996). Work is needed to bring out and clarify the criteria people actually use to make judgments about effectiveness.

A lot of work has been done both within and outside the NHS over the last decade or so to address this issue (Tyson and Fell 1986, Collins 1991, 1992, Guest and Peccei 1992). Much of this work has been concerned with the need to make HRM activity relevant to the goals of the organisations. A recent survey by the NHS Confederation (NHS Confederation 1997) underlines this aim – 73 per cent of the 361 responses to a pay and reward survey said the most important point was that HRM strategy should support overall service objectives. What appears to be less clear is how this can be achieved in practice.

No doubt part of the problem continues to be the relative lack of certainty and long term focus on key policy goals and priorities in the NHS. HR strategy is usually about changing patterns of work, skill and behaviour on the part of the workforce which require timescales of 5 years plus, backed by sustained effort. Political timescales are much shorter.

Additionally, there is a sensitivity in the NHS about being seen to be putting too much resource into the development of effective managers or management processes. The level of development activity for senior HR staff appears to have dropped off, compared to the early 1990s.

It seems that the NHS is going to look again at effectiveness in HRM. This could result in the development of a set of national criteria for monitoring and managing HRM performance. Existing and known measures, such as unit labour costs, absenteeism/sickness, turnover and staff survey results could be adopted. But how would they aid the fulfillment of the three strategic aims suggested (Figure 9.3)? Some work would have to be done to identify the three or four criteria critical to each of the strategic goals of change capability, workforce flexibility and employment security. What is measured is what gets done. If it is possible to develop a national set of criteria, and they are taken seriously, then they would become a focus for action in developing/increasing the capability of the HRM function to lead and deliver against the criteria. In order not to lead to a lot of misplaced or even harmful activity they will need to be developed carefully, so that what is measured is what matters.

The discussion around the infrastructure supporting the delivery of HRM in Health Service organisations underlines the fact that there is really no common model. The balance between line and staff involvement varies from one organisation to another with varying degrees of centrality. Much reference is currently made to the 'GP' consultancy model within organisations whereby the central generalist department is based on very low staffing levels, with a clear responsibility for the day to day management of the organisation's human resources resting with line managers. The strategic direction, OD and Change Management aspects of HRM are managed centrally through the director, but often involving the use of external consultants.

At the other end of the spectrum there are centralised departments undertaking many activities on behalf of line managers. Sometimes this

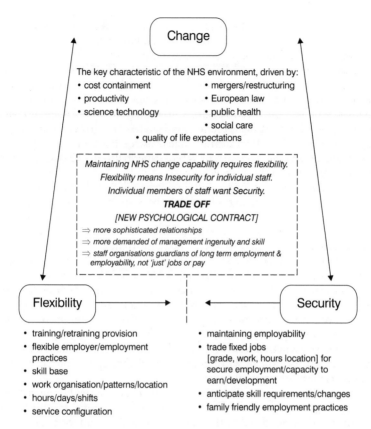

Figure 9.3 The key drivers and goals of HR strategy in the 21st century

stems from a view about economies of scale, the capacity and skills of line managers or history. There is no obvious correlation between apparent effectiveness of the HRM function and a particular model.

There is an increasing sense that there is a risk management aspect to effective HRM in terms of removing, or at least reducing to an acceptable level, risks to the organisation that might arise from litigation, disruption and conflict, poor employee relations imbalance in supply and demand within the workforce, skill in patient communication etc. Views about how this is best achieved may dictate decisions about who handles many of the routine aspects of HRM, including training. Putting critical, but routine tasks in a central department which has expertise, and therefore becomes more expert, is a way of reducing risk.

Technology is used to both centralise and decentralise some basic HRM functions such as recruitment and workforce information. The rationale behind local decisions on technology-based infrastructure can be a function of the preference of the director, the willingness/unwillingness of line managers to operate IT-based systems or, as before, unchallenged history.

Perhaps rather surprisingly, a number of senior HR people raised fundamental questions as to what HRM really is and in particular what Strategic
Human Resource Management is. This perhaps relates back to the first
point about concern over delivery and outcomes in HR and the balance
between the hard and soft aspects and the inherent uncertainty about NHS
priorities which results in a task based approach to managing. It is difficult
to be strategic without addressing organisational software issues and without taking a long term perspective that matches the growth and learning
timescales required to effect fundamental changes in workforce and configuration and behaviour. The current White Paper talks of a 10 year time scale
which makes sense in this respect.

There is clearly a grouping around those who take a task based view of the
HRM agenda and those who take a more process-orientated view. In general
terms, task-based activity without effective process is likely to have little substantial result, whereas heavily concentrating on process without identifying
clear task outcomes is likely to be of little value to the organisation.

It is almost engaging when some of the most senior and able HR directors
in the NHS come clean in this respect, some would say it is worrying. But
HRM is the most complex aspect of management in organisations, the least
understood and therefore the most difficult. Therefore, those who say they
are not sure are probably the most honest. Concentrating on the techniques
and tasks of management makes it easier to handle, but we may be kidding
ourselves about whether we are really making a difference. Much of the current debate (at the time of writing) about NHS strategy reflects task based
thinking rather than strategic thinking.

There appears to be a general consensus that there should be an enabling
strategic framework in HRM for the whole of the National Health Service
and that for these involved in this survey, the policy framework should be
based on the three key issues of change, flexibility and security identified at
the beginning of this chapter (Figure 9.3).

The national strategy framework should enable and not prescribe,
should concentrate on policy outcomes and results and should be monitored in terms of the effectiveness of local delivery of the policy outcomes. Within the latter point there should also be some focus on and
monitoring of the effectiveness with which outcomes are delivered, ie
effective process.

Many practitioners now feel that the NHS has become much better at
managing change. At local level the technical aspects of managing change
are often extremely well handled. However, there is a feeling that some of
the foundations of HRM, such as concern for the welfare of staff, have
been rather overlooked. This is not to suggest a return to the traditional
welfare model, but to achieve a better balance in terms of managing change
effectively both in human as well as in resource terms.

References

Audit Commission (1997) *Finders Keepers* Audit Commission/HMSO,
    London

Audit Commission (1994) *Trusting in the future, Towards an Audit Agenda for NHS Providers* Audit Commission/HMSO, London

Black Country Personnel Consortium (1997) *A Revised Approach to NHSPay* Report prepared by the consortium

Collins, M (1991) *Human Resource Managemeent Audit* North Western & West Midlands RHAs

Collins, M (1992) *Evaluating the Personnel Department* West Midlands RHA

Corby, S and Higham, D (1996) Decentralisation of Pay in the NHS: diagnosis and prognosis *Human Resource Management Journal.* **6,** No. 1

Flanagan, H (1990) *Managing the human resources of the NHS in the 1990s* In the changing face of the NHS Spurgeon, P (ed.) Longman, Harlow

Flanagan, H (1993) Managing the human resources of the NHS in the 1990s In *The new face of the NHS* Spurgeon, P (ed.) Longmans, Harlow

Flanagan, H (1997) What chance a caring management culture *Health Manpower Management* **23,** No. 5

Flanagan, H, and Spurgeon, P (1996) *Managerial effectiveness in the public sector* Open University Press, Milton Keynes

Fredman, S, and Morris, C (1989) The state as employer: setting a new example *Personnel Management,* August 1989

Gratton, L (1997) Tomorrow people. *People Management* **3,** No. 15 (from: *Human resource strategies in transforming companies,* to be published by Oxford University Press 1998)

Guest, D, and Peccei, R (1992) Measuring effectiveness in NHS personnel *Health Manpower Management* **18,** No. 4

Handy, C (1989). *The age of unreason* Century Hutchinson, London

Hendry, C, and Jenkins, R (1997) Psychological contracts & new deals, *Human Resource Management Journal* **7,** No. 1

Hiltrop, M, and Despres, C (1994) Assessing the performance of human resource management *Journal of Strategic Change* **3,** 113–142

McHenry, R (1997) Spurring stuff *People Management* **3,** No. 15

NHS Confederation (1997) *Pay & reward systems in the NHS – survey* Summary paper circulated to members

Parker, D (1995). Privatisation and the Internal Environment: Developing Our Knowledge of the Adjustment Process *International Journal of Public Sector Management* **8,** 49

Patterson, M, Malcolm, G, West, M, Michael, A, Lawthorn, R, and Nickell, S (1997) *Impact of People Management Practices on Business Performance* IPD, London

Thornley, C (1996) Poor Principals: the realities of local pay determination in the NHS. *Pay Review Body Report* Unison, London

Tyson, S, and Fell, A (1986) *Evaluating the Personnel Function* Hutchinson, London

Wall, A (1997) Motive Power: What Motivates Managers. *Health Service Journal* 24 April 1997

10 Developing managers for the late 1990s

David Thompson

Managers and development

One of the first actions of the incoming Labour Government in May 1997 was to fix a target for NHS management cost reduction of £100 million, which could then be available for frontline patient care. Health secretary, Frank Dobson, was quoted as announcing:

> Health Authorities, health boards and trusts in England, Scotland and Wales must save GBP80 million on management in 1997–1998, although this does include GBP46 million already identified. A further GBP20 million of management cost is to be saved by deferring for a year the next [eighth] wave of GP Fundholding.
>
> (Limb and Chadda, 1997)

The Institute of Health Services Management deplored the Government's 'knee-jerk targeting of management'. The NHS Confederation claimed that cuts in bureaucracy 'must not be made at the cost of high quality managers' *(ibid)*.

There was concern that the cuts would aggravate the impact of the proposed abolition of the internal health market in the UK under Government plans and lead to a wave of Trust mergers and job losses.

These political proposals have enormous implications for NHS managers and their development. They can be seen to illustrate the central theme of this chapter: that the challenge of developing managers for the NHS is posed by the pressures on, and the changing nature of, NHS management itself. While management development can, and should, influence management, it will only be successful if it responds to the present state of management.

This vital factor was first recognised by the policy makers of the 1980s:

> If management is clear and confident about its purpose and tasks, the climate for management development is favourable. If management is confused or harassed, tired or demoralised, management development is an uphill task.
>
> (Williams 1988)

In this context, management development can be seen to be any learning experience undergone by those holding managerial roles in an organisation. Such experience may be a highly visible educational programme, with recognised qualifications although no specific organisational outcome; it may be a training event focused on particular skills and understanding; it may be an almost unrecognisable flash of insight at the workplace, prompted consciously or unconsciously by others. It is beneficial to share this perception that learning is at the heart of development because, even after three decades of activities in the NHS, development is still associated by many managers with 'going on courses'. There is much more to it than that.

If development is the heart, the managerial organisation forms the skeleton. As the NHS approaches the end of the 1990s, its organisation can be seen to be facing a 'fourth wave' of change. The first wave occurred after 1974, when a comprehensive change established an integrated structure within which the service could be efficiently administered. The intention was that managers should provide a positive and supportive climate for professionals to deliver health care. This traditional view has been summed up as follows:

> *The efficient control of expenditure is the cardinal management virtue. Those who pursue this approach tend to be relatively unconcerned with changes in the social and economic environment. They will implement policies but take few initiatives themselves. Their view of management rests on values and priorities within the Service.*

> (NHS Training Authority 1986)

The Griffiths report published in 1983 heralded the onset of the second wave. This was characterised by the assertion that management is concerned with:

> *levels of service, quality of product, meeting budgets, cost improvements, productivity, motivation and rewarding staff, research and development, and the long term viability of the undertaking.*

> (DHSS 1983)

Griffiths found that the absence of 'general management support' meant that there was no driving force 'seeking and accepting direct and personal responsibility for developing plans, securing implementation and monitoring actual achievement'. This constituted an altogether more active management, which had to concern itself with professional matters.

These two waves were not, of course, neatly divided in time. The general management approach of the second wave was recognised and practised by some managers some time before the appearance of the Griffiths recommendations, especially after the structural 'tidying up' of 1982.

The flood tide of the third wave has now surged through the NHS as we approach the end of the 1990s. It is now possible to evaluate its main features and to identify the implications for the development of managers, which are likely to remain current until the full force of a possible fourth wave is felt from the new Labour Government.

A revolutionary decade?

Arguably, the most crucial event for the NHS in the 1990s was the re-election of the Conservative Government in April 1992. It seems unlikely that the election of the Labour Government in May 1997 will result in such momentum for change. The result of the earlier election confirmed that the reforms proposed in the White Paper *Working for Patients* would continue to be implemented (DoH 1989). NHS managers who had nailed their colours firmly to the fence before the general election now had to plan changes within a framework whose main features were known. This news was good in so far as it reduced some of the political uncertainty surrounding the early 1990s. Further good news came from the Government's anxiety to minimise disruption by ensuring a steady state and a smooth lift off in the early part of the implementation period. This gave some time to prepare an infrastructure. News which was less unqualifiably good was the lack of detail about important aspects of the proposed changes. This constituted an opportunity for energetic managers to create their own response to the proposed internal market while at the same time posing problems, as policy makers and managers at all levels made their, sometimes contradictory, contributions to the debate.

During the decade there has been experiment with real change at all levels of the NHS. National politicians and policy makers have at last grappled with the problems of London's health care provision and world class medical centres. In fundholding practices throughout the land general practitioners (GPs) delivered measurably better services to their patients. In between, NHS managers indulged in the game of managerial musical chairs which has been played during the restructuring of the 1970s and 1980s. The difference third time round was that when the music stopped, there were fewer chairs for them to sit on. One of the growing and worrying features of the decade has been the damaging loss of senior managerial talent, as these managers failed to convince their chairmen or chairwomen that they were performing adequately; or they just lost heart and turned their talent to other fields.

With the advent of the new Labour Government in May 1997, the nagging doubt was heard more loudly that all the turmoil and change had not added up to the promised revolution. There have been signs that the internal market has been working, albeit in the crude way of all markets: senior managers and medical staff in many big city hospitals have been coping with a dramatic shift in their traditional markets. But in retrospect, this can be seen as shifting the deckchairs on the secondary and tertiary decks of the NHS liner. Nearer the waterline, on the primary care deck, there are fewer signs of substantial change. Enterprising GP Fundholders have led the way, but their existence has remained controversial, not least because of widespread dislike of signs of a 'two-tier' service. They have always been inhibited financially and managerially by the traditional forces of 'accountability'.

What follows, then, should be read with the caution that the third wave has not carried us on its crest to the end of the millennium. It is about to be overtaken by a fourth wave whose firm features are not yet clear. The new

Government has yet to make specific proposals, but two aspects are emerging: as has been noted above, one is the early attack on NHS managers themselves, under the guise of 'bureaucrat-bashing' and complaints about 'red-tape'; the other is the commitment to make structural changes by abolishing the internal health market, including GP Fundholding, to be replaced by 'local commissioning'. Notwithstanding this caution, the third wave of change has altered the face of the NHS management and management development in many ways. Six of the most significant are now discussed.

Provider development

The most striking feature of NHS management in the 1990s was the introduction of the purchaser–provider split which took effect in April 1991. This constituted yet another attempt, following on those in 1974, 1982 and 1985, to delegate decision-making downwards. Previous efforts had always foundered on central insistence on 'accountability upwards', which effectively throttled any real autonomy. This time round there were signs of greater success.

An increase in local autonomy has come from the mechanism of the NHS Trust which could be established by any hospital or hospitals or community services previously directly managed by a District Health Authority. After an uneasy couple of years, all NHS units became Trusts by April 1995. There was a gestation period, unusually long even by NHS rates of change, because of the uncertainties of national politics and of the need to prove financial and business viability.

The fog covering this 'provider' landscape eventually cleared, and some of the challenges for developing managers in the rest of the 1990s became evident. Much remained the same as in the old days of 'management development' in the 1970s and 1980s. Hospitals did not change overnight in April 1991: they still consumed great quantities of capital and revenue; they continued to employ the majority of NHS staff and to have a voracious appetite for supplies and information. They still required traditional skills of financial, human and information management: salaries and wages had to be paid and accounted for; patients had to be discharged and categorised. The skills to accomplish these important tasks – the life blood of the institutions – had to be maintained and managers had still to be developed to manage them.

These and additional competencies, however, were soon seen to inhabit the valleys of the provider landscape. The high ground looked very different. It was not now a world of management in the old hierarchical sense, of a chain of command stretching from the ward sister and charge nurse to the Secretary of State. It was a world of the internal market. To be sure, this was not a market that the purists like Kotler would recognise: it was not composed of two equal parties who are willing and able to trade something of value to each party (Kotler 1988). Le Grand has described it as a quasi-market, but a market nonetheless, in which consumers tended to be represented by agents and competition was not always between equals (Le Grand 1990).

Even the quasi-market has been slow and hesitant to arrive on the NHS scene. It has been prevented from operating by the political imperatives of public expenditure control and fierce 'provider' and community lobbying. But the impact has undoubtedly constituted the most important challenge to developing managers in this decade. It has demanded a whole new mind map for managers to navigate over the new landscape. They have had to be able to cope with a more fragmented world and one which recognised that the business of the NHS was now a business. The language of business was foreign to NHS managers at the beginning of the decade, but now it has percolated through even to many professionals who were accustomed to viewing their job as providing patient care to exact scientific standards with little attention to cost.

The language of business embraced the fact that NHS trusts have had to operate in a fragmented NHS market, albeit with national and regional regulation. The focal point has become the business plan, which has demanded a consciousness of costs which transcended previous drives for value for money. At the same time, the trend towards the emphasis on quality has been absorbed into the business planning process. This must be an improvement on professional paternalism and the legacy of postwar austerity welfarism but, again, there has remained the feeling that there is some way to go before the drive to improve quality becomes internalised within managers. All too often it has arisen from a response to external stimulus, such as the Patient's Charter. The quality assurance 'movement' in some ways has revealed, and in other ways obscured, a greater awareness of the consumer – the patients, relatives and public of yesteryear. There have been some strides towards a better deal for the consumer: shorter waiting lists and waiting time, better physical surroundings. But there have remained severe conceptual and practical difficulties. The consumer has been seen to be both the payer – purchaser – and the user – the patient – and the interests of these parties have often not been identical. Indeed, they have often not been known, because providers have been accustomed to provide what provider professions deemed appropriate, and they have had only a rudimentary idea of what their users needed, wanted and demanded.

The market and its language has shown how a new reality in the outer world had to become internalised into a new mind set. Old ways of thinking were clearly not sufficient: beds and budgets no longer mattered; gaining the competitive edge was becoming all-important. This has not been comfortable for managers developed in the old, pre-1990s NHS. Without mental adjustment, they have found it difficult to absorb and use the related skills of market research and definition, negotiating and contracting.

The language of the market is now better understood. Ironically, it may soon be necessary to learn a revised language which reflects the values of the new Government. The task of developing managers to interpret and implement what this stands for will be formidable. This constitutes the agenda for the remainder of the decade and beyond. Harrison and his colleagues pointed out that the process of altering the mindset once is a development skill in itself; one that may be employed again in a further alteration to adapt to an ever-changing world. (Harrison *et al.* 1994).

A further challenge for managers has been converging and may come to dominate the final years of the decade. This will be the way in which the people – the NHS employees – are managed. The market has brought a cultural revolution which profoundly affected chief executives and their directorial teams (for the most part). It impacted on professional practice. But the effect on managers in the middle and the staffs they have traditionally managed has not always been fully appreciated. Some outline features are clear:

- The business drive has predominated: people have taken second place to the preservation of the business. Tough decisions have been taken on 'downsizing' ie making people redundant.

- The middle manager has become an endangered species, in the NHS as in other large organisations such as banks. Hierarchies have been 'flattened' with fewer links on the chain of command. For some, this has empowered those at the bottom; for others it has increased the workload and strain.

- In spite of, or because of, the ill-fated struggle to institute local bargaining, employment conditions have become less secure and more individualised. There has been less protection available from national terms and conditions from the collective actions of the trade unions and professional associations. Again, for some, a greater individualism and insecurity has struck terror into their hearts; for others, there has been a great sense of liberation and the opening up of opportunity after a stifling regulation.

These trends, from top to bottom of the organisation, suggest that new ways of managing people must be found and managers developed to cope with them. The NHS is already beginning to conform to Handy's 'shamrock' of organisation – a tripartite structure consisting of core full time workers, part-time, temporary workers and contract workers (Handy 1989). Each segment requires a different management approach. Flexibility is being demanded from the workforce: flexibility will be necessary in managing its various parts. The 'people' item will rise up the business planning agenda in the remainder of the decade as managers learn how to take more seriously the development of their greatest asset. One of the first steps of the Labour Government was to reverse the painful drive towards local bargaining; this may be a symbol that it recognised the rock-bottom morale of many NHS managers and staff.

Purchaser development

As the reforms of the early 1990s were implemented, it became apparent that the purchaser function was potentially the most innovative aspect of management in the reformed NHS. Much effort went into understanding it and constructing a whole new management infrastructure. It was from this work that a whole new syllabus for developing managerial skills emerged.

As a result of work commissioned by the then NHE Management Executive, the hallmarks of what made an effective purchaser were established. These included: a strategic approach; being open and accessible to the public; assessing health need more systematically; obtaining professional advice; involving GPs; working with other agencies; using contracts more effectively; having a mature relationship with providers; building structures and skills (Ham *et al.* 1993a). Perhaps, sadly, it could be recognised that this agenda was just what senior NHS managers should have been addressing since 1948, or at least since 1974. And indeed, they have given some attention to them. But the reforms have brought a fresh emphasis and intensity.

As is usual with NHS reorganisation, much energy initially went into new structures, as senior managers secured their personal positions. This provided an important foundation for approaching new tasks. An interesting variety of management infrastructures appeared around the country, often reflecting the character of the original, now defunct, regions, from the formalised orderliness of Wessex to the eclecticism of the West Midlands.

This is an area where organisation development and traditional management development blur. Structures tended to evolve from the existing pattern, but the new purchasing authorities were a new kind of institution, where functions roles and competencies had to be understood before new structures were cemented in place. They were small but powerful, in an NHS more used to equating size with power – size of budget, staff and premises. Purchasing staff have been characterised by being few in number, but more highly specialised and senior in proportion to provider staffing.

Organisational development in the broad sense has had to be matched by the acquisition of key managerial skills. The process of developing purchasing skills is likely to continue for a number of years, as the function evolves into, or is replaced by, the local commissioning bodies proposed by the Labour Government. A range of these skills may now be reviewed.

It was rapidly recognised among purchasers that they must be able to assess health need. This has largely become the province of public health medicine specialists, whose annual reports have supplied the building bricks for the purchasing plan. But it also became clear that there was a history of neglect in this area, and that more expertise was required to impact on the material. Existing specialists have often been hard pressed to produce more than a good demographic and epidemiological survey and an analysis of a selected number of conditions or services, such as coronary heart disease or diabetes.

Second, the acquisition of such hard information has had to be matched by the search for softer intelligence. The challenge here has been to seek the views of the (tax-paying) public, who were largely ignored for 45 years. It has been pleasing to see a variety of methods attempted around the country: surveys in-house and by polling firms, public meetings, telephone interviews etc. Managers and their advisors have developed the skills of direct contact quite rapidly where there was a will. But there remained a feeling of dabbling daringly in dangerous waters. Expectations could easily be aroused which had no hope of being met. Worse, the public sometimes expressed preferences which did not conform to professional priorities, such as the closure of long stay hospitals and the opening of sheltered accommodation. There remain problems for managers in handling such issues with confidence and credibility. However, soft intelligence has undoubtedly enriched the purchasing plan: for example, it has revealed whether the public has been prepared to travel further to reduce the waiting time for treatment.

A third skill area has embraced the process of establishing a strategic vision, setting priorities and contracting with providers. These have required both creative and analytical intellectual efforts and a tactical capability. The purchasing plan must be coherent and credible to a greater extent than has been demanded before from senior NHS managers. The capabilities required for producing were discovered by purchasers learning by doing. They were not clearly envisaged in the original White Paper formulation, which saw only as far as the contracting element. It was an area where best practice needed to be captured and disseminated to other purchasers. The NHS has never been markedly good at learning from its own demonstrations, but there was an urgency about this element of purchasing which demanded an unprecedented opening of minds to what was discovered elsewhere.

The final aspect of developing purchasing management has been arguably the most crucial. It is on the purchasers that the burden of creating real change has fallen. The challenge has been to make a real shift in the historical pattern of dominance of professionally driven, high technology secondary and tertiary care, which swallows the lion's share of resources to treat a minority of patients. Purchasing managers have contemplated the task of managing change on a scale not seen before. There has been some interesting work on altering the balance of care within specialties or care groups, eg putting more resources into preventing stroke and less into 'curing' it. The detail of service contracts has enforced this pattern, where soundly monitored. The real challenge has come with proposals for a more fundamental shift in the pattern of care from secondary to primary. The London health care scene has been the cauldron for this debate, following the publication of the Tomlinson Report in November 1992 and the Government's calculated response in the face of fierce opposition from the elite medical institutions. This debate has been repeated in microcosm throughout the NHS.

The new twist in the tail of purchaser development comes, of course, from the commitments of the incoming Government. It has confirmed that the purchaser–provider split will remain but become 'less competitive'. Contracting will be replaced by 'three to five year agreements'. The 'costly' internal market will be scrapped, but there will be no return to

'top-down management'. It seems likely that the skills developed by purchasers will be put to good use in the new locally planned and commissioned NHS.

Involving doctors in management

The continuing saga of attempts to involve clinicians in management is a
refrain reverberating through both provider and purchaser development.
Overt attempts to involve clinicians date back at least to the Cogwheel
Reports of 1967–1969. It was a central plank of the Griffiths recommendation of 1983 and the evidence suggests that success was only fitful and
scattered (Hunter and Williamson 1989). It remains the greatest challenge
facing management developers – and others, of course – in the late 1990s,
and as such will be examined in more detail here.

The case for clinicians' involvement has been rehearsed many times and
is taken as already established. The fundamental problem appears to lie in
the balance of power within the NHS as an organisation. Clinicians have
been accustomed to having prime influence over the deployment of
resources and to enjoying considerable freedom to pursue their professional activities. As agents of Government, managers have been gradually
given more 'structural' power to control the 'expert' power of the professional. Among wise men and women, there is a respect for the contribution of clinicians and managers. Among the unlucky and foolish, there is
the potential for damaging conflict.

The question of the balance of power will be debated and decided ultimately at a political level. For managers, the issue manifested itself initially
at a more procedural level, revolving around resource management. This
issue was the subject of the previous chapter and will not be discussed
here, except to identify implications for the management development.

These turn, in part, on a conceptual question: who are the managers? To
what extent are the managers those with an identifiable managerial
responsibility, such as general managers, senior managers and indeed clinical directors? Or are they all those who 'manage' resources, which must
include all senior clinicians. It would seem only prudent and realistic to
adopt the wider definition, otherwise the management developer risks
ignoring substantial numbers of powerful people who 'make things happen' in health care. The management developer must now contemplate
two powerful groups of clinicians in management. One is familiar, the
other rather newer.

The familiar group – a rose by any other name – consists of clinical
directors. These have now assumed the traditional burden of the senior
hospital doctor in management. As officially envisaged, they emerged as
powerful managerial functionaries: line managers, deployers of a wide
range of medical, nursing and supporting resources, purchasers of other
services, able to influence policy. A national survey of 702 directors in
1996 found that they have experienced difficulties in living up to these
managerial expectations while maintaining a considerable clinical practice.

The time they can devote is strictly limited: usually two sessions a week and as much spare time as they can stand. In the survey, most directors reported that they were spending double the contracted hours on management tasks (Simpson and Scott 1996). The result for many has been a disillusionment and compromise. Some have been shifted *de facto* or even *de jure* from line responsibility which is assumed by their business manager and sometimes their senior nurse: their title becomes 'clinical co-ordinator'. Many have not been able to establish managerial authority over their clinical colleagues; some have given up even trying.

In spite of considerable national and local effort devoted to developing them as managers, the directors have usually not enjoyed much development beyond basic skills for these demanding managerial roles. The national survey found that 61 per cent had received some training, which they judged to be of value. However, most development lasted only one or two days. Directors reported that they would welcome more advanced training in handling complex changes and in dealing with difficult colleagues *(ibid)*.

As in all aspects of an organisation as big as the NHS, good practice can be found: there are many examples of successful clinical directors. But there are too many NHS Trusts which did not implement the approach soundly. The result has been a hole at the centre of the management structure: a discontinuity between higher management and service deliverers. This suggests a massive need for organisational and manager development. Structures need to be kept under review and made credible; managers, including clinical directors, require continuing opportunities for individual and team development. All too often both types of development have been squeezed by day to day priorities and crises. Elsewhere, Thompson has reviewed the research evidence and drawn a balance between development for directors on a uni-professional basis and multi-professional development for them (Thompson 1994).

Many NHS Trust chief executives have reported a tension with their clinical directors, a lack of support in achieving the business plan. Many clinical directors complain of being kept in the dark, of being denied in practice what freedoms they were initially promised. This lack of mutual confidence, sufficiently widespread, has been a major problem of development.

The second group of clinicians who entered the wider management arena were the GP Fundholders. They constituted arguably the most exciting newcomers to arise from the purchaser–provider split. They have been worthy of attention from management developers, because it is from them that many have hoped for real change: the aggregate of many small improvements which GP funds may purchase. Like gravel thrown into a pond, the ripples of many small purchasing decisions would not create a big wave, but would none the less lap on many shores. It has been seen how an active and well-organised GP Fundholding practice with real money to spend can force new responsiveness on their local provider hospitals. The doors of once supercilious consultants have been opened. It can also create a stir in the traditional NHS bureaucracies, not yet wedded to the entrepreneurial culture. Officials at regional offices, at district purchasing, have cried 'accountability' and argued for greater integration of fundholders in 'strategic' purchasing plans. This is logical and reasonable. But it was George Bernard Shaw who said in 1910 that 'all progress depends on the unreasonable man'.

Each fundholding practice can give examples of real health gain for individual patients which could not have been secured without the availability of real and ready money. The impression given by a brief survey of first wave fund holders (Ham *et al.* 1993b) suggested that they were among the most able and organised of GP practices: close to their patients, up to date with best clinical practice, on top of their information requirements, and well financed. They held many lessons for management developers faced with later waves of fundholders, or even non-fundholders, whose development needs were seen to be greater.

In 1997, fundholders constitute 56 per cent of all GPs; as was noted above, an eighth wave has been delayed until 1998; budgets will be reined in under new guidelines issued in mid-1997. At this time, it is not confirmed by the Government whether it will go ahead and replace GP Fundholding with GP Commissioning, which is intended to adopt a wider perspective and embrace the development of all services for a local population, not just to focus on the purchase of secondary care.

As in the case of district purchasers, GP Fundholders have now become involved with the planning and purchasing of services. It seems equally likely that the skills and experience will be transferable to GP Commissioning. But more may be required, if pioneering experience in Birmingham and elsewhere is an indicator: there are more complex funding mechanisms and a greater range of options to challenge even the best of GPs.

The infrastructure issue

In the world of purchasers and providers, which has dominated the 1990s, there have clearly been several great development tasks to be addressed. What are the implications for management development infrastructure and roles? The first edition of this book noted the tensions inherent in the balance between centralised and localised infrastructure. Since the early days of management development in the NHS, in the 1960s, there were always valuable initiatives at the centre and in localities. Activities were, as always in NHS management, varied as to geographical spread and personal commitment but, in the main, there was a clear division local effort for local benefit, and central sponsorship for the general good. For example, university-level NHS National Education Centres offered general development programmes at middle and senior levels for which any suitable manager could be nominated. Junior and first line managers tended to be provided for locally by Health Authority specialists and/or local colleges.

The advent of the NHS Training Authority in 1985 gave a great boost to management development nationally. The publication of *Better Management, Better Health* (BM,BH) in 1986 was an occasion of great significance. It constituted the first comprehensive review of management development since the mid-1970s, and was the first time that management development requirements were discussed nationally in the context of an explicit notion of 'management'. The major achievements of BM,BH were to move 'development' closer to the central concerns of 'management', and away from the province of the management development specialist. This was asserted in its definition of management development as: *'any influence or experience that helps to improve management effectiveness'* (*NHS Training Authority 1986*).

Additionally, each Health Authority had to identify a local person with responsibility for implementing management development strategies. Stimulated by this policy initiative and other favourable encouragement, there was an apparent upsurge in development activity. New programmes were launched nationally: Individual Performance Review, National Accelerated Development Programme etc. The enduring problem of preparing clinicians to participate in management was tackled. It was estimated that more than half of the 200 Health Authorities in England and Wales designated a responsible officer, and that there was a greater volume and variety of activity than ever before: traditional courses were supplemented by a new range of imaginative options, to which more managers than ever before had access (Thompson and Edmonstone 1988).

However, there was a serious contradiction in the Training Authority's approach. In keeping with the emerging philosophy of the NHS, there was a concern to obtain better value for money by encouraging a 'market' among management development suppliers. From September 1987, the traditional 'block grants' to a cartel of National Education Centres was withdrawn and the market was thrown open to any suppliers to compete for contracts. At national level, the Training Authority could thus ensure that its contracts were led to suppliers who would work to tightly drawn specifications. Locally, Health Authorities were encouraged to buy what specialist management development they felt fitted their needs, and to meet the full cost of their requirements. Programmes would wither away if they did not command sufficient local support.

The essential contradiction lay in the incompatibilities of 'command' policies and 'market' practice. Nationally-endorsed policies suggest a need for consistency and co-ordination in implementation. Consistency was difficult to achieve if the policies were in competition with other priorities at local level. In practice, management development proposals found it hard to claim managers' interest in the face of demand for improved patient care, professional training etc. So the manager or 'customer' chose to not to buy on many occasions.

At the supplier end, education providers were encouraged to behave commercially, with the penalty coming from lack of co-ordination. They naturally sought competitive advantage and were reluctant to share their experience and expertise with their 'rivals'. With prices honed to the bone, very little surplus was available for ensuring a solid infrastructure and the means of continuity.

A central organ such as the Training Authority naturally found it difficult to relax its hold completely but, unless it could 'command' the situation, it fell to the mercies of the local 'market' economies. A notable example of this occurred when the Authority attempted to implement a process of 'accrediting' management centres and 'recognising' Health Authorities who had met appropriate standards. In 1987 a working party produced a very worthy report for the Training Authority outlining a six-step process involving self-appraisal, a review team visit and adjudication by an accreditation/recognition panel. This scheme found no favour with either purchasers or providers of management development. The process seemed to be too cumbersome and costly to provide much useful guidance to purchasers, who, in any case, preferred to back their own judgement. Providers felt that a good 'product' or service would be bought with, or without, the Training Authority's stamp of approval.

Unless the Training Authority backed its proposals with hard cash, it found itself drawn increasingly into the market in a rather ambiguous purchase/supplier role. A further and more complex instance of this was the National Accelerated Development Programme (NADP). The merits of the programme itself are debated below, but it spite of considerable resources expended, the programme never took on its comprehensive scope. While many of the components came into existence, they were never co-ordinated in a proper national programme. Thus the NADP became synonymous with three General Management Training Schemes (GMTS) and never deployed the full range of intended options, especially the use of 'designated posts'. The processes of Individual Performance Review and Personal Development Planning only functioned fitfully, and were distorted by their association with Performance Related Pay. While many individuals gained from GMTS programmes, others were inhibited by the inexperienced use of assessment centres to identify 'fast track' potential. The national impetus became diffused into regional effort, with consequent fragmentation and inconsistency of standards.

At the other end of the management hierarchy was the ambitious Management Education Syllabus and Open Learning (MESOL) project sponsored by the Training Authority and devised by the Open University and the Institute of Health Service Management. Later entitled Managing Health Services, the aim was to invest in a distant learning system and materials appropriate for some 70,000 NHS managers at the threshold of their careers, with a take up of 3,000 participants per year, at a cost of between £100,000 and £300,000 for initial development. The Training Authority controlled the development of system and materials through direct funding but it had to be marketed to the NHS in competition with a multitude of alternatives, many of which were long established and closely adapted to local needs. By mid-1994, 6,500 managers had been through the programme. The then chairman of the steering group, Mr Ken Jarrold, noted this as 'a very satisfying achievement'. It was not easy, but it succeeded because it suited the market, rather than because it was implemented as national policy.

In the first edition of this book, this review pointed to the confusion in the Training Authority's role: either it had to be strengthened as an effective arm of central policy, or it should be abolished so that the market – created by itself – could have free play. By the time of the second edition of the book, two years later, the market had won. In April 1991, the Authority was replaced by a Training Directorate under the control of the NHS Director of Personnel.

Towards a 'demand-led' strategy?

In this review in the second edition of this book, it was suggested that the traditional 'supply-led' strategy for management development should move towards a 'demand-led' strategy. It is pleasing to observe that, in the intervening four years, the trend has been in the latter direction. It was argued that there were three parts to a 'demand-led' strategy.

First, there was seen to be a continuing need for policy guidance for development from the centre. At the very minimum, the NHS Executive needs the availability of skilled advice. This need was given sharp focus when, in April 1996, the NHS Training Directorate was disbanded and its central functions split into two parts:

- a development unit at the Leeds headquarters with responsibility for overall policy and strategy;
- a new, self-financing Institute of Health and Care Development, based like its predecessor, the Training Authority, at arm's length in Bristol; an NHS trading agency to provide consultancy for human resource development and to act as an award body in conjunction with the Open University.

This formally removed the enduring confusion in the role of the NHS Training Directorate, which had combined a policy and strategic function with a major function as a commissioner and indeed supplier of training 'products'. It has reversed the direction set by the *Management Development Strategy for the NHS*, published in October 1991, which set out national policy in terms of the then Management Executive's values and expectation at that time (NHS Training Directorate 1991). It was in the action plan that the weaknesses became apparent. The plan assumed a unitary organisation in which national and regional levels 'support' the local implementation of the strategy. Such a world had now disappeared, as the timescale for the eight key measures clearly demonstrated. All the target dates were missed with very little achieved, except perhaps some practices which were a little more 'women friendly'. Even the establishment of a national management centre did not seem to have survived its principal sponsors. All this seemed to endorse the history of the 1970s and 1980s which suggested that a 'supplier-led' strategy would have a very limited success.

The second edition of this book suggested the alternative – and theoretically the more sound – approach of a 'demand-led' strategy, in which the chief executives and general managers are committed to investment in development because they can see its importance to the achievement of the business plan. Given their commitment, resources will be found and expertise deployed where it is wanted by them and not where remote policy makers or self-interested specialist would prefer.

A further step towards this approach was also taken in the April 1996 changes, with the establishment of a network of local training consortia, working under regional groups – Regional Education Development Groups (REDGs). These groups are made up of purchasers, providers, both NHS and non-NHS, and GPs. Their purpose was to fulfil part of the strategy to make workforce planning and development an employer-led responsibility. This seems a substantial move towards a 'demand-led' approach.

The third element of this approach was seen to be a focus on what might be called the 'competitive policy': the necessity to decide on the amount of resource to invest in management development, and what mechanism should be used to control these resources. In 1993, it was recognised that the reins of central control in management development had slackened, and the provider units and NHS trusts – where most managers were found – were freer to decide for themselves. This faced management development proposals with hard competition from patient care, business and professional imperatives. The generalised and long-term values of the former were always likely to be seen at a disadvantage against the more immediate and more publicly 'acceptable' benefits of the latter.

It is for the NHS Executive to consider the merits of investment in NHS managers and, as necessary, to ease this competitive situation locally. The temptation is to establish a structure which attempts to control and direct resources and which relies on the initiatives of experts – Training Directorate, Regional Training Departments, Management Development Advisors. This largely constituted the road that the NHS Training Directorate went down in the five years of its existence. This served to confuse its role in the purchaser–provider world, and has sometimes diminished the impact of its valuable policy statements.

The new, more 'demand-led' approach has been in existence for a year, at the time of writing. The timetable has slipped, so that the consortia will not have real money to commission non-medical education and training until April 1998. From a recent review, the signs are that only big and urgent priorities, such as nursing manpower, will get on agendas (Snell 1997). Management development may not claim a hearing. The idea of consortia, representing various interests, funded by a levy, suggests the inertia of a bureaucratic structure. The jury is still out deliberating whether both the principal and the practice are improvements on the earlier 'supply-led' command approaches.

To what extent is the re-focus from 'supply' to 'demand' a threat to the management development specialist, the traditional supplier? In the short term, it may upset established practices. But in the longer term, it promises to move the specialist closer to the levers of power, which have often eluded his or her grasp, leaving a sense of being on the periphery of events.

Nor need specialists be passive spectators during any transition in strategy. They can and should influence events. One of the challenges is to engage more convincingly in the process of evaluation, especially in relation to the business plan. This has always constituted something of an Achilles heel: it has been impossible to prove the value of development activity in most cases. It remains an act of common sense or even faith. The problems of evaluation are well known, and a number of approaches are available in the writing of Easterby-Smith and others (Easterby-Smith 1986). The task for the NHS developer is to be more careful in evaluating learning and to make the findings more visible to policy-makers.

Formal and informal development approaches

The 1970s and 1980s witnessed a striking growth in the range of development options available to NHS managers. The traditional short, off-the-job course, first used in the mid-1960s, became a flexible and sophisticated tool, joined by a host of less formal techniques.

In the late 1980s, the predominance of the short, 'continuing education' event gave way to a polarisation between formal 'educational' programmes, such as Certificates in Management Studies and MBAs, and informal workplace, problem-solving learning, often associated with consultancy. The former approach offers the student a continuity of learning, although within an academic rather than a practical framework. The value of the latter often comes from relevance to managerial concerns, but its immediacy can often drive out its usefulness as a source of learning.

Between the mid-1960s and the mid-1980s, there was a range of centrally funded short development courses available on a national basis to eligible managers from all disciplines at middle and senior levels. The were sponsored successively by the DHSS, NHS National Training Council and the NHS Training Authority. The latter body intended that the programmes would become self-financing, but the National Education Centres who were the major providers found that employers were not attracted by full-cost funding. At best, these courses integrated the twin goals of relevance and continuity by providing a set of learning experiences over 4–6 months which enabled thousands of NHS managers to have their first and, in many cases, only systematic opportunity for development.

With the almost total demise of these courses, the running has been taken up by the education sectors with an increasingly comprehensive variety of accredited programmes. Academic barriers to learning in the form of 'gateway' qualifications have been increasingly diminished until even the most hidebound institution have evolved 'open-access' programmes. Recent evidence suggest that more NHS managers than ever before are studying by one mode or another for certificates, diplomas, graduate degrees and postgraduate degrees in relevant managerial sub-jects. Since many of these are financed by their NHS employers, there is at least *prima facie* evidence that these employers will be looking for out-comes in terms of enhanced performance.

At the end of the spectrum, learning opportunities have crept even nearer to the workplace. All too often, however, progress depends on the energy of individual managers and the support of their superiors. Techniques such as Individual Performance Review and Personal Development Plans have helped, but will not guarantee any action. But, just as there is less and less surprise at managers studying for masters and doctoral qualifications, there is an equally diminishing resistance to infor-mal learning events involving learning sets, time out reviews, even one-to-one coaching.

Perhaps the demand for high-calibre and competent managers in the late 1990s will guarantee the continuation of this 'twin-track' strategy of formal and informal development, guided by politics and monitoring from the centre. There is, however, a strong case to be made for the reten-tion of management development expertise available to the NHS. Much of the 'provision' can be, and is being, bought in from independent or semi-independent contractors. But there is a need to ensure a capacity for expert advice which will depend on the continuous involvement of experts with the complexities and problems of the NHS. There is a central role for specialists who can integrate the formal with the informal, who are able to influence the centres of power, and are committed more closely to the mission of the NHS than just financial reward.

References

Department of Health (1989) *Working for patients* The White Paper HMSO, London

Department of Health & Social Security (1983) *NHS management inquiry* The Griffiths Report DHSS London

Easterby-Smith, M (1986) *The evaluation of management education and development* Gower, London

Ham, C, Honigsbaum, F and Thompson, D (1993b) *Priority setting for health gain* DoH, London

Ham, C, Thompson, D and Tremblay, H (1993a) *Effective purchasing* HSMC Birmingham

Handy, C (1989) *The age of unreason* Business Books Ltd, London

Harrison, J, Thompson, D, Flanagan, H and Tonks, P (1994) Beyond the business plan *Journal of Management in Medicine* 8, 1

Hunter, D and Williamson, P (eds) (1989) Perspectives on general man-agement in the NHS *Health Services Management Research* 2, 1

Kotler, P (1988) *Marketing management analysis, planning, implementa-tion and control* Prentice Hall, Englewood Cliffs, New Jersey

Le Grand, J (1990) *Quasi markets and social policy* SAUS Publications, University of Bristol, Bristol

Limb, J and Chadda, D (1997) News feature *Health Services Journal* May 29 1997

NHS Training Authority (1986) *Better management, better health* NHS Training Authority, Bristol

NHS Training Directorate (1991) *Management development strategy for the NHS* NHS Training Directorate, Bristol

Simpson, J and Scott, T (1996) *National survey of clinical directors* British Association of Medical Managers, London

Snell, J (1997) Shaping up: special report on the NHS training reforms *Health Services Journal,* March 6 1997

Thompson, D (1994) *Developing managers for the new NHS* Longman, Harlow

Thompson, D and Edmonstone, J (1988) *Resources for management development* NHS Training Authority, Bristol

Williams, D (1988) Have we achieved better management, better health? *Health Services Manpower Review,* March 1988

11 Of confidence and identity: the doctor in management
Michael Tremblay

Introduction

Doctors in the UK have always been involved in the management of clinical resources. Over the past few years, the changes in the NHS have put doctors, often precipitously and precariously, into the front-lines of health care management. General practitioners too have not been immune from these changes, having gone from running small independent businesses, to large and complex fundholding practices, and even larger multi-funds, of some 100 or so other doctors. Many consultants have retained private medical practices, while others have invested in private hospitals or work with larger commercial enterprises.

The NHS, though, as the public health system, has appeared to disenfranchise hospital doctors in particular from management roles since the 1948 nationalisation of most UK hospitals. Today, we are now facing heightened concern that doctors are not properly represented in health care management or, when present, that they are inadequately prepared for these responsibilities.

This chapter considers the various factors which need to be taken into account when looking at the broader issue of doctors and management. The chapter will consider a variety of factors, or forces, which have an impact on doctors and on management, and thereby provide a framework for considering the two together. The chapter will be divided into the following sections, each dealing with a corresponding core question:

1 Terminology: what do we call a doctor in a management role?

2 Role Change: what are the factors which are active when a doctor takes on managerial responsibilities?

3 Career Structure: what are the characteristics of a doctor's career which affects their exposure to management ideas and may influence their thinking about management?

4 Educational Opportunities: what courses and other educational activities are available to help a doctor who is interested in developing as a manager?

5 Competency: what does it mean to be a good manager and is that incompatible with being a good doctor?

6 Peer Relationships: how do doctors in management relate to their colleagues who are not managers, particularly if they have managerial responsibility for other doctors?

7 Why Bother? What incentives/disincentives influence a doctor interested in a managerial career path?

Terminology

It is important to get the terminology clear. These days we often speak of front-line management, devolved management, empowerment etc to describe the pattern of cascading managerial responsibility down the organisational hierarchy. Middle managers in these organisations are at risk as management responsibility from above is given away to those below them; these managers, in turn, are challenged to prove that they are needed. Increasingly, organisations are finding that they are not needed, at least not in abundance. And, as organisations flatten, and become less hierarchical, the diffuse sharing of managerial responsibility empowers more people with management responsibility, decoupling the role of manager with the tasks of management.

To some extent, the recent past and the anticipated future, has demonstrated a preference for new managerial roles to embrace a service component as well. For example, managers who also go out on sales calls, repair equipment, or doctors in management who maintain a case-load. While dedicated middle managers may become an endangered species, the tasks of management, such as budgeting, staffing, planning and so on become tasks undertaken by increasing numbers of people, often but not always closely associated with management.

This process can be considered as either adding management tasks to a person's job, or as rethinking the organisation so that dedicated management roles become fewer as management tasks are shared out. The former for some represents 'just more work', while the latter for others represents a fundamentally new way of configuring management in modern organisations. Happily, the latter is becoming recognised as the right approach; sadly, too many organisations engage in the former.

From a traditional doctor's perspective, managers have not always been viewed kindly. Indeed, it might be characterised with considerable hostility, if not antipathy. So why would a doctor want to become a manager, this creature which causes doctors so much grief, concern and problems (at least from the doctor's point of view).

Doctors, though, are always actively involved in management. They managed the earliest hospitals, and in most parts of the world take a close and important role in hospital management. Advances in clinical technology and the expanding role of other health professions has challenged this role, and generally relegated doctors more towards a purely clinical role, management functions to be assumed by a new breed of specialist health care managers. Developments such as general management in the 1980s in the UK, further disenfranchised doctors by proposing that management required managers to be effective.

It is unfortunate, though, that general management thinking was introduced at the expense of a more robust concept of management involving clinicians. Industry, for example, draws its general managers from within its own staff who have had many years of management development, through schooling and experience on the job, and possess a thorough understanding of the business. Dropping general managers into health management as though health were just another product appeared to show little insight into the complexities of management of health service organisations as distinct from other types of organisations.

We are now paying for this, to some extent; doctors, who have an informed inside understanding of clinical priorities, for example, often clash with managers who are perceived to have little appreciation of the values of the health service.

Doctors can often be perceptive in their suspicion of accountancy-driven health care when governments need to create wholesale reforms to ensure that patient services and needs are paramount – through patients' charters and elaborate contracting systems.

So who is a doctor in management? The options include:

1   a doctor who is a manager;

2   a manager who is a doctor;

3   a manager who used to be a doctor;

4   a doctor who does management.

The terminology does little justice to the complexity of management and medicine. A doctor who does management engages in an activity which others might view with some consternation: can he/she be sincere; after all, there are other people who are full-time managers who do little other than manage. What if the doctor wants to get *good* at management?

Doctors do go through rigorous selection and education to become doctors, which requires well-developed numeracy skills, judgement (such as in working with incomplete information on a patient), attributes which are looked for in managers and which often underpin competency models of management.

The ambiguity in how to describe a legitimate management role for doctors does little to foster an interest in it. This may be partly because of the poor definition of the management role in the evolving NHS itself, but also because of a perception that management is not a particularly challenging or difficult activity.

So what terms might be better. I would suggest the following terms for doctors: 'medical manager' or 'medical executive'. In the United States, people such as this are called 'physician managers' or 'physician executives'.

The medical manager is the more generic term, while medical executive refers more precisely to board level medical director, and heads of clinical directorates. We must, however, be judicious. When these senior roles are filled by other health professions, similar terms will need to apply: nurse executive, or health executive, otherwise we risk replicating unhelpful hierarchies amongst the health professions.

The identity crisis, therefore, reflects profound problems for doctors in how they describe themselves to others in the managerial structure.

Role change

It is a general characteristic of career development of professionals such as lawyers, accountants etc that in due course management roles become career possibilities. Some people, pursuing specialist qualifications in management, such as MBA degrees, arrive at management roles sooner than others; while some professionals increase the likelihood of filling management roles by acquiring specialist qualifications such as these. Doctors need to consider themselves no different from their other professional colleagues, with the exception that the career structure of doctors makes the development of management competency less certain.

However, for a significant number of professionals, the role change which occurs as they assume greater management responsibility, and thus provide less direct service (as an accountant doing the books, or engineer building bridges) will influence how they describe themselves, and how they represent themselves to their colleagues and to the public.

For hospital doctors, who arrive at the possibility of management roles after many years in a subordinate training role, for instance, which has unacknowledged management responsibilities, this presents unique problems. The career structure of doctors, culminating in a consultant post, also confers the necessary positional responsibility to undertake formal management responsibilities such as a clinical director. However, the management responsibility will usually involve responsibility for the actions of a peer group, and may involve management purview over clinical competency and clinical autonomy.

Doctors in clinical directors' roles have described their relationship with their peers as one of the most challenging aspects of clinical management. Others have indicated a concern about appearing too eager to embrace their management role for fear of alienating the necessary support of their consultant colleagues.

However, doctors do successfully undertake management responsibilities throughout their medical career. That formal recognition of this occurs rather late in their career, usually only really being recognised upon appointment as a consultant, does little to encourage doctors to develop an interest in management at an earlier stage. Indeed, for doctors pursuing specialist training towards a consultant appointment, their postgraduate training is characterised by a highly academic and research-focused period of study, with often onerous service responsibilities. An interest in management is not the same as doing clinical research, and reflects a prejudice in postgraduate training towards highly specialised clinical roles, and not a wider responsibility within health care decision-making.

To be fair, junior doctors now enjoy access to many short courses in management, and related subjects, but are usually disconnected from becoming involved in managerial activity by the demands of clinical work. This disconnection means that a role change for a doctor moving into management is made all the more difficult by the failure of the career and training structure to recognise it, and anticipate it.

The role change is more fully understood by considering the career structure of doctors as it appears to look in the UK in 1997. Doctors, in summary, while experiencing some understandable anxiety, also face resistance and stigma from their colleagues as they consider or assume a medical manager role. This role is one which creates an inequality among doctors who see themselves as a peer group.

Career structure

The career structure for doctors has very specific characteristics, which reflect the interest society has in the medical profession. The career structure also reflects the historical reactions to changes and developments in medical staffing and medical hierarchies, and may be again changing in the UK in response to influences from membership in the European Community.

Particular European influences include ensuring that doctors can move freely within the Community (or more precisely the Union), and have their qualifications recognised for the purposes of establishing themselves to practise medicine. There are also background studies being undertaken within the European Commission focusing specifically on the trainee and employee status of junior doctors, and suggestions that junior doctors should fall under the control of the Working Time Directive, limiting their work week to 48 hours.

Various organisations also take an interest in the career of the doctor. The General Medical Council sets the standards and expectations for medical education and licensing, with the Royal Colleges taking on the responsibility for specialist credentialling. The other groups are concerned with general practitioners and still others are concerned with the postgraduate education of doctors.

Within this network of interests lies a doctor who, upon graduating from medical school, undertakes a year of work prior to registration, and then makes or follows through particular career decisions.

These decisions lead our young doctor into one of the following paths:

1 hospital medicine not leading to a consultant position;
2 specialist medicine leading to a consultant position;
3 general practice.

The general approach these three career paths involve reflects distinctions between the training grades and the non-training grades of medical staffing.

The career choices, though, are daunting. Following registration, a doctor can pursue a career in general practice or begin basic specialist training. For those opting for general practice, a course involving work as a senior house officer which will lead to independent practice as a general practitioner. Some doctors, however, may not choose the GP vocational training programme, and may enter directly into general practice.

General practitioners who want to maintain an interest in hospital medicine, can become clinical assistants. This clinical assistant position can in some cases lead to a staff grade position in a hospital. Staff grade positions are newer and subject to numerical limitations. Thus, the doctor interested in general practice, can choose a route which also provides an opportunity to take on a non-training staff grade position in a hospital.

Doctors whose interests are different, pursue a five-year specialist registrar training programme. The Specialist Training Authority (STA) has been designated by the various Royal Colleges as the competent body in the UK (a condition which satisfies wider European Union requirements) and which is responsible for ensuring standards in postgraduate training. Individual Royal Colleges maintain their own training programmes to meet their specialist requirements, but upon completion of this training, a doctor applies to the STA for a Certificate of Completion of Specialist Training (CCST); the awarding of a CCST indicates the completion of specialist training and it was this procedure which was necessary to bring UK law into line with European law. The CCST means that a doctor is now eligible for appointment as a consultant.

The system implemented in March 1996 (see *A Guide to Specialist Registrar Training 1996*, also called 'The Orange Book') introduced a system of matching training posts in NHS trusts with individual specialist registrars [SpR], all SpRs have National Training Numbers, and only SpRs can undertake postgraduate training for a CCST. When the CCST is awarded, the SpR ceases to have a training number and can therefore no longer occupy a training post. This eliminated the old system whereby senior registrars could hold training posts for years while awaiting a consultant appointment, and restrict access to training by more junior colleagues.

Importantly, then, this recent reform means that CCSTs are only awarded to SpRs who have completed a substantive (approved) training programme in the required time period and therefore that training posts are occupied only by trainees pursuing CCSTs. Training now has an end.

The introduction of SpRs has also welcomed flexible training offering part-time training opportunities. The main purpose of flexible training for CCST qualification is to keep doctors within the NHS who might otherwise leave if full-time commitment was not possible. Perhaps of greater importance, is that flexible training is covered by European law, specifically EC Directive 93/16/EEC which requires that part-time training, if available, must meet the same requirements as full-time study. The perceived lower status of part-time training notwithstanding, flexible and full-time SpRs will earn equal CCSTs.

The Specialist Workforce Advisory Group (SWAG) advises the Department of Health on the numbers of different specialists that are needed, and represents the formal planning machinery which determines how many SpR trainees there will be, and therefore how many trainee posts there will be within NHS trusts.

Eligibility for a consultant appointment cannot occur until the CCST has been awarded. It is a legal requirement that a doctor be on the GMC's Specialist Register before being appointed.

For some doctors, academic medicine is another opportunity, with its own hierarchy of lecturer to professor alongside that of registrar to consultant. The General Medical Council in its *Recommendations on the Training of Specialists* (1987, p. 15), state: 'Training in essentially non-clinical subjects should include components of appropriate clinical experience'.

This report, though, does not mention management training and development as a formal competency of the independent practitioner, apart from the following components (p. 6):

understanding and appreciation of the roles, responsibilities and skills of nurses and other health care workers.

the ability to lead, guide and coordinate the work of others.

Acquisition of experience in administration and planning, including:

1 *efficient management of the doctor's own time and professional activities;*

2 *appropriate use of diagnostic and therapeutic resources, and appreciation of the economic and practical constraints affecting the provision of health care; and*

3 *willingness to participate, as required, in the work of bodies which advise, plan and assist the development and administration of medical services, such as NHS authorities, Royal Colleges and Faculties, and professional associations.*

Figure 11.1 represents the various career roles of doctors. It is important to add that management roles for doctors are actually undertaken throughout their career, both in and out of training. The regret is that the due recognition of these activities for career development is not readily forthcoming.

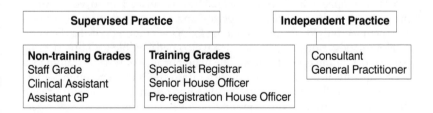

Figure 11.1   Medical career structure

The challenge for health management is developing ways to legitimise the acquisition of appropriate management competencies alongside the development of clinical competency. This would make the subsequent selection of candidates for senior management roles one of selecting from a larger and probably better prepared talent pool than is currently the case. Certainly, the doctors who aspire to or have attained management roles reflect the best management talent available; but the uncertainty of its development by doctors makes it problematic that as health service organisations seek to become better managed they will be able to find a ready source of expertise when they need it.

This last point is a general problem for health service management, ie the identification of managerial talent. Encouraging the medical profession to recognise management as a legitimate competency of some doctors would go some way to helping address the shortage of highly skilled managers which will become more acute as the reformed health service places greater and more sophisticated demands on people with management responsibilities, including doctors.

Figure 11.2 shows the career structure in general as it appears in 1997. In due course, changes may occur which reflect responses to the recent reforms of medical training which cannot be anticipated at this time.

Educational opportunities

The difficulty for doctors developing management competency is the overriding concern for clinical skill development during their training years. There are many and varied courses generally available to develop management aptitudes which would bring aspiring physician-managers into contact with others similarly disposed, but from different backgrounds.

Fitzgerald and Sturt (1992) suggest that doctors should not be developed in isolation from other types of managers. This sound advice would ensure that doctors developed appropriate understanding of how other people view their own responsibilities and problems. Doctors who have attended courses with managers from the private sector have indicated that it was helpful to share insights and learn from others new ways of looking at similar problems.

At present, there is available a wide array of courses in management in the UK, ranging from courses on television from the Open University, to self-study management texts, to short courses, to full-time postgraduate management degrees. There is also a tendency to look at the management development of doctors as occurring away from the development of other managers. It is difficult for doctors to organise their work to attend part-time MBAs, or to undertake a short course programme.

Certainly, doctors with an interest in management can find an increasing array of formal and informal opportunities. In the past few years, too, many doctors have moved comfortably into medical executive positions, such as chief executives of NHS trusts, as medical directors with board

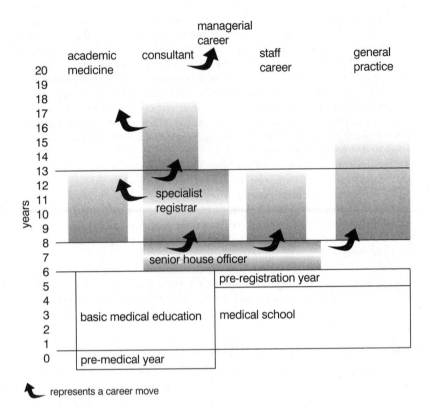

Figure 11.2 Medical career structure

level responsibilities, and have become much more firmly committed to leadership of clinical directorates, and other clinical structures.

That numbers have grown suggests that new opportunities for training are possible. Indeed, mentoring of doctors by doctors in executive roles is a well established practice in the private sector, and offers a very-high level entry to managerial learning.

But how can they practise what they are learning? What if they want to undertake significant clinical management responsibilities; how might this be matched against the existing career structure which puts consultants into these roles? And there is the additional issue that junior doctors rotate from place to place. Rotation through different organisational systems provides an important opportunity for the doctor to learn how other people do things, and thus bring a broad perspective to each new employer. But is anyone interested?

These questions, though, provide the basis for developing substantial learning opportunities for doctors. We need talented doctors in management and we need these doctors to assume these managerial and executive roles with confidence.

Competency

Doctors are concerned with competency: to them, managers appear not to be working with structured models. Doctors and managers must be developed together. It is not uncommon to hear doctors speak critically of managers. From the doctors' perspective, managers seem to get in their way, and be concerned only with financial matters. When managers speak, they use ordinary language in special and coded ways. For many people, including doctors, this 'management speak' often sounds like it ought to mean something, but a lack of familiarity with management models can make access to the meanings difficult.

It is in fact the use of management models that might be surprising to many non-managers. Indeed, the past 100 years have seen the development of many models of management, from Frederick Taylor's scientific management through various schools of thinking to today's ideas. Today, many of these models and ideas of management may appear to some to lack scientific rigour, to be a product of a popular management culture, an issue of management fashion and trend and not rational thought.

Much of management thinking, though, does rest on simple truths about how to treat a fellow human being, about basic notions of ethical conduct, as well as researched work on human motivation and behaviour, financial controls and information technology.

For doctors who have undertaken a fundamentally scientific programme of study, and who work with data, dealing with the softer issues of human relationships in the workplace and motivation challenges their own well-developed methods of analysis.

Certainly, there is no reason why a doctor should not be able to comprehend financial accounting, statistical and other data. Working with data is part of their own medical education. Similarly, doctors should be able to use this information to inform decision-making and planning about allocation of health resources.

The important difference for a doctor and a manager is that while the doctor is concerned about this or that particular patient, managers are concerned with types or groups of patients. A doctor faced with dealing with a patient for whom a recommended procedure is unavailable has a human problem of their relationship to each patient; a manager faced with the same problem, is dealing with rationing, and the efficacy of the intervention in patients of similar type.

There are many models of competency, and competency models have sprouted most often as long lists of items. Competency, though, is not just knowing *how*, but knowing *why*. It is about knowing rules, and knowing when to break the rules. Doctors know and understand clinical competency and respect colleagues on that basis. Managerial competency is different, but no less worthy of respect. Doctors who are both bring an important perspective, of blending two sets of rules, with enhanced judgement across the wide canvas of health care management.

The challenge for doctors, managers and indeed everyone concerned with health care in the UK, is developing a model of competency that works here, and reflects the complexity of clinical and managerial priorities. Doctors interested in management should exercise critical caution and ensure that the managerial skills and abilities they embrace are appropriate to their managerial role and are based on acceptable ethical and value considerations.

Peer relationships

Peer relationships within medicine for doctors in management are complex, and challenge traditional notions of peer and professional relationships. A medical executive among other doctors is *primus inter pares* – first among equals. The medical executive or manager faces significant new responsibilities which could imbalance the peer relationships:

1 the management of resources such as money, support personnel, clinical equipment;

2 the management of terms and conditions of employment including increasingly being involved in hiring new consultants or being involved in decision-making about who is hired, and the contractual expectations of the position;

3 the responsibility for ensuring that the other staff, including the medical staff, are carrying out their responsibilities which may involve simply ensuring that the clinical services are provided, but may involve formal review of clinical performance and a veto role over the use of junior medical staff or others by consultant colleagues.

Wanting to maintain a balanced clinical relationship with colleagues may present challenges to the medical manager or executive. Participative and democratic management styles are preferable to high-handed and authoritarian approaches but present greater challenges when times are difficult.

Managing professionals, like doctors, by other doctors, will always involve these challenges; it is hardly a reason to avoid the responsibility.

Why bother?

Of course, thinking about doctors in management involves asking the question 'why bother?' Why bother encouraging doctors to become involved in management? It is not sufficient that doctors play a significant role in the health of people and the resources to help them, is it not sufficient that it does not make much sense to suggest that doctors needed a particular rationale for wanting to become involved in management, is it not sufficient that organisations should want to identify all their talented people for management, and not make certain assumptions about fitness to be a manager? After all, such assumptions often have the effect of discriminating against talented people for failing to have certain characteristics and not others.

There is an argument from self-defence: if doctors do not fill these management roles, others will, and they may not deal with the issues doctors feel are appropriate. However, medical executives are not in these roles to acquiesce to their colleagues' interests either, and their managerial responsibilities extend to encompassing other health professionals, support staff, premises, and indeed the needs of the local population.

There is an argument from ability: doctors are capable of learning about management and being good at it. This adds to and challenges the doctor's repertoire of talent and may arguably be a good thing in itself.

There is an argument from added value: a doctor brings to management an important perspective that is often missing around the board room table. By being involved, the doctor ensures that management processes reflect broader concerns and interests. Importantly, as key decision-makers in the allocation of clinical resources, medical managers and executives are able to integrate clinical accountability for effective resource use with the management of the use of that resource.

Conclusions

This chapter has addressed key factors concerned with the doctor in management. Specific conclusions are appropriate in light of this discussion.

Terminology

While what we call things is often arbitrary, words have meaning and it is important to develop a language we are comfortable with to convey important meaning. Legitimising specific terminology for doctors in management, such as medical executive, or medical manager, moves us towards words evocative of what we are talking about. The effect of acceptance of these terms by other doctors and managers will be to empower doctors as managers to assume the role and titles with the support and respect of their colleagues.

Role change

It is appropriate to support doctors in their pursuit of managerial and executive responsibilities. We need to address important concerns at the transitions within their careers, and ensure support from colleagues, such as other doctors and managers.

Career structure

The identification of managerial talent remains the one most important weakness in the present system of medical careers which is focused exclusively on clinical development in a highly academic and research-oriented framework. Indeed, some of the more recent short courses in management, and some of the more heavily funded initiatives, may have actually done more to trivialise the importance of managerial competency, and managerial roles within the medical career structure. Doctors 'do' management throughout their training, but it must be acknowledged and made explicit. Career development for those seeking a place in management should incorporate suitable expectations of ability, interest and aptitude. The managerial role expectations need to be much more explicit and pervasive throughout, and certainly not formally identified only at the time of consultant appointment.

Educational opportunities

Doctors will need to practise their budding management talents. We need to know how they can do this and have it recognised as an important part of their professional development. This is not for all doctors, but it must be for those who will fill executive and managerial roles in the future.

Competency

It is probably time that a more formal system of accreditation of health service managers be considered in the UK. Possession of academic qualifications is one thing; recommendations of friends for membership in an association another. Rigorous assessment of basic competency is long overdue. The responsibilities of management are more complex and demanding than in the past. The NHS is no longer administered (one hopes) to central dictat, but is guided and developed, indeed managed, by capable people acting properly in the public interest. For doctors interested in management, recognition of competency would ensure their credibility and warrant enhanced peer support – from doctors, and from other managers.

Why bother?

Recognition of a proper role of the medical executive is timely and appropriate. The effective use of scarce resources in health has heightened society's awareness of the difficulties associated with meeting limitless demand for health care. The medical executive or manager can bridge this gulf between public understanding and the setting of health service priorities into the proper context. It is time for the medical profession to recognise this important role and to ensure that interested doctors can pursue meaningful career paths leading to leadership roles.

References

Curry, L (1989) Identification of functionally necessary knowledge and skills in the practice of Canadian health care management *Journal of Health Education Administration* 7, 47–69

Department of Health *A Guide to Specialist Registrar Training* March 1996, currently under revision

Ellis, R (ed.) (1988) *Professional Competence and Quality Assurance in the Caring Professions* Chapman & Hall, London

Fitzgerald, L and Sturt, J (1992) Clinicians into management: on the change agenda or not? *Health Service Management Research* **5**, 137–146

General Medical Council (1987) *Recommendations on the Training of Specialists* October 1987

Harrison, S, Hunter, DJ, Marnock, G and Pollitt, C (1989) General management and medical autonomy in the National Health Service *Health Service Management Research* **2**, 38–46

Johnson, JA and Boss, RW (1991) Management development and change in a demanding health care environment *Journal of Management Development* **10**, 5–10

KET Foundation Inc. (1984) *The Business of Managing Professionals* TV Ontario: Toronto, Canada

Matheson, K and Tremblay, M *The Value of Assessments* The National Association of Clinical Tutors, London, 1996 *(a guide to assessing SpRs under the new training regulations)*

Pollitt, C *et al.* (1988) The reluctant managers: clinicians and budgets in the NHS *Financial Accountability and Management* **4**, 213–233

Sternberg, RJ and Killigian, J (1990) *Competence Considered* Yale University Press, Yale

Stewart, R and Dopson, S (1988) Griffiths in theory and practice: a research assessment *Journal of Health Administration Education* **6**, 503–514

Tremblay, M (1993) *Evaluation Report of Clinicians in the Senior Executive Course at Manchester Business School* HSMC, March 1993

Tremblay, M Physician – Teach Thyself *AUPHA Newsletter* September 1995. Chicago, USA

Willis, SL and Dubin, SS (eds) (1990) *Maintaining Professional Competence* Jossey-Bass, San Francisco

12 Managing stress in health care organisations

Peter Spurgeon

Introduction

Stress has become a popular term, if an unpopular experience, through the 1980s and 1990s. It is widely used and is offered as an explanatory concept in a great variety of situations. It is a term that seems to appeal to scientists and researchers, appearing to offer a technical definition of something in particular, whilst at the same time appealing to the public at large as a common sense way of describing situations and experiences. Inevitably when a concept is used in such a diverse manner variations in meaning develop and one is uncertain as to whether it is always referring to the same thing. Indeed some authors have almost begun to advocate a movement away from stress and a search for a more precise terminology. Fleming *et al.* (1984) comment that 'There are so many uses of "stress" that it may be more confusing than anything else', and Pollock (1988) says 'the term has become so vacuous that it represents an obstacle rather than an aid to research'.

Perhaps typical of the appealing nature of a generalised use of the term stress is a recent survey of 1,200 staff in a variety of industries (Guardian Financial Services 1996) suggesting that health care and the pharmaceutical industry have experienced almost unparalleled increases in levels of reported stress. A total of 40 per cent of staff in this sector claim that they currently work under high or very high stress, and 74 per cent believe stress is playing an increasingly significant role in causing ill–health, with one in three stating that they had recently suffered ill-health as a direct result of excessive stress (migraines, headaches, ulcers, irritable bowel syndrome, digestive problems and heart disease top the list of stress-related conditions). Health services are actually at the head of a list of industries whose workers believe stress levels have increased in the last few years (75 per cent of health care staff feel this to be the case).

At first glance this suggests a clear problem in the health sector. There is though the slight worry about the consensus with which all respondents understood and were using the same concept of stress in such a survey.

But does it matter? If people feel this, then it could be argued the problem exists. Here we have a simple statement of one of the key dilemmas of stress research – is it to be based upon individuals' psychological perceptions (self-report) or should it (must it) be supported by more external objective evidence of the experience of stress?

This chapter has an applied orientation with a particular focus upon the health sector and it is not appropriate to engage in a lengthy debate about the technical niceties of stress research. Nonetheless it would be equally remiss to fail to offer the reader an awareness of the basis of the conceptual uncertainties relating to studies of stress. Evans *et al.* (1997) offer a succinct review of some of these more technical aspects. The classic model of the operation of the stress chain may be described as individuals experiencing stress which affects the immune system leading subsequently to ill-health. Evans *et al.* state that 'there is now absolutely no doubt in scientific circles that our psychological experiences can influence the activity of our immune systems'. But they also suggest that it is not possible to define stress solely in terms of objective events that happen to people, since different people react differently to different stressors. Nonetheless these authors quote a review of 38 studies by Herbert and Cohen (1993) which confirms fairly conclusively that there is a link between a broad range of stressors of many types and an effect upon the immune system. The greater difficulty comes in linking such experiences to particular changes in the immune system, or indeed to a particular illness such as cancer where the precise point of onset is often impossible to determine. This is further complicated by physiological evidence that stress is a fundamental part of normal life and that the operation of the immune system is part of our natural adaptation, such that exposure to short term stress can also have a positive activating impact upon our immune systems (Herbert and Cohen 1993).

Thus we can see that there are a set of complex interactions at work in the dynamic of the stress process. Indeed, one of the more cynical authors in this area (Briner 1994) attempts to warn against the over-inclusive and unicausal use of the term stress as a means of explaining everything and explaining nothing. He suggests there is no such thing as a general stress response. Reactions are in fact differentiated specific affective and physiological states. Therefore although it may be possible to establish a general link between stress and illness it is likely to vary across individual situations and disorders and this complexity has not been incorporated into current thinking.

Recognising this cautionary note, the rest of this chapter will attempt to examine how the issue of stress in the workplace has been studied, and what practical information exists as to sources of stress and means of counteracting the consequences of stressful experiences.

The nature of the stress process

Approaches to the study of stress have taken different forms. Briefly, these approaches may be described as follows:

- as an organism's response to a demand or to events that challenge it (Seyle 1976);

- as an event external to the individual that places demands upon him/her (Kahn 1964);

- as a characteristic of the environment that poses a threat to the individual (Caplan *et al.* 1975);

- as a state that results from a misfit between a person's skills and the demands placed upon him/her (McGrath 1976).

Stress is seen either as something external to the individual, or as an internal state or as an interaction between the two.

Early attempts to examine stress concentrated on the physiological aspects of the stress response, although in time psychological components were increasingly incorporated in stress models. However, the wide range and variability of the reactions of different people to apparently similar situations have constrained the development of a simple universally acceptable model of stress. Cox (1978) added a useful insight in suggesting that 'stress has to be perceived or recognised by man'. From this stance has emerged the consensus view that understanding stress requires that an interpretative element is introduced into the process by which different individuals respond to their environment.

Newton (1989) saw this interpretation as the subjective appraisal of the demands made on the individual and argued that it is a vital aspect in understanding stress. From this perspective, it becomes easier to understand why people react differently in certain settings. Life without stimulation or challenge would be intolerably boring and reasonable amounts of pressure heighten our arousal and performance. It is only when an individual feels that the amount of pressure being applied is excessive that the outcome becomes potentially damaging (BMA 1992).

This notion of positive enhancement is described by Quick and Quick (1984) as a process by which individuals attempt to maintain a balance in ongoing variations in stress levels. This occurs not only when the demand on a person exceeds capability or the desired level, but also when capability exceeds demand; in other words, when boredom arises. Clearly, the individual is not a passive component in the stress process since he or she can conceptualise surrounding events and situations in many different ways.

From this perspective of the individual as an active component in the stress situation, several approaches arise by which the individual may attempt to manage stressful environments. A key factor in the negative impact of stress is the perceived control, or more accurately the lack of perceived control, over the provoking situation (Landsbergis 1988). Similarly, individual strategies such as defence mechanisms, aimed at improving the 'fit' of the individual to the environment, are active attempts to restructure the stress environment.

However, the person-environment fit approach to understanding stress is not without its critics. Handy (1988) and Hobfall (1989) both suggest that the emphasis on the perception or appraisal process merely leads to a view that everyone is different and shifts the emphasis of research to defining individual personality characteristics that allow some people to thrive while others suffer. They are also concerned that an overemphasis on appraisal mechanisms has the potential danger of detracting attention from the proper consideration of the sources of stress within organisations. These stressors may be conveniently ignored since experience of them is always mediated by the individual.

This interactive model is presented in Figure 12.1.

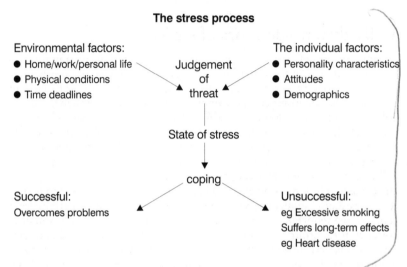

The stress process

Environmental factors:
- Home/work/personal life
- Physical conditions
- Time deadlines

Judgement of threat

The individual factors:
- Personality characteristics
- Attitudes
- Demographics

State of stress

coping

Successful:
Overcomes problems

Unsuccessful:
eg Excessive smoking
Suffers long-term effects
eg Heart disease

Figure 12.1   (after Furnham 1997 p.323)

Within this process framework one may see stress arising when certain individual factors lead the person to see particular circumstances to be threatening. Once threatened, coping mechanisms may come into play but may be more or less successful and the application of an inappropriate coping strategy may actually exacerbate the problem.

McGrath's (1976) definition of stress is perhaps as acceptable as any. He describes the situation as follows:

> *A potential for stress exists when an environmental situation is perceived as presenting a demand which threatens to exceed the person's capabilities and resources for meeting it, under conditions where s/he expects a substantial differential in the rewards and costs for meeting the demand versus not meeting it.*

The main components of the stress process can thus be seen as:

- subjective appraisal of a demanding environment (stressors);
- recognition that demands of the situation may outstrip the resources available;
- the individual experiences the anxiety of not coping.

These processes are then mediated by a whole variety of cognitive processes and personality variables. This dynamic, highly interactive situation is well illustrated by a study conducted by Cooper *et al.* (1986) who attempted to explore the link between experienced stress and breast cancer. They reported that although some of the patients found to have breast cancer tended to have experienced fewer stressful life events in total they did almost without exception rate the events as more severe, ie stressful. The patients with cancer also used different (presumably less effective) coping behaviours.

Individual moderators of stress

A range of potential stressors may be present within an organisation to varying degrees, but the way in which individuals perceive these situations will be modified by a variety of individual and social factors. The current opinion is that environments are not inherently stressful although it is probably self-evident that some situations will be perceived as more adverse by more people and therefore might be classified as potentially very stressful. Nevertheless, there has been considerable research effort directed to finding why some people react to stressors in markedly different forms.

The obvious concern with stress generally is, of course, based largely on the predicted link to poor health. However, even this relationship is subject to potential moderation by other factors. For example, Paffenbarger *et al.* (1966) reported that personality scores on levels of anxiety and neuroticism for a group of students were predictive of future fatal coronary heart disease. More generally, other personality characteristics identified as modifiers of response to stress include introversion-extroversion (Brief *et al.* 1981), anxiety (Chan 1977) and tolerance of ambiguity (Ivancevich and Matteson 1980).

Perhaps the most significant of the personality-based modifiers is the evidence accumulated about the Type A and Type B personality and its link to vulnerability to stress. The area was defined in the 1950s by Friedman and Rosenman (1959) who noted a distinct behavioural pattern within their coronary heart disease patients. The typical Type A personality is described as a work-oriented, high achiever who is very competitive and impatient. Of course, this is a pattern of behaviour that many organisations might value and indeed such individuals are often very successful. Also, it may be that Type A individuals also seek out stressful work environments that meet their personal needs for challenge and achievement. Nonetheless, there is a general view that there is a difference between Type A and Type B individuals with Type As being more disposed to suffer negative stress outcomes. Of course, if this were consistently the case, we could identify Type A personalities and conclude that they have an enhanced risk of stress-related illness. However, recent evidence suggests that the Type A/Type B distinction is not quite as clear-cut as it once seemed. There appears to be a strong link between social class and whether an individual is Type A or B, while Haynes *et al.* (1981) only found a link with coronary heart disease with white collar groups. Johnston *et al.* (1987) in a six-year study failed to find any distinction in levels of heart disease between the two groups.

Another stress moderator is the 'locus of control' construct. This is essentially concerned with the degree of control that individuals perceive they exercise over events. Those with an internal orientation are motivated by their own actions and believe life events are under their control, while those with an external orientation believe that other forces influence events and consequently have a greater tendency to feel helpless. Clearly it is natural to see such a dimension as a moderator of stress. In general, individual orientation provides a much greater chance of dealing with stressors (Blaney 1985, Payne 1988), while Perrewe and Ganster (1989) argue that control is important to various positive health outcomes.

Finally, there is evidence that some very specific individual characteristics may interact with experience of stress. Research evidence suggests that women suffer psychological and physiological stressors in the work environment on a rather greater scale than their male counterparts (Hall and Hall 1980). However, a recent review of the stress literature by Mavtocchio and O'Leary (1989) has fuelled renewed debate in the area since they were unable to detect any gender-based differences in susceptibility to stress. Osipow *et al.* (1985) found that older employees reported less stress than younger employees and used more coping strategies to deal with stressors.

Quite recently two intriguing personal qualities – optimism and hardiness – have emerged as mediators of the stress process. Optimists seem to be much more resistant to stress than pessimists. For example Seligman and Schulman (1980) report optimists are much less likely than pessimists to report physical illness and symptoms during highly stressful periods such as final exams.

Kobasa (1989) describes a concept of hardiness as having three components:

- level of commitment (involvement in activities);

- level of control (belief about the ability to exert influence);

- level of challenge (change as opportunity rather than threat).

Individuals high on these characteristics seem to have a high resistance to stress. Further research is required to understand the operation of hardiness since there is a hint of a tautological argument in this definition: ie those who feel least stress are hardy, and hardy individuals experience less stress. The danger Handy (1988) identified earlier in this chapter is perhaps most evident here – should organisations seek to recruit individuals high on hardiness and thereby deal with problems of stress?

Experience and consequence of stress

We have seen that it is possible for the individual to act upon the person-environment fit and, if successful, adjust the situation appropriately.

However, this may not succeed and the individual may then become subject to longer term strains and may start to demonstrate the symptoms of stress. There is a danger in simply listing sets of symptoms, partly because individual reactions are so different and partly because it might suggest that specific symptoms have a specific one-to-one relationship with a source of stress.

Nonetheless, there are some crude classifications that are useful. The first category is really a short-term response to stress: 'the fight or flight response' is well understood physiologically. The release of adrenaline and steroids associated with stress causes various physiological changes, such as:

- increased blood pressure;

- increased muscle tension;

- increased sweating;

- release of glucose and fats into the blood;

- dry mouth.

These physiological changes can be directly related to the observed outcomes of stress in individuals.

The second category traverses both short and long-term responses, being primarily psychological: here we find such symptoms as anxiety, depression and job dissatisfaction. A final level is behavioural: where performance is adversely affected in some way. For example, behavioural problems can be manifested as absenteeism from work or difficulties within personal life.

Despite the earlier comments in this chapter about the impact of stress on individual health, there is less clear-cut evidence about the links between the effects of stress and longer term illness. However, studies have suggested an association between stress and the following illnesses:

- long-term depression;

- ulcers;

- allergies;

- headaches;

- coronary heart disease;

- cancer;

- asthma.

While there is controversy about the precise causal link between stress and particular illnesses, it may be useful to look briefly at two conditions where stress is acknowledged as a primary cause; 'burn-out' and post-traumatic stress disorder (PTSD). Although individuals may adopt superficially successful methods of coping with stress, it might be that the very act of coping exacts a toll upon the person so as to impair professional functioning.

The term 'burn-out' was first used by Freudengerger (1984) to describe a syndrome especially common among health workers. The syndrome, although lacking a precise definition, is usually seen as having three components:

- emotional exhaustion (tiredness, irritability, depression);

- depersonalisation (poor relationships with others);

- low productivity (with accompanying feelings of low achievement).

The initial link with health workers is interesting and will be discussed more generally later in this chapter.

Post-traumatic stress disorder is a specific anxiety disorder that occurs following a stressful or traumatic event. The key component seems a re-experiencing of the traumatic event at a later date. The syndrome is particularly associated with direct experience of major disasters but it can occur with apparently less significant everyday events. In the long term, sufferers tend to manifest social and occupational dysfunctioning as well as psychiatric illness. It is again of special interest to the medical world because of their exposure to the victims of disasters.

Margolis *et al.* (1974) did take the time factor into account with regard to health outcomes, usefully pointing out that stress can lead to both short-term subjective conditions, such as anxiety and long-term, chronic symptoms such as depression. Schuler (1980) puts forward additional health outcomes such as tension, boredom and mental fatigue and also includes job dissatisfaction. Beehr and Newman (1978) ably describe the health consequences of stress in the human consequences section of their six-part facet analysis of stress. The psychological health consequences are listed as: anxiety, tension, depression, dissatisfaction, boredom, somatic complaints, psychological fatigue, feelings of futility and alienation, inadequacy, low self-esteem, psychoses, anger, repression, suppression of feelings and ideas and loss of concentration. The physical consequences of stress put forward include: cardiovascular disease, gastrointestinal disorders, respiratory problems, cancer, arthritis, headaches, bodily injuries, skin disorders, physical/physiological fatigue or strain, and the ultimate way that nature advises slowing down, death.

Stress at work

Illnesses such as mental health, coronary heart disease, stroke and cancer are acknowledged killers in the western world and they have been increasing dramatically over the past 30 years (Kasl and Cooper 1987). Concern and study of this trend has led to two key factors being identified:

(a) The role of psychosocial factors in the development of physical illness.

(b) The relationship of work to individual stress.

A number of powerful statistics underline these statements.

Table 12.1: Mental health, stress and its consequences

- During one year 1 in 10 of the population will suffer some form of mental illness
- 80 million working days were lost in the UK due to certified mental illness in 1989
- 15 per cent of all occupational disease claims in the US are linked to job-related stress.
- Sickness absence costs UK employees an estimated £13 billion in 1992 – costing NHS over £1 billion
- 30 per cent of sickness absence is due to stress, anxiety and depression

Main source: HEA 1994.

In addition to these calculable costs there are the hidden more insidious costs to human lives – the impoverishment of relationships and the quality of life, not to mention the potential for error from stressed staff.

It is clear that reaction to perception of stressful environments is affected by individual differences. This makes the listing of sources of stress at work a hazardous business. However, Cooper *et al.* (1986) have provided a helpful general categorisation of five major types:

1 Factors intrinsic to the job:
   - poor physical working conditions (due to noise, vibration, temperature, ventilation, humidity, lighting, hygiene and climate);
   - work overload and underload (qualitative and quantitative);
   - time pressures;
   - responsibility for lives.

2 Role of the individual in the organisation:
   - role ambiguity/conflict;
   - image of occupational role;
   - boundary conflicts.

3 Career development:
   - overpromotion;
   - underpromotion;
   - lack of job security;
   - thwarted ambition.

4 Relationships at work:
   - poor relations with boss, subordinates or colleagues;
   - difficulties in delegating responsibility.

5 Organisational structure and climate:
   - little or no participation in decision-making;
   - restrictions on behaviour (budgets etc);
   - office politics;
   - lack of effective consultation.

Noise is typically associated with fatigue, headaches, irritability and inability to concentrate, whilst shiftwork (a significant element in the NHS) tends to be related to fatigue and gastrointestinal troubles (Barton *et al*. 1995). However, the interaction between individuals, context and symptom is very complex, and rather than see these sources as having a direct one-to-one relationship with specific variables, it may be more sensible to see these as a set of general factors including a variety of symptoms.

Warr 1992 has elaborated on the previous list somewhat by identifying additional job features likely to produce stress. Perhaps of particular interest of the additional factors are:

- high uncertainty – both lack of feedback on how one is performing and the security offered of future job prospects;

- low pay;

- low value in society.

It may well be argued that the public sector is susceptible to a range of more general pressures that serve to exacerbate other sources. Payne and Firth-Cozens (1987) argue that the nature of the work within the NHS – the demands of the job itself, dealing with patients and relatives, and the emotional spillover of the job into family and private life – make health care workers especially vulnerable. More specifically, the expectation from the public on nursing staff to live up to the 'vocational calling' behaving with dedication and extreme professionalism can produce great tension when nurses perceive a reality of low pay, staff shortages and poor working conditions. Hingley *et al*. (1986) however, report that only bereavement is a patient-related source of stress for nurses. More organisationally based sources were cited as more significant, such as:

- workload, particularly relating to time pressures, and staff shortages;

- relationships with supervisors, especially lack of positive feedback;

- home/work conflict, typically a female professional with additional pressures created by working unsociable hours and still trying to manage a home and family;

- physical resources, relating to unsuitable and inadequate equipment;

- change, resulting from major and continuing upheavals in the structure and management of the NHS.

Litwinenko and Cooper (1995) examined the impact of organisational changes on health care workers. They found that for particular occupational groups there were negative consequences in terms of rated job satisfaction, perceptions of control, job security, health status and self-reported absences.

For staff affected by such pressures, the level of stress can feel even worse where the culture of the organisation fails to recognise with any sympathy the nature of the problem. George (1990) reported the NHS as experiencing a culture of cynicism as far as stress was concerned. He cited reactions such as:

- Macho management; the tough guy approach. 'If you can't stand the heat, get out of the kitchen'.

- I'm all right Jack; 'I didn't get where I am today by not handling stress'.

- Task is paramount. Process is unimportant. This is the pressure of relentless task forms.

- We don't discuss things like that around here. Stress is seen as a character weakness.

Haynes and Jackson (1996) examined the impact of managerial style on health care staff. They report that staff who reported better mental health also rate their managers as being considerate, aware and responsive – particularly with regard to helping with personal and work related problems.

Other health workers, particularly GPs, have also been the focus of study. Chambers *et al.* (1996) report that for GPs the most potent sources of stress were family–job conflict, patients' unrealistic expectations and disruption to social life. Spurgeon *et al.* (1995) identified 10 independent factors as being the basis of GP stress (Box 12.1).

Box 12.1 Factor analysis of work stressors for GPs

Factor 1: new contract demands
- NHS organisational management changes
- Altered professional priorities (eg targets, health promotion clinics etc)
- Government direction of professional matters
- Communicating with FHSA staff
- Dealing with paperwork/administration
- Communicating with health service managers

Factor 2: balancing work and other demands
- Dividing time between work and home life
- Demands of work on home/family life
- Effects of job on social life
- Workload demands

Factor 3: coping with challenging patients
- Caring for the terminally-ill and their relatives
- Dealing with behaviourally difficult patients
- Dealing with medically challenging patients
- Taking medical responsibility for relatives, friends and colleagues

Factor 4: worry about making mistakes
- Fear of possible litigation
- Fear of making a mistake
- worry about complaints from patients/relatives

Factor 5: extra demands during surgery
- Emergency calls during surgery
- Interruptions during surgery consultations
- 'Time pressures', eg Running late during surgery
- Late requests for home visits during surgery hours

Factor 6: working with practice staff
- Working with employed practice staff
- Communicating with partners in practice
- Liaising with attached nurses in the primary health care team

Factor 7: unrealistic patient demands
- Unrealistically high expectations of GPs role (eg contact for trivial matters)
- Little personal appreciation of GPs work by patients
- Patient demands for non-medical (eg social matters)
- Demand by patient or relative for a 'second opinion'

Factor 8: 24 hour responsibility/night calls
- Accepting 24-hour responsibility for patients
- Night calls
- Remaining alert while on call
- Interruption of family life by telephone

Factor 9: hospital liaison
- Contacting hospital doctors
- Arranging hospital admissions/referrals

Factor 10: non-clinical routine
- Repetitive aspects of GP work
- Dealing with new information technology
- Financial management issues

More generally, health care staff have been felt to be particularly vulnerable to the concept of burnout, emotional exhaustion, depersonalisation and lack of personal accomplishment. Thornton (1992) examined the concept with professional mental health workers and found that for those experiencing burnout, their overwhelming desire was to get away from the situation – hence the consequent high levels of absenteeism, and early retirement in the health sector.

Finally, in terms of individual experience of stress, not only is the issue complicated by how people perceive stress but also how they attempt to cope with it. Individuals learn to react and cope in different ways, which may be more or less successful. These strategies may be emotionally-based (trying to reduce the impact) or problem-based (trying to alter the source of the stress). Carver *et al.* (1989) have identified 15 potential strategies:

1 Positive reinterpretation and growth.

2 Active coping.

3 Planning.

4 Seeking social support for emotional problems.

5 Seeking social support for instrumental problems.

6 Suppression of competing activities.

7 Religion.

8 Acceptance.

9 Mental disengagement.

10 Focus and venting emotion.

11 Behavioural disengagement.

12 Denial.

13 Restraint coping.

14 Alcohol use.

15 Humour.

It may be that individuals can be assisted to adapt and develop better strategies as a means of minimising the impact of stress. However, the discussion to date has sought to describe the nature and sources of stress as experienced by the individual. This approach has tended to reinforce the concept of stress as a problem for individuals – whether the source of stress is work-related or not. More recently there has been a move to see organisations as shaping this responsibility. The final section will consider how stress and its impact have been tackled.

Managing the effects of stress
Individually-based interactions

The experience of stress at work might be described as a 'psycho-social hazard' in contrast to more common work-based hazards of a physical, chemical or biological nature. Even though there has been an increasing awareness of the organisation's contribution and responsibility for stress at work, the majority of work-based initiatives still turn upon improving the ability of the individual to cope. This remains the case despite criticisms of such approaches as addressing the symptoms rather than the cause.

Individually-based approaches essentially involve training in techniques which enable employees to respond more positively to the stressors they encounter. The techniques most frequently used are:

- relaxation (muscular relaxation);
- biofeedback (helping the individual to develop self-control over physiological activities);
- coping strategies (problem-focused v. emotion-focused);
- counselling.

A number of research studies have attempted to demonstrate the efficiency of those approaches. Murphy and Sorenson (1988) compared workers trained in biofeedback with a group trained in muscle relaxation, and with controls on a range of outcomes including absenteeism, performance ratings, equipment accidents and job-related injuries. Multivariate analysis indicated small but statistically significant effects on absenteeism of muscle relaxation, but no other significant relationships. As in many such studies, groups were small (17 and 21 in the respective groups, and self-selected. Ingledew *et al.* (in press) examined the behaviour of psychiatric workers facing redundancy. They report that use of coping strategies (problem- and emotion-focused) did have some impact on mediating the stressors, whilst avoidance behaviour had a deleterious affect.

The majority of studies of individual programmes tend to report small but positive effects. However, the methodological quality of the studies is very variable with many of the studies exhibiting the following faults to varying degrees:

- subject selection bias (virtually all subjects are volunteers and very few studies report drop out rates);

- lack of control groups;

- lack of adequate follow-up;

- lack of standardisation of the method and quality of support given;

- lack of standardisation of outcome measures;

- small groups;

- lack of assessment of specific approaches (there is a tendency to use different approaches simultaneously).

While such weaknesses make firm conclusions difficult, individually-based programmes have a role – not least because they are minimally disruptive to work, are generally popular and can contribute to problems outside the workplace. However, increasingly there is a concern to focus stress reduction initiatives upon the organisation rather than the individual.

Organisational interventions

One of the main strands of thought here is that of increased employee participation in decision-making. This builds upon the notion of control and influence over events being critical to perceptions of stress factors (Karasek 1979). Jackson (1983) reported that such participation increased feelings of control but did not translate into a sustained reduction in emotional distress. However, positive outcomes for participation approaches are by no means universal.

Wall and Clegg (1981) in a well designed study, demonstrated that well managed job redesign (emphasising greater job autonomy) was associated with improvements in employee well-being. Moos *et al.* (1987) have studied a range of workplaces in terms of the interplay between the actual events and qualities of the organisation and the individuals, values and beliefs. He argues that the work environment can be organised into three underlying dimensions:

1 the relationship between employees;

2 goal orientation which includes factors such as autonomy, task orientation and work pressure;

3 system maintenance and change, which refers to the amount of structure, clarity and openness to change.

Using a scale to measure these variables with a group of health workers, he demonstrated that a problem-solving session narrowed the gap between the actual environment and the preferred work environment. Schweiger and De Nisi (1991) examined the effects of communication during a proposed merger. The negative effects of the merger – measured in terms of perceived uncertainty, stress, job satisfaction, organisational commitment, intention to leave, work performance and absenteeism – occurred in both of the organisations studied, but were markedly reduced in the plant which experienced the communication programme, both immediately after the merger and four months later.

The evidence on organisational interventions is not large but what does exist suggests they can be effective. However, they are rather more difficult to implement than individually-based approaches and require a high degree of commitment at all levels of the organisation.

The key issue would appear to be a change in the corporate mind of organisations to recognise:

1 stress that affects individuals leads to negative and costly consequences;

2 organisations have a responsibility to deal with the sources of such stress.

This change in approach might be classified as seeking to become healthy as opposed to unhealthy organisations. The 'hard' edge of healthy organisations is that through reducing the impact of stress, the associated negative costs are reduced and performance level enhanced. At the 'soft' level the organisation also needs to commit to maintaining the good health of its staff and providing a collaborative and supportive environment. An unhealthy organisation will experience:

(a) mortality – high levels of disruptive turnover;

(b) morbidity – uncooperative, unmotivated staff;

(c) higher costs – repairing and replacing the impact of (a) and (b).

As Sutherland (1990) argues, the requirement is to make explicit the link between healthy, non-stressed staff, the reduced cost of maintaining good health and the increased productivity of non-stressed individuals. Acceptance of this model may well provide the impetus for more organisationally-based approaches to stress which would appear to offer the most fruitful approach to managing the impact of stress in the future.

References

Barton, J, Spelten, E, Totterdell, P, Smith, L, Folkard, S and Costa, G (1995) The standard shiftwork index; a battery of questionnaires for assessing shiftwork related problems. *Work & Stress* **9**, 4–31

Beehr, M and Newman, A (1978) Job stress employee health and organisational effectiveness: a facet analysis, model and literature review *Personnel Psychology*: 31, 665–699

Blaney, PH (1985) Stress and depression in adults: a critical review, In Field, TM, McCabe, PH and Schmiedeman, N (eds) *Stress & Coping* Earlbaum, New Jersey

Brief, AP, Sculer, RS and Van Self, MC (1981) *Managing job stress* Little Brown, Boston

Briner, RB (1994) *Stress as a trivial concept and modern myth: some alternative approaches to stress phenomena* British Psychological Conference, Brighton

British Medical Association (1992) *Stress and the medical profession* Chameleon Press, London

Caplan, RD, Cobb, S and French, JRP (1975), *Job demands and workers health* US Govt Printing Office, US Dept of Health, Education & Welfare, Washington DC

Carver, CM, Scherer, J and Weinstrab, J (1989) Assessing coping strategies: a theoretical based approach *Journal of Personality & Social Psychology* **56**, 267–283

Chambers, R, Wall, D and Campbell, I (1996) Stresses, coping mechanisms and job satisfaction in general practitioner registrars *British Journal of General Practice* **46**, 343–348

Chan, KB (1977) Individual differences in reactions to stress and their personality and situation determinants *Social Science & Medicine* **11**, 89–103

Cooper, CL, Davies-Cooper, RF and Faragher, EB (1986) A prospective study of the relationship between breast cancer and life events, type A behaviour, social support and coping skills *Stress Medicine* **2**, 271–277

Cox, TC (1978) *Stress* Macmillan, London

Evans, P, Clow, A and Hucklebridge, F (1997) Stress and the immune system *The Psychologist* July 1997, 303–307

Fleming, R, Baum, A and Singer, JE (1984) Towards an integrative approach to the study of stress *Journal of Personality & Social Psychology* **46**, 939–949

Freudenger, HJ (1984) Staff burn-out *Journal of Social Issues* 30: 159–65

Friedman, M and Rosenman, RH (1959) Association of specific overt behaviour patterns of blood and cardio-vascular findings *Journal of American Medical Association* **169**, 1286–1296

Furnham, A (1997) *The psychology of behaviour at work: the individual in the organisation* Psychology Press, Guildford

George, J (1990) Why stress is a management issue *Health Manpower Management* December 1990, 11–16

Guardian Financial Services (1996) *Stress soars in the healthcare and pharmaceutical industry, causing sickness among staff* Guardian Royal Exchange Group, London

Hall, DT and Hall, FS (1980) Stress and the two career couple, In Cooper, CL and Payne, P (eds) *Current cancers in occupational stress* Wiley, New York

Handy, JA (1988) Theoretical & methodological problems within occupational stress & burnout research *Human Relations* 41, 351–369

Haynes, C and Jackson, P (1995) *Management styles, social support & mental health in the NHS* British Psychological Society, Lancaster University

Haynes, SG, Feinlieb, M and Eaker, ED (1981) Type A behaviour and the ten year incidence of coronary heart disease in the Framingham heart study, In Rosenman, RH (ed) *Psychosomatic risk factors and coronary heart disease: indication for specific preventative therapy:* Hans Huber, Berne

Health Education Authority (1994) Health at work in the NHS *Working well: a guide to success* HEA, London

Herbert, TB and Cohen, S (1993) Stress and immunity in humans: a meta-analytic review *Psychosomatic Medicine* 55, 364–379

Hingley, P, Cooper, CL and Harris, P (1986) *Stress in nurse managers* King's Fund Centre, London

Hobfall, S (1989) *The ecology of stress* Hemisphere, New York

Ingledew, DK, Hardy, L and Cooper, CL (1997) Do resources bolster coping and does coping buffer stress? An organisational study with longitudinal aspect and control for negative effectivity *Journal of Occupational Health Psychology* Vol 2 No 2 pp. 118–133

Ivancevich, JM and Matteson, MT (1980) *Stress at work* Scott Forestman, Glenview, IL

Jackson, SE (1983) Participation in decision making as a strategy for reducing job-related strain *Journal of Applied Psychology* 68, 3–19

Johnston, DW, Cook, DG and Shaper, AG (1987) *Type A behaviour and ischaemic heart disease in middle aged British men* Society of Behavioural Medicine, Washington DC

Kahn, RL (1964) *Role stress: studies in role conflict & ambiguity* John Wiley, New York

Karasek, RA (1979) Job demands, job decision latitude & mental strain: implications for job redesign *Administrative Science Quarterly* 24, 285–308

Kasl, S and Cooper, CL (1987) *Stress & health issues in research methodology* John Wiley, New York

Kobasa, S (1989) Stressful life events, personality, health; an enquiry into hardiness *Journal of Personality and Social Psychology* 37, 114–128

Landsbergis, PA (1988) Occupational stress among health care workers, a test of the job demands – control model *Journal of Organisational Behaviour* 9, 217–239

Litwinenko, A and Cooper, CL (1995) The impact of trust status on health care workers *Journal of Managerial Psychology* 10, 12–16

Margolis, B, Kroes, W and Quinn, R (1974) Job stress an unlisted occupational hazard *Journal of Occupational Medicine* 1(16) 659–61

Mavtocchio, JJ and O'Leary, AM (1989) Sex differences in occupational stress: a meta analytic review *Journal of American Psychology* 74, 495–501

McGrath, JE (1976) Stress & behaviour in organisations, in Dunnette, MD (ed.) *Handbook of Industrial & Organisational Psychology* John Wiley, New York

Moos, RH and Schaeffer, JA (1987) Evaluating health care work settings: A holistic conceptual framework *Psychology & Health* **1**, 97–122

Murphy, LR and Sorenson, S (1988) Employee behaviour before and after stress management *Journal of Occupational Behaviour* **9**, 173–182

Newton, TJ (1989) Occupational stress & coping with stress: a critique *Human Relations* **42**, 441–461

Osipow, SH, Doty, RE and Spokame, AR (1985) Occupational stress, strain & coping across the life span *Journal of Vocational Behaviour* **27**, 98–108

Paffenbarger, RS, Wolf, PA and Notkin, J (1966) Chronic disease in former college students *American Journal of Epidemiology* **83**, 314–328

Payne, R (1988) Individual differences in the study of occupational stress, In Cooper, CL and Payne, R (eds) *Causes, coping and consequences of stress of work* John Wiley, Chichester

Payne, R and Firth-Cozens, J (1987) *Stress in health professionals* John Wiley & Sons, Chichester

Perrewe, PL and Ganster, PC (1989) The impact of job demands and behavioural control on experienced job stress *Journal of Occupational Behaviour* **10**, 213–229

Pollock, K (1988) On the nature of social stress: production of a modern mythology *Social Science & Medicine* **26**, 381–392

Quick, JC and Quick, JD (1984) *Organisational Stress & Preventive Management* McGraw-Hill, New York

Schuler, R (1980) Definition and conceptualisation of stress in organisations *Organisational Behaviour and Human Performance* 24:115–130

Schweiger, DM and De Nisi, AA (1991) Communication with employees following a merger a longitudinal field experiment *Academy of Management Journal* **34**, 110–135

Seligman, M and Schulman, P (1980) Explanatory style as a predictor of productivity and quitting among life insurance agents *Journal of Personality & Social Psychology* **48**, 832–840

Selye, H (1976) *The stress of life* McGraw-Hill, New York

Spurgeon, P, Barwell, F and Maxwell, R (1995) Types of Work Stress and Implications fot the role of General Practitioners Health Services Management Research 8(3), 186–197

Sutherland, V (1990) Managing stress at the worksite, In Bennett, P, Weinman, J and Spurgeon, P (eds) *Current developments in health psychology* Harwood Academic Press, London

Thornton, PI (1992) The relation of coping, appraisal & burnout in mental health workers *The Journal of Psychology* **123**, 261–271

Wall, TD and Clegg, CW (1981) A longitudinal field study of group work redesign *Journal of Occupational Behaviour* **2**, 31–49

Warr, P (1992) Job features & excessive stress, In Jenkins, R and Coney, N (eds) *Prevention of mental ill-health at work* HSMO, London

13 Future patterns of primary health care

Jonathan Shapiro

The notion of primary health care has served the National Health Service well, but it may now be reaching the end of its useful life. In this chapter, we will briefly describe the history of primary care since 1948, review the current developments in the area, and consider what the future has to hold. In following this path, we shall be able to see why the whole concept is now being called into question, and what sort of NHS is likely to emerge if there is radical change to the way in which services are delivered.

Origins

Primary care is so called because it marks the primary point of contact with the health service. Illness has been defined by the World Health Organisation as an absence of well-being in either a physical, social or psychological sense (WHO 1978); the vast majority of people who perceive themselves to be ill will either treat themselves, will consult their family, informal networks (friends, work colleagues, and so on), or will seek help directly from commercial agencies such as community pharmacists. In the United Kingdom, only about 10 per cent of 'ill' people will seek formal medical assistance from the NHS, and in 90 per cent of these cases, they will access such help through their general practitioner, who is thus contracted to deliver 'primary health care'. These days primary and community care is provided in a much more multidisciplinary manner than it was in 1948, but in the next few paragraphs, we shall be referring mainly to the GPs when we consider the origins and progress of primary care in the NHS.

The role of the GP

Precisely what was originally contained in primary care in 1948 was never defined; in practice, it consisted of the care which a GP felt competent to deliver, and it was up to that GP to decide his or her own levels of competence in any particular areas. Whilst such a definition seems very woolly in today's climate of measurement and visible accountability, it was originally applied in days when professionals (of whatever occupation) were trusted to do their best for their clients, and when self regulation was considered adequate control over clinical standards.

In reality, GPs in those early days of the NHS were less likely to be vocationally inclined towards community work, than to be doctors unable to gain employment as hospital specialists. The prestige jobs were perceived as those within the walls of the hospital, and those where specialised knowledge ruled. In the words of the street saying, 'those who could, did; and those who couldn't, did general practice'.

So the hapless GPs saw the hordes of patients who presented at their doors, did what they could for them, and referred onto hospital those patients whose illnesses exceeded the limits of their self-perceived medical capability. Since most illnesses which presented to the GPs were (and still are) either self-limiting, amenable to reassurance and advice, or remediable by straightforward medical therapy, the doctor came to be an effective filter, dealing with the 'simple' illnesses, and passing the 'complex' diseases to the 'real' doctors.

Such a reductionist approach is, of course, only applicable to straightforward physical disease, such as trauma or appendicitis; it makes sweeping assumptions about the nature of illness, and does not take into account any of the complex links between the physical and psychosocial aspects of disease. This has always been a common preconception which has, if anything, become more marked in recent years. Be that as it may, the notion of having GPs controlling access to hospitals came to be seen as offering many advantages to the health service:

1 First, it meant that scarce hospital resources could be used more rationally and effectively. Then, as now, hospitals were limited in their capacity; the supply of services (beds, operations, nurses) is the limiting step to their activity, whereas general practice has always had to be geared up to deal with demand, with no such luxury as waiting lists. Having built-in triage in this way was a priceless asset, now being copied by most other health services in the developed world.

2 Moreover, and this is the second advantage, those carrying out the triage also provided most of the services. As we have already noted, only 10 per cent or so of the patients who enter the medical system pass onto the hospital, and so the person doing the triage is also able to deal with the patients not referred onwards.

3 Third, such a system provides patients with somebody to act as an 'interpreter' of the medical labyrinth; GPs, with their broad base of general medical knowledge, and (usually) a grasp of communication skills, could help their patients understand what was happening to them, keep them informed, and enable them to make more informed choices than they might otherwise be able to do. Whether this was in choice of specialist clinician, or an interpretation of a hospital letter, or in filling in an application for a new truss, capable GPs had a useful and powerful role as their patients' guides.

4　The final advantage offered by this 'gatekeeping' approach to health services is that GPs have developed a role as co-ordinators of their patients' care. In some health services, patients direct themselves to the specialists of their choice, and there is no single point of co-ordination for care. Thus, investigations may be repeated, channels of communication between clinicians not used effectively, and inappropriate consultants used to deliver care. In the British system (in theory, at least), it is the GP who makes the referrals, links the decisions, and acts as the linchpin of the system. The notion of care management is much discussed these days as a mechanism to make best use of resources, but informally it has always been a part of the NHS.

GPs' position in the NHS

Before we move onto the current picture of primary care in the NHS, it is worth briefly mentioning the manner in which GPs were originally employed and their relationship with the service. In the earlier days of the NHS, GPs were paid largely for *being*, as opposed to gaining remuneration for *doing* lots of things. They were given a relatively small capitation fee for each patient registered on their 'list' (which mounted up to about half their total salary), and a number of allowances for age, seniority, and so on. There were also a number of regulations which governed their employment of staff, purchase of equipment, use of premises, etc.

There were relatively few 'items of service', although exceptions included night visits, supply of contraceptive advice, maternity care, and so on, but in total they contributed comparatively little to the GPs' incomes.

This made for a primary care sector which was relatively cheap and predicable for a Government to fund, and which created no perverse incentives for unnecessary extra activity by the doctors. However, there was a risk that the system might encourage some lazy doctors, who received their income whatever happened to their patients.

As far as employment is concerned, GPs have always sat slightly awkwardly in the NHS, since they are self-employed entrepreneurs who happen to have a contract with the health service. The original medical negotiators who worked with the post-war Labour Government to create the NHS gained a unique dispensation, so that GPs (but no other NHS doctors) are not actually employed by the NHS, and are therefore entitled to do other work in addition to their work for the health service; they also have a particularly advantageous tax status.

Prelude to the present

If the system described above was apparently so effective, why has it been changed? Where were the problems, and how have they been addressed? From a general practice perspective, there were two main problems, each recognised at different times: the first concerned general practice itself; while the second involved the wider health service.

As we have already discussed, general practice in its early days was not held in particularly high regard, nor did it generally attract the cream of medical graduates. As time went on, the problems of quality in general practice, and of the recruitment and retention of GPs, became more and more severe; working conditions were not good, payment was considerably below that of hospital doctors, and the job itself was perceived as being unrewarding and dull. The foundation of the Royal College of General Practitioners in the 1950s was driven at least partially by the desire to improve these aspects of the profession, and to improve the standing of general practice, and this campaign culminated in the so called 'GP Charter' of 1966.

This document changed some of the terms and conditions of service for GPs, altered their standing in the medical hierarchy by encouraging a more vocational approach to general practice, and in so doing signalled the rebirth of the whole concept of primary care. The rise of practice nursing, for instance, can be traced back to this time, and the improvement in the calibre of recruits to the speciality. Progress continued with the introduction of vocational training, voluntary in its early stages, but made compulsory by Act of Parliament in 1981. General practice was now recognised as a speciality in its own right, and the independence and lack of constraints placed on the way GPs practised made it the speciality of choice for the following decade.

Within the wider NHS, there were other problems, many of which will have been discussed elsewhere in this book. From the primary care perspective, they can be summed up in three points:

- Hospital activity was rising inexorably, and with it the costs of treatment
- New technologies were accelerating the rate of increase of those costs
- Community services were being starved of resources to feed the acute sector

These tensions were shown in the inexorable rise of waiting lists, an informal and unaccountable means of health care rationing used across the country, and one which tended to affect the more disadvantaged areas of society, particularly those without a public voice or the money to obtain treatments privately.

The 1990 changes to the health service

Combine these issues, catalysed by a political imperative (fed by pictures of children dying in hospital before they could obtain treatment) to demonstrate progress, and a Government always keen to apply market principles, and the origins of the 1990 reforms can begin to be seen. Add to the brew the increasingly consumerist attitudes of society generally, and the potential power of the GPs' hospital gatekeeping role, and the picture of the reforms emerges almost fully fledged. Put simply, the 1990 *Working for Patients* (DoH 1990) changes can be summed up as follows:

1 The procurement of services for patients was separated from their provision. This 'purchaser–provider split' was intended to prevent confusions of interest, or collusion between those who paid for services (who were now to think purely about the needs of their local population) and those who provided services, who could concentrate on providing the maximum amount of high quality care at the lowest price.

2 Large provider organisations were to become self-governing, autonomous trusts, each of which was intended to be self-financing, and able to respond to the needs of its local purchasers. By and large, trusts were divided into those which delivered acute and those which delivered community services, although there were a few trusts which combined both. In addition, services for mentally ill people and people with learning difficulties were delivered by trusts specialising in these areas (although again, there were a few which combined these with other services).

3 Trusts were to be funded on the basis of the work they actually did, rather than on an historical precedent; the 'money should follow the patient'.

4 Cognisance was to be taken of the fact that it was the GPs' referrals which largely determined how many patients (and hence how much business) reached each Trust. The creation of GP Fundholders, with the power to purchase certain services for their patients directly from trusts, without the intervention of Health Authorities, was intended to link the four advantages of general practice (triage, provision, interpretation and co-ordination) with the resources to implement them more effectively.

5 The manner in which GPs as providers related to their purchasers was to change; their contract would no longer be administered merely by means of rules and regulations, it would be managed, with purchasers having discretion over the manner in which resources were to be allocated, and practice performance managed.

GPs in purchasing

Let us focus more closely on these last two changes: the introduction of fundholding explicitly took account of the mixed role of GPs as providers of some services, and procurers of others. It was intended to give GPs considerable executive flexibility in the way that they obtained services from their providers, and in this way persuade trusts that they had to be responsive, or risk losing their 'business'. It was intended to provide incentives to GPs to treat more patients at their practices, and refer fewer to hospitals. It was perhaps also intended to provide a goad to the Health Authorities to be more assertive in their purchasing.

While the services covered initially were limited, and the list size required for fundholding relatively large, over time the range of services has expanded to cover virtually all routine hospital and community referrals and procedures, for list sizes down to 5,000 patients. Community Fundholding, introduced in 1996, was applied to lists as low as 3,000, but for a narrower range of community-based services.

In principle, these ideas sounded fine, and the move away from the rigidity of a tightly administered bureaucracy to a more flexible managed system was very attractive. Over the following six years, the theory was progressively turned into practice, and the strengths and weaknesses of the new 'managed market' were able to be assessed.

On the positive side, there is no doubt that cultural attitudes have changed enormously; clinicians of all sorts, whether they be GPs (fundholding and non-fundholding), hospital consultants, or paramedics, are all much more resource conscious. In the early days, there was resentment amongst many non-fundholding GPs about the fact that they were being forced to think in terms of the costs of services, and about making choices for their patients. As time has gone on, it has become normal to think in those terms, to consider the implications of clinical actions beyond the immediate 'I want to do the best for my patients', and it is those who refuse to do so who are now the exceptions.

This culture has also percolated through to the hospitals, where dynamic trusts have encouraged their consultants to 'market' themselves and their services to the local GPs, in an attempt to generate more referrals and hence more income. It seems to have had less impact on consultants' ability to make prioritising decisions about which patients to treat or what treatments to use.

In service terms, the GPs' new found ability directly to influence other providers' services has shown itself mainly in the movement of community-based service contracts (physiotherapy, community nursing, chiropody etc.). In the first few years of fundholding, community trusts were often reluctant to modify the way in which they delivered their services (to make them more practice based, for instance), and the more assertive fundholders used their muscle to set a precedent by moving their contracts from one trust to another.

Where this had been done once, it was often easier to negotiate with the trusts, and many contracts were moved back to the original providers at the next contracting round. Clinical staff who were actually delivering the services rarely changed, it was the managerial arrangements around them which were modified. Once the principle of contestability was established, then the threat of a contract move was often all that was required to gain provider compliance. This idea worked fairly well for community services where there was a choice of providers, but was much harder to implement where there was a monopoly provider (and hence a dearth of choice) or for acute services where trusts were often able to ignore fundholding GPs: the total contract values for all local fundholding practices often amounted to a small fraction of the total trust turnover, which was itself split among many tiny contracts whose contradictory effects often cancelled each other out.

In addition, GPs generally did not seem to have strong opinions about services beyond their immediate horizons; most fundholders tried to influence community services, which directly affected their practices, but fewer were keen to change the nature of services in acute hospitals, which had less obvious effects within their practices. They were happy either to accept the service *status quo*, perhaps modifying a price or quantity detail, or they focused on waiting times for their patients. There are relatively few examples of fundholding GPs trying to change the nature of a service offered by their local acute trust, or of introducing a new one at their behest. The exception to this rule is in the introduction of hospital out-reach clinics, at which hospital consultants saw GP referred patients in a practice setting, often more quickly than they would have been seen at a hospital clinic.

Outreach clinics highlight the key shortcoming of the fundholding system, its inequities. GP fundholders generally appeared in the more prosperous areas of the country, where health care needs were known objectively to be lower than average, but where current funding for ser-vices (historically based) was higher than average; they catered for middle class patients, many of whom had private health insurance to augment weaknesses in the NHS, and they sought differential services for their patients at the expense of others in the system.

The counter argument to this was that such differentiation provided the stimulus for others to catch up (the 'levelling up' approach), and there is some evidence for this: Health Authorities have followed fundholders in encouraging outreach work, and in modifying trust contracts more assertively, but the issue of funding remains, and will only be overcome by a move to some form of nationally recognised health care needs-based capitation formula (not a popular option with those fundholders who stand to lose funding). Thus, doubts still persisted about the equitable provision of resources, as well as misgivings about the cost:benefit ratio of fundholding. With a management allowance of nearly £40,000 per fund-holding practice, extra investment in information technology, and addi-tional management capacity needed at Health Authorities, studies such as those from the Audit Commission (1996) suggested that the degree of change or service improvement to have emerged as a result of fundholding may not have been worth the investment in it. Having said that, it is clear that such studies have concentrated largely on measurable service changes, and may not have taken enough note of the cultural changes which have taken place throughout the NHS as a consequence of fundholding.

Whatever the misgivings, the notion of GP led purchasing grew during the 1990s, and fundholding developed to encompass examples of total purchasing, whereby GPs held a budget for all hospital and community services (rather than selected ones), as well as the simpler community fundholding.

In parallel, other models of GP involvement developed, some simulat-ing fundholding, and others working more in the planning and strategy areas. Locality purchasing (in which Health Authorities worked with groups of practices to develop a more population based approach to GP based purchasing) tends towards the former, whilst GP commissioning, whereby GPs have a significant input (it varies between Health Authority areas) into the service planning intentions of the Health Authority, is a strong move towards the latter.

Despite the new White Paper on the NHS, published in December 1997, the future of GP based procurement is slightly uncertain; the new Government's rhetoric still maintains the centrality of general practice (and indeed, could not do otherwise without a complete overhaul of the way in which patients access hospital services) but there is a feeling that the focus of attention has moved, and that co-ordination if not control of major service reconfiguration may revert to Health Authorities, whilst GPs and community trusts work hard to reshape the nature of primary and community care, with a varying input to the major commissioning divisions.

GPs as providers

The 'new contract' of 1990 also affected all GPs in their provider capacity, and further developments since then have emphasised the changing nature of GPs' relations with the NHS. First, although GPs have retained their 'independent contractor' status, they now have much stricter terms and conditions of service laid down: surgery times and services have to be explicitly stated; funding for staff and premises is now cash limited, and so its distribution is in the gift of the Health Authorities; prescribing patterns are monitored closely; and an increasing focus is being put on the place of evidence in medical decision making.

In general, it feels as if the whole of general practice is being increasingly scrutinised, and needs to justify itself more explicitly. Whilst there is nothing wrong with this in principle, it is worth remembering that decisions in such a complex area of work often depend on an enormous number of variables, each difficult to pin down precisely, and that the GPs on whom the system depends are still fiercely independent. There are always risks in trying to turn an inexact art with some logic, into an exact science with answers to everything, and the risks grow if one tries forcibly to corral self driven professionals in a direction which feels wrong to them.

Those Health Authorities which have tried to impose a performance management framework onto their GPs have found the task painful and unproductive; none of us likes suddenly to be measured in areas in which we feel competent. Those authorities which are succeeding in developing performance management for the provision of primary care are doing so by working in conjunction with the GPs, and linking measurement to new activity, new accreditation, and new incentives. In those circumstances, the GPs have been very receptive to new ideas.

This is clearly vital, since the nature of the services which are delivered at a general practice level has been changing quite radically, and there is a risk that changes may occur on an *ad hoc* basis if performance management is not built in. Services which would have required a referral a few years ago are now being carried out routinely in general practice, by GPs, their employed staff and the wider 'primary health care team' (including in the best examples both practice employed staff and practice attached clinical staff such as district nurses, midwives, health visitors, community psychiatric nurses and even social workers). Diseases such as hypertension, diabetes and ischaemic heart disease are often assessed and treated entirely in a practice setting, and even physical interventions such as gastroscopies, vasectomies and simple lumpectomies are carried out without reference to any other organisation. With the introduction of ever more effective drugs and of cheaper 'near patient' equipment and procedures, this evolution in role looks set to continue, if not to accelerate.

The preceding paragraphs suggest that the provision of general practice and procurement from general practice are two disparate activities which may easily be considered separately, but this is patently not so. Not only do the boundaries between the two depend on external variables such as the type of patient, type of illness, and the local availability of services, but it also varies with the doctor's skills and interests, and even with the time of day and doctor's degree of ennui.

Is there any way then that the two may be linked, and the overall performance of the practice or doctor be assessed? This is an important question in the current development of the NHS, and may be the key to its future progress. Before we address it, we shall briefly consider the function of community Trusts, and the way in which they fit into the NHS community.

Community trusts

Community trusts were created as part of the 1990 reforms, and are intended to provide all community services in the NHS apart from those provided by general practitioners (medical, dental, optometric and pharmacist), mental health trusts, trusts for people with learning difficulties, and a few specialised 'high tech' services. In most cases, they stand alone, rather than existing in combination with a provider of other services.

In particular, there are few combined community and acute service trusts; while the 'seamlessness' of such an arrangement is appealing, and it would appear that patients would be able to obtain all their institutional services from one organisation, in reality the financial and political pressures put on acute hospitals usually mean that resources get sucked out of the less visible, less contentious community sector. Even when community trusts exist on their own, they are generally less well funded, and carry less 'clout' than their acute cousins. Such organisational boundaries, such grit in the machinery, such obstacles to flexibility, are apparently necessary to prevent organisational imperialism from occurring. What a sad reflection that is on the conflict between service needs and organisational politics.

Within community trusts, it is usually the paramedical clinical specialities which predominate; community nursing (district nurses, health visitors, and community midwives in some cases, but not practice nurses), and the 'therapies' (physiotherapy, occupational therapy, speech and language therapy and chiropody).

In addition, there are various combinations of community dental services, paediatric health services, services for the elderly, and so on, which may or may not employ medically qualified staff. Indeed, some community trusts have acute beds, accident units, and technical procedures to rival many a district general hospital.

Community trusts have largely been seen as augmenting the services offered by general practice, either by providing support (as for the community nurses), or by offering a safety net to cover gaps in the general practice network (as in paediatric surveillance services). In addition, their potential management capacity is only now beginning to be recognised. The average community trust is vastly larger than a general practice, and is therefore able to offer able to offer an economy of scale in financial, organisational and service terms which could never be obtained at a single practice level.

Thus, staff employment, provision of specialist nursing services, management support in areas such as training and human resource development, and financial risk management could all potentially be carried out at a trust level, with financial as well as clinical benefit to the whole system. This idea does not obviate the need for general practice itself, whose small and disparate organisational nature brings a local sensitivity and flexibility which would be difficult to match at a larger level. The knack would seem to be to combine these separate features in a way which maximises the benefit of both, whilst minimising the costs (financial, clinical, and human).

Despite such an optimistic scenario, the position of community trusts, sandwiched between general practice and the acute sector, seems to sit uncomfortably with many of them; rather than seeing themselves as the bridge between the two sectors, with the potential to expand in either direction, the more passive of the community trusts feel that they are being squeezed out between the rock of growing general practice and the hard place of outreaching acute trusts. This is a pity, since the potential reconfigurations in the NHS over the next few years are likely to benefit flexible, proactive, community based organisations.

The 1997 Primary Care Act

The NHS is an organic organisation, and is never static. Since the 1990 *Working for Patients* reforms, there has been a steady progression of further changes, and an increasing focus on the role of primary care in the system. More GPs have become involved in the procurement of services from other agencies; Health Authorities have begun to incorporate GPs into their planning and commissioning processes; alliances have sprung up between practices, initially on fundholding/non-fundholding lines, but latterly beginning to ignore some of this demarcation; and trusts (particularly community trusts) have begun to work much more closely with their local GPs.

Such iterative progress was encapsulated in the 1997 *Primary Care Act* (DoH 1997), which was passed in March 1997, with cross party support, as one of the last Acts of the old parliament. The Act sought to explore some of the remaining organisational barriers within the NHS, and to offer ways of experimenting with service provision in a relatively 'safe' way. In particular, it encouraged GPs to work in new ways, outside the confines of the existing paradigms. When it appeared in March 1997, the Act suggested that GPs could be salaried, and not always be self-employed; it offered trusts the option of offering traditional general practice, perhaps in competition with GPs; it gave GPs the opportunity to control the entire health service budget for their local population (and not just the hospital element, as is the case in any of the fundholding models); and it looked at models of contract which did not depend on national agreements, but gave patients the chance to 'sign on' with an organisation, rather than an individual GP.

It offered a 'facilitative framework' for all these developments, and impressed observers by its contrast with the bombastic tone of the 1990 Act, full of directives and certainties, with no room for questioning or genuine experimentation. For all that, the new Act was probably no less radical than its earlier counterpart, although some of it edges have been honed off by the change of Government in May 1997. At the time of writing, the experiments in provision of community services look set to run, but those which encompass a combination of all funding streams at a practice or locality level have been deferred and now look set to be incorporated into some of the changes mooted in the new White Paper *The new NHS: modern, dependable.*

Future scenarios

We have seen how the nature of primary care provision has changed over the years, and how the gatekeeping function has been formalised. We have also discussed some of the problems which still beset both these roles, in terms of costs, equity and effectiveness. On this last, we have noted that the purchaser–provider split has worked well where fundholders and community trusts are concerned, but has had little impact on the way in which acute services are provided. Even Health Authority purchasing, with its enormous potential leverage, has not been able radically to alter the way large acute service trusts, with their vast fixed overhead costs and degree of political leverage, and this may be seen as the major failure of the 1990 health service changes.

It may be that GP Fundholders should have been given more freedom to be even more iconoclastic; it may be that the market should have been allowed to work more naturally, with less central protection; or it may be that the generation of large institutional change requires more central management, that tiny little dinghies can never influence the course of a large liner, which requires powerful tug boats and a confident pilot.

Suffice it to say that the change of Government that took place in May 1997 has allowed a stocktaking process to take place, which looks set to lead to a change in direction.

The New NHS: modern, dependable

The newest White Paper (published in December 1997) introduced a number of important changes to the concepts of primary care. First, on the provision side, the distinction between general practice and community trusts will get more and more blurred. There is a recognition that members of the primary health care team need a common physical base, and that it makes sense to have it at a local level, where it is most accessible to patients. Thus, the practice is emerging as a common denominator, not only for community trust and general practice employed staff, but also for others such as community psychiatric nurses and social workers, and this trend looks set to continue. Conversely, there is also a realisation that economies of scale may be beneficial for some functions. Thus, those more mechanical operations such as superannuation, payroll, discipline, sick leave cover, as well as the more specialised clinical activities (the stoma nurse, renal dialysis support, and so on) may well be provided more effectively through a larger organisation than a single practice. So we may begin to see practice nurses employed by the local community trust, and practices pooling resources to pay for a share of a specialist nurse.

The new White Paper encapsulates these notions in the idea of the Primary Care Group (PCG). Such groupings are seen to include a number of GP practices, covering geographically defined localities with populations of around 100,000 people. There is room in the definition for a range of models and population sizes, but the implication is that there will move over time towards the defined 'norms', probably coterminous with local authority boundaries of some sort.

The groups are seen at four different levels:

1. supporting the health authority in commissioning care for its population, acting in an advisory capacity;

2. taking devolved responsibility for a healthcare budget, as part of the health authority;

3. becoming established as freestanding bodies accountable to the health authority for commissioning care;

4. as 3. but with added responsibility for the provision of community health services for their covered population.

In all cases, the PCGs will continue to function as providers of traditional general medical services (ie general practice). What is not prescribed is the manner in which these separate activities will be delivered: the emphasis is on the **functions**, and not on the **form**.

As the boundaries begin to blur, so we will see GP practices working more closely with each other, and reinventing the functions of a community Trust themselves, thus obviating the need for such an organisation in their area; we may see them setting up and running services which mimic more and more the functions of a traditional community hospital, or even a small DGH. Conversely, we will begin to see community trusts move into the business of providing general practice itself. In some instances, particularly where it is difficult to recruit and retain high calibre independent doctors, it makes sense to provide a more structured environment, with premises, more clearly set hours and less administration to attract doctors into the area on a salaried basis. That model is unlikely to displace entirely the independent self-employed GP, since there advantages to both practice and NHS in having small, disparate, individualistic organisations working around the health service. They provide innovation and flexibility, as well as a level of service which would be far more expensive if it were bought any other way.

However, as a way of providing services in a deprived inner city, or where standards of existing services are poor, or in a newly developing area, such schemes have some clear merit.

Now we can begin to see why the term 'primary care' is beginning to look faded and irrelevant; when GPs run inpatient beds, and carry out their own operative procedures, the notion of 'first point of contact' becomes an inadequate definition of their activity, and a new term becomes necessary. As a term, 'community services' has its own connotations, and conjures up visions of elderly and social care; it may be that the newly coined phrase of 'personal medical services' (DoH 1997) fits the bill well, without any implication of organisational boundaries, but with its emphasis on care for people, and not just for diseases in abstraction.

The manner in which the original 1997 Primary Care Act is being enacted already allows the development of these models of providing primary and community care; by April 1998, all the different types of examples mentioned above were running somewhere in the UK, and each has some form of built in evaluation; the lessons learned from these pilots should then be ready to be disseminated to the rest of the service, and the evolution of personal medical services continued.

That Act, as it is being applied, does not allow for the full integration of hospital and community health services (HCHS) funds with general medical services (GMS) funds. These two separate funding streams each support a different part of the NHS, and help to prevent funds which should be used for GP type services being diverted to hospital activities, and vice versa.

Whilst such a 'ring fence' has obvious benefits, it has in recent years also prevented the development of new services, and the shift of resources from one sector to another. Suggestions have therefore been made in the new White Paper to end, or at least to loosen, this ring fence. Some of the pilots which were originally put forward included a complete abolition of the separation, and put all the NHS resources for the pilot area into the project, effectively giving GPs control of the entire service. The level 3 and 4 PCGs will have this capability; what remains is unclear is whether the GMS elements under their control will include GP's own salaries, or whether such an action would signal a move too far in the direction of commercial provision of NHS services.

As well as the risks entailed by trying to lan services for small populations, many GPs themselves have misgivings about finding their own pay out of this resource, particularly when resources are tight. The whole of health care is moving into a more fluid, less efined phase, in which organisations are beginning to be defined by their function, rather than by their structure, or the strengths of their vested inerests.

Fifty years of the NHS, and eight years experience of a quasi-market suggest that we have developed a set of soun underlying principles which can be carried forward into the newer modes of co-operation and collaboration replacing competition and the notion of 'market'. We want our system to offer universal access, in an equitale way, to services of consistent, high quality. It should subdivided into wo basic functions: the procurement of health services (by the NHS Executive, its outposts, and the Health Authorities, representing the needs of their patients), and the provision of care (by general practice, community trusts, secondary and tertiary care trusts, and all the other provider organisations).

We should not be too anxious about the precise way in which either group is configured, but we should insist that both groupings have a responsibility to deliver all care to their registered population. In addition, our guarded gateway between patients and expensive technical services seems to be effective, and should probably be preserved. Beyond this, all should be open and flexible; the days of structured solutions are over. Even if they can be made to work, society changes and its requirements of its health service change with it. Any structural solution will be out of date as soon as it is implemented, whereas a generic approach to services, whether based in the community or an institution, will be amenable to appropriate change. In the words of Tony Blair, 'Let us stick to ideals, and not to ideology.'

References

Audit Commission (1996) *What the doctor ordered: a study of GP fundholders in England and Wales* HMSO, London

Department of Health *Working for Patients* (1989) HMSO, London

Department of Health *Primary Care Act* (1997) HMSO, London

The New NHS: modern, dependable (1997) Secretary of State for Health, HMSO, London

World Health Organisation (1978) *Alama Ata declaration*

14 General practice: natural buildingblock for a population-focused NHS

Andrew Willis

Introduction

As the NHS celebrates its 50th birthday it is as if we have at last understood and accepted the vision of its creators. Until now, many within the service have smiled indulgently at Aneurin Bevan's idea that illness might actually be reduced by preventive measures. Others have argued vigorously that the interests of the individual patient should at all times reign supreme and not be influenced by the implications for others. The idea of 'clinical freedom' has been held as sacrosanct, allowing clinicians to do whatever they like, free of accountability to anyone.

However, to realise the founding vision of the NHS requires a more sophisticated approach. It requires recognition that it is a service where the intention is to provide the best possible care to every individual, while adopting the same approach to everyone else, working within the constraints of the available resources. That ideal is not contradictory but it does require compromise. As such it will appear heresy to some, but a moment of reflection can demonstrate how health economics and equity of access already play a part in everyday clinical practice. Why do doctors prescribe drugs generically? Why do they constrain the duration of an appointment when more time would be beneficial to a particular individual? Why do GPs not seek an urgent specialist appointment for every patient they refer to secondary care, or indeed for every patient who consults them? Why do consultant surgeons not operate personally on every single patient requiring surgery, as they might in elective private practice? The answers to such questions are all the same. The NHS is a population-based service founded on the concept of fairness and equity. Such an attitude recognises that resources are finite and that they must be used wisely in order to provide high quality services that are clinically effective, appropriate to the needs of local communities, and yet delivered efficiently and effectively according to individual clinical need. The differing weight given to these two aspects of the service helps explain the variety of opinions about its future development.

The introduction of a competitive, internal market in 1990 produced a direct contradiction of fairness and equity. The very function of a market is to use competition to raise quality and value to some consumers to the detriment of others. While the intentions to raise quality and sensitivity to the needs of patients were to be applauded the method and consequences were not. A logical justification for an internal market within health care would require the goal of equity to be sacrificed on the altar of crude economic efficiency. That would have proved unacceptable to the British people and was wisely denied at the time by the Prime Minister (Gilmour 1992). An unconstrained market economy is incompatible with the NHS as it is understood and valued by the public.

This chapter considers the further development of the NHS as a population-focused service consistent with its fundamental principles. It does so from the perspective of general practice and in ways that are compatible with the stated views of the Labour Government. It was written before this Government published its White Paper in December 1997.

What are we trying to achieve?

The development of UK health and social care should support relevant, fundamental values of our society. Unless we establish those values first, and let them be the foundations for our policies and plans, we are in danger of eroding aspects of our society that are cherished by the public.

The incoming Labour Government of 1997 lost no time in reaffirming its commitment to the central themes of the NHS, set out as broad aims by the 1979 Royal Commission (Merrison 1979):

- Equality of entitlement
- Provision of a broad range of services of a high standard
- A service that is free at the time of use
- A service that satisfies the reasonable expectations of its users
- A service that remains a national service responsive to local needs

These were really no more than a considered reaffirmation of the founding principles of the NHS set out in 1948. However, there are at least two reasons why the aims expressed by Merrison are central to any discussion of the future development of the NHS and the role to be played within it by General Practice. First, they describe the fundamental characteristics of an NHS that is, despite its limitations, a deeply rooted and highly valued part of British society. Second, they illustrate how the NHS is different from many other health care systems, notably those in the USA. The US has no pretensions of providing all its citizens with access to services according to relative clinical need, within a comprehensive system funded largely out of taxation and free at the point of delivery. Even Health Maintenance Organisations do not have such a broad remit for their focused, catchment-populations as does the NHS for its non-discretionary, resident ones.

The broad character of the NHS described by Merrison was endorsed by seven criteria defined by the new Secretary of State to be used to validate approaches for developing the service: the pursuit of fairness, efficiency, sensitivity, effectiveness, integration, flexibility and responsiveness (Dobson 1997).

These basic principles and validation criteria also find support amongst professional bodies. For example in 1994 the National Association of Commissioning GPs was formed with the singular purpose 'to promote and support the involvement of all GPs in the equitable commissioning of high quality care for their patients in the context of wider populations' (NACGP 1997). The important distinction made by NACGP between commissioning and purchasing is discussed later. Resolutions at the 1997 annual conferences of the Local Medical Committees and British Medical Association called for the application of equity within the NHS and implementation of the locality commissioning approach (LMC 1997, BMA 1997).

Some groups of GPs adopted similar aims even earlier. For example the Northampton GP Core Group had formed in April 1990 as a response to the White Paper *Working for Patients* (DoH 1989a) and was in effect a prodrome of GP Commissioning Groups (Willis 1992, Ham and Willis 1994). Since its inception the intentions of the Northampton Core Group have remained unchanged – to work with the Health Authority and local providers to strive for:

- effective, high-quality, cost-effective services sensitive to the needs of local communities;

- equitable resource allocation within local services;

- the most economical use of administrative resources, thereby maximising the funds available for direct patient care.

These aims are similar to those of an ever-increasing number of GP Commissioning Groups, of which there were at least 135 by mid-1997. They involved over 11,000 GPs covering 22 million patients (NACGP 1997). Although Commissioning Groups initially operated against the flow of Government policy they have seen other approaches steadily adopt many of their ideas, such as GPs coming together to work both together, and with the Health Authority concerning the totality of services.

Collectively, therefore, there has been a political and professional confirmation of the fundamental principles of the NHS as a fair, comprehensive and population-based public service available to all. It continues to aspire to the global, socialised medicine archetype of managed care described by an international conference in 1997 (Smith 1997). Set upon that foundation of principle, the overall task can be seen to be that of raising quality, effectiveness and cost-effectiveness while constraining growth in costs. General practice is well placed to take a pivotal role in those processes and act as the building block of a population-focused service.

The role of general practice

General practice already holds the key role of providing overall care to a registered list of patients. What is required now is a co-ordinated structure for effective general practice involvement in developing local services.

It should continue as the main provider of acute primary care, for within this is the gatekeeper, resource allocation role necessary for the co-ordinated care of Locality and District populations. For similar reasons it should also continue to offer preventive care services to its registered population, and the continuing management of chronic conditions. General practice is characterised by providing this amalgam of acute care, preventive care and chronic disease management for a population sufficiently small to support a personal service. In this way it addresses the twin objectives described earlier of personal and population-focused services. However, it is likely to operate under renewable contract as a provider of Primary Medical Services. It should be alive to the challenge from organisations such as Community Units and the private sector.

General practice will also take on a significant role in the planning of all local services at both practice and locality levels, and the review of those services as they are delivered. It will have an expanding function working across the interface with its patients concerning their self-help at home and their views about what they want and need from the local health service. Not only does that encourage self-reliance but it also facilitates effective use of resources. Furthermore, general practice will increasingly work with secondary care providers to develop efficient and effective clinical management pathways that cross the blurring primary–secondary care interface, as well as with Social Services concerning patient management across health and social care.

Finally, some practices will have a variable involvement in procurement under licence from the health authority. This should be voluntary.

What would help?

Key elements of future development are now considered.

An acceptance of nested populations

Planning and review should take place at the appropriate population size for the relevant service (Fig. 14.1). For example, this will clearly differ for planning a Health Visitor's Developmental Assessment Clinic for children (Practice), hip replacement surgery (Locality) and bone marrow transplants (District). Yet all three are inextricably related in terms of overall resource allocation; more of one means less of something else. Commissioning is concerned with making the critical decisions about the correct balance of services for given populations. Thus multi-level commissioning is not an optional luxury for the NHS but rather a central element of its development.

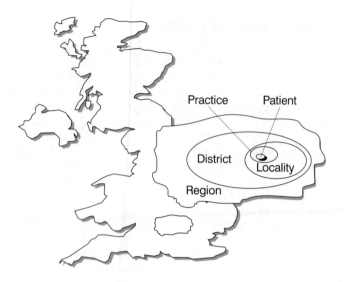

Figure 14.1 Nested populations

For many services the appropriate population will be greater than the size of a single practice and for this reason practice populations should aggregate to form appropriate localities. These will themselves be combined within health districts. The base currency of such groupings should usually be the lists of patients registered with individual general practices, rather than geographical areas such as districts or boroughs. Some statutory bodies will contest this assertion, but it is essential if health services are to be provided equitably. It is consistent with, and supported by, the precedent established by the fundholding scheme.

The distinction between planning, procurement, provision and review

Government policy and legislation since 1990 has recognised two processes in managing the NHS, those of purchasing and providing. Such thinking ignores the importance of planning and review to any generic model of service development (Fig. 14.2) That failure may come to be seen as the single greatest error in the Health Service changes of 1989/90. The following definitions have been used by the National Association of Commissioning GPs since 1994 and are implied throughout this chapter (NACGP 1997).

Commissioning
'The process of gathering and analysing the wants and needs of a population for which services are to be procured and of monitoring those services as they are delivered'.

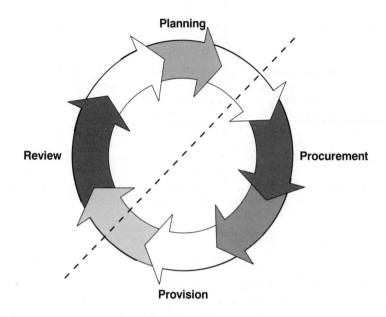

Figure 14.2 A generic model of service development

When fully developed, commissioning is a multi-agency activity that includes the public and social services. It is an activity that should take place in a co-ordinated and equitable manner at practice, locality and district levels. Commissioning plans are strategic, free of resource consideration but indicating the path that could be followed, as resources permit, from the current position to a desired goal. Commissioning is more concerned with the 'what' than the 'how', and as such transcends such barriers as the interfaces between primary and secondary care, and between health and social care. The setting of priorities is a part of commissioning.

Procurement
This term refers to the process of service acquisition. Procurement has always been necessary within the health service whether or not it has embraced a market economy. 'Purchasing' is a specific form of procurement that was introduced in 1990. NACGP defines procurement as: 'The conversion of commissioning plans to time-related procurement plans and the arrangement of the services required to undertake them.'

Procurement is a tactical, operational activity that seeks to optimise the use of resources made available through the administrative structure of the NHS. It is more concerned with the 'how' than the 'what'. It includes the disbursement of a finite budget against agreed priorities, and the contracting processes of negotiation, agreement and monitoring of contracts with providers. Procurement plans may aggregate the requirements of a number of smaller populations to benefit from scale. The extent of this aggregation will vary from place to place and from subject to subject. Rationing of services is an inevitable component of purchasing.

In 1990 the Government incarcerated its failure to distinguish commissioning from procurement within primary legislation. It was an error that at the time of writing has yet to be corrected and unfortunately hindered NHS development by excluding the majority of general practitioners from taking part in what was to be termed a 'Primary Care-led NHS'. By early 1997 the result of seven years of intense promotion and pecuniary incentives had only resulted in little over half of all GPs adopting the Conservatives' preferred option of GP Fundholding. Many of those had done so reluctantly (Francome and Marks 1996), with the Audit Commission finding a surprisingly few bringing about significant change in their use of hospital services (Audit Commission 1996).

Equity
'The appropriate use of resources within a given population, based upon individual clinical need and agreed priorities that apply throughout that population.'

Equity of access to services is one of the most important defining qualities of the NHS, and one that is revered by the public. No Government has obtained a mandate to rescind it; none has dared seek one. Equity does not necessarily imply equality. Indeed for optimal effect it may on occasion require inequality.

Equality
There is a national policy of equality of resource distribution to districts (with a few, exceptional weightings, for example concerning London).

In contrast to equity, equality is defined as: 'The distribution of resources throughout a population on an equal, unitary basis regardless of differential need.'

Multi-agency, multi-level commissioning

It took the development of GP Commissioning Groups to illustrate the benefits of GPs working with the Health Authority in a co-ordinated manner that is both multi-level and multi-agency in approach. More recently the fundholding movement has moved in the same direction to obtain the same benefits. If general practice is the basic unit for a population-based service then local practices should combine to work cohesively at Locality and District level, though the precise mechanism for that co-operation will vary according to local circumstances. It is difficult to see how a cohesive primary care-led commissioning framework could operate effectively without such communication. At the same time, to greater or lesser extent, all other agencies will need to work at these different levels in order to co-ordinate services appropriately.

The plurality of procurement

Within the framework of the Merrison principles and Dobson criteria there is room for a plurality of procurement approaches. It matters less by whom the procurement is done than that it conforms to the values and operational boundaries of the service. Certainly, the involvement of practices in developing local services should not depend upon their taking a purchasing role.

The separation of purchasing from provision was an aspect of the 1990 changes in the NHS that has received widespread commendation. It is therefore ironic that both the major political parties contested the 1997 General Election with policies that sought to disseminate budgets and purchasing to general practitioners, for these are independent contractors to the NHS with a current monopoly on providing primary medical services. In the interests of accountability and public probity it would seem desirable to separate procurement from provision and to maintain ultimate control with the Health Authority as the local statutory body.

The plurality of provision

The 1997 Primary Care Act provides threats as well as opportunities for the cohesive development of local services. The task is to counter the former while promoting the latter. The co-ordination of GPs within a district is a valuable function of local medical committees that may not be fully appreciated until it has been lost. It should be developed and protected from being undermined. What is required is a means for ensuring all providers of primary medical services are accountable to their own patients as well as collectively to the local community. The method should neither be so cumbersome as to stifle innovation within the delivery of primary care, nor so lax that it permits individual practices to ignore the interests of the locality as a whole.

The need for cultural shift

As with anything else, appropriate incentives and levers will have to be put in place for change to occur. The current culture of the NHS requires a shift towards one in which there is a greater acceptance of the value of health economics. There is a need to promote a culture of planning, of making informed choices between competing demands, of evaluation, and of working towards shared goals. The idea that this means an overwhelming focus on money and a dogmatic adherence to narrow, 'evidence-based' decision-making is erroneous. Both would run counter to the instincts of many working within the health care professions and have an uphill path to committed acceptance. Clinicians are increasingly prepared to consider how they can make the best use of resources but this should be done in ways with which they are professionally comfortable. Their disciplines are founded upon a scientific approach to the determination of appropriate practice. Educational pathways are likely to be more effective at bringing about sustained change than are those based on crude accounting. Similarly, over-emphasis on evidence-based decision-making is unhelpful and counter-productive as it distances its disciples from the clinical experience of many practitioners. It should be remembered that, from the patient's perspective, the central hub of general practice is the consultation. Here characteristics such as accessibility, empathy, time to listen, inter-personal skills, kindness and attentive personal service shine out as matters of importance to patients. In numerous surveys these have commonly been given higher priority than clinical skills themselves (Allen 1989). They are the 'intangibles' Stanley Davis refers to when writing about the management of service businesses (Davis 1988). The identification of valid markers for such aspects of quality is as difficult as it is important. It is work that needs to be done so that the results can take their rightful place amongst the evidence that informs thinking and decision making. This author is unaware of any scientific evidence that justifies the use of kindness within medicine. As it is time consuming, and therefore expensive, should we not practice it?

The need for appropriate information

For general practice to take such a central, co-ordinating role within the NHS requires an appropriate information system that makes full use of modern technology to help plan, deliver and review services. There is an urgent need to start developing the cohesive, multi-level information systems necessary to support such a service. This should extend to a formal replacement of the paper-based medical record for general practice. That system remains essentially unchanged since its introduction before the First World War and is, not surprisingly, quite inappropriate for the NHS as it moves into the highly computerised next century.

The pivotal role of primary care

This is clear: for primary care is the services' first interface with the public and the one where both the greatest number of interactions take place and where the initial decisions concerning resource distribution are made. It is here that resource management is likely to have the greatest beneficial effect. General practice alone contains the clinical generalists responsible for, and accountable to, a registered population of patients. Their practices form the natural building block for a population-focused NHS. For all these reasons the raising of quality within general practice, and the encouragement of its involvement in developing local services can be seen as a key investment for the NHS. A danger is that the insatiable appetite of acute hospitals will make that investment difficult to achieve. It is a statement of the obvious that GPs can only help increase efficiency and effectiveness if they receive the resources and incentives to do so.

What have we learned so far?

Prior to 1989 there were five events that had particular fundamental significance for future general practice. These were:

1   1911 The National Insurance Act
2   1948 The formation of The National Health Service

3 1952 The foundation of The Royal College of General Practitioners

4 1965 The Charter for the Family Doctor Service

5 1980 The availability of microcomputers

Of these the first was the most important, for the National Insurance Act laid the foundation stones of general practice by introducing the registered list of patients (albeit only for some people), the referral system, capitation payments, and the self-employed status of the GP. As Richards observes, once these key elements had been created, the formation of the NHS in 1948 merely represented their formalisation and development (Richards 1988).

The Royal College of General Practitioners has led the fields of research, education and the development of information systems, and by so doing has raised the standing and credibility of general practice. For example, for many years prior to 1989 it had been undertaking research into improving quality (Buck *et al.* 1974, Irvine 1983, RCGP 1985, Buckley 1989).

The advent of commercially available microcomputers heralded the most significant change in clinical information systems since 1911, though the true potential of computer technology has only in recent years been explored on anything like the required scale. Regrettably, there is still no cohesive national policy for providing the appropriate information systems required for co-ordinated planning, procurement, provision and review within the NHS.

Nonetheless, it was the action in 1965 of the General Services Committee (GMSC) of the British Medical Association (BMA) that had the greater initial effect on the development of General Practice. At a time of 'profound malaise and disorder within general practice' (BMJ 1965) members of that committee produced a Charter for the Family Doctor Service. This called for assistance with obtaining appropriate practice premises, the attachment of community staff to practices, support for postgraduate education, help with the employment of receptionists and secretaries, the reduction of the average list size to 2,000 patients and trials of different methods of payment for GPs.

As a result of the Charter a new contract was negotiated by the GMSC, the result being the birth of modern general practice with embryonic Primary Health Care Teams working from appropriate premises. Remarkably, in practical terms the contract placed no restrictions upon the level of resources available, but unfortunately provided inadequate motivation for most practices to alter their behaviour to make good use of them. The profession's failure to seize that opportunity for development proved to be the seed-corn for the Government's move, some 23 years later, to introduce a further, more prescriptive, contract (DoH 1989b).

Conversely, the changes following 1990 provided motivation for behavioural change (albeit some of it coercive) but relatively few additional resources, other than those made available within the fund-holding scheme. Partly because of the internal market, clinicians from primary and secondary care were working together through fundholding or

Commissioning Groups to improve local services in a way that had not happened before. GPs and hospital clinicians were being made accountable for their expenditure by one method or another and so the thrust for cost-effectiveness was supported. This sea change in attitudes towards effective cooperation at a local level is an undoubted success of the changes of 1990. Purchasing, by whatever means, has been increasingly concerned with quality, value for money, and sensitivity to the needs of local communities and individual patients. One theoretical effect of purchasers considering cost effectiveness was intended to be a long-needed shift of resources away from the acute hospital sector into clinical care within the community. In reality not even fundholding has brought about much significant change in this way (Audit Commission 1996).

An important lesson since 1990 is recognition of the innate ability of GPs to act as pragmatic and effective agents for their patients in planning and procuring services. This is hardly surprising since the clinical consultation in general practice is itself very much a commissioning exercise. While the GP Fundholding scheme has had a variable level of impact in terms of innovation and clinical effect, it has certainly demonstrated how GPs, given the appropriate incentives, can work both at practice and supra-practice level to bring about change. It is the provision of incentives within that scheme that requires emphasis here.

On the other hand, the fundholding scheme has demonstrated the weakness of simply focusing upon the relatively small unit of a single practice and on the purchasing of secondary care. There is a need for Government to apply a similar commitment to involving all apropriate organisations in multi-agency planning and review at practice, locality, district and regional levels. A further lesson from the GP Fundholding scheme has been the demoralising and divisive effects of providing incentives for GPs to act in ways that are alien to their professional principles.

The internal market has thrown up perverse incentives which have weakened its overall effect and indeed undermined it in the minds of many observers as well as those working within the service. The hurried implementation of the market inevitably relied on crude units of measurement and accounting. It is not surprising that these have been found wanting when set against a multitude of complex, interwoven medical decisions. The Finished Consultant Episode and Efficiency Index are two of the more obvious examples of this inappropriate simplicity that concern the hospital sector. There were similar examples within the imposed GP contract of 1990. Of these, the requirement to measure the height of all adults every three years was perhaps the most widely ridiculed. It was subsequently withdrawn.

GP Commissioning originated in the early 1990s as an informal response to what many saw as unacceptable Government policy. These GPs and Health Authority managers saw a need for the population-focused cohesion that is the subject of this chapter. They also saw the Government's focus on market forces as creating difficulties within a service striving to adhere to the principles of equity and co-ordinated healthcare planning. That GP Commissioning survived and prospered despite a hostile political climate and sparse resources is testament to its strengths and values. Its greatest achievement was to keep the flame of equity alight until there was a change of Government to one more in tune with its values. In seven years GP Commissioning moved from heresy to Government policy, demonstrating the profession's powers of constructive innovation when faced with unacceptable pressures. In these ways the GP Commissioning movement is reminiscent of the GMSC's 1965 Charter Group.

Two conclusions arise from this brief historical review. First, it illustrates how the medical profession tends to respond in a reactionary manner to proposals from outside. The 1911 Act, the negotiations preceding the Charter and the changes of 1990 were all associated with hostility from the profession towards the Government, with threats of mass resignation in 1911 and 1965. However the College, Charter, development of microcomputer systems and GP Commissioning were all successful results of initiatives by the profession responding to unacceptable circumstances.

Second, in order to bring about optimal change the profession requires appropriate resources as well as the motivating forces to make use of them. One is little use without the other. The 1965 contract provided unlimited resources but little motivation. The 1990 legislation provided motivation for some aspects of general practice but little more than contractual coercion for others. The GP Commissioning movement now has support from Government policy, but at the time of writing there is no sign of the necessary new resources being made available to support it!

How can we move forward?

The models described here provide global cohesion and local flexibility. They support the following concepts.

Matters of principle

- Support for the principles of the NHS set out by The Royal Commission in 1979.

- Compliance with the seven development criteria established by The Secretary of State in July 1997.

Operational matters

- Acceptance that primary care in general, and general practice in particular, has a leading role in the planning and review of local services.

- A distinction between planning, procurement, provision and review.

- Support for cohesion in planning and review, and co-ordinated plurality in procurement and provision.

- The need for all four processes to take place at different population sizes for different activities.

- An acceptance of the need for different agencies to work internally in a co-ordinated way at the different population sizes of practice, locality, district and region.

- An acceptance of the need for different agencies to work together on matters of mutual interest at the different population sizes of practice, locality, district and region.

- An acceptance of the need for an appropriate, multi-agency information structure.

It is possible for GPs to work as peers with the Health Authority in commissioning *all* services whilst avoiding the role of purchaser, and yet to contract with the HA as providers of primary care. This is the only way in which policy can truly support a purchaser–provider split.

For this to happen requires some form of two-way, vertical communication between practices and their locality structures, and between localities and a district-wide representative GP structure (Fig. 14.3). The LMC and HA would together construct localities based upon GP lists, which would in sum cover the entire area of the district. While specific arrangements would vary from place to place, each democratically representative locality GP Commissioning Group would be elected under LMC supervision and work with other agencies at locality level, and collectively at district level. It is acknowledged that this model would need significant adjustment for many inner-city areas where boundaries are more fluid than elsewhere. Many of its concepts, however, remain valid.

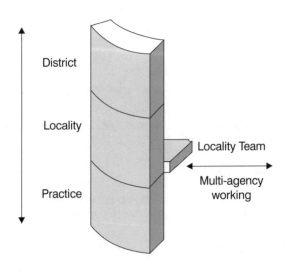

Figure 14.3

Other agencies such as the Health Authority, hospitals, community units, and social services will need to work in a similar fashion, both vertically within their own structure and horizontally with other agencies at each of these levels. Within localities much of this communication will take place through small multi-agency teams.

Figure 14.4 shows different agencies working in a co-ordinated manner at different levels of population. (The segment representing patients has been removed from the front of the diagram for clarity.) This model envisages the main engine of commissioning being GP locality groups and multi-agency locality teams (Webster and Willis 1993). Such a model of commissioning is a robust structure for developing the NHS. However, for it to be successful it will require appropriate resources to be made available by Government with comparable vigour to that which accompanied previous strategies.

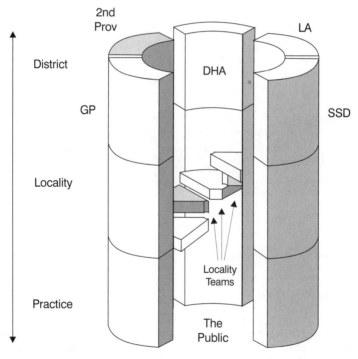

Figure 14.4

The service development cycle

Figure 14.5 considers how the generic development cycle shown in Figure 14.2 can be interpreted within the context of the NHS.

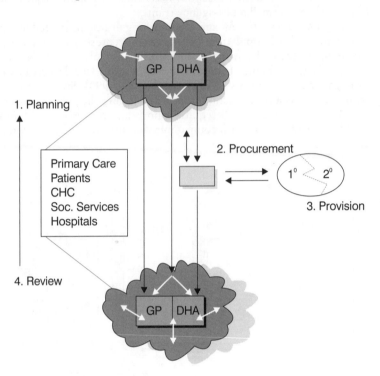

Figure 14.5

Planning and review

The model envisages joint power-sharing within commissioning between GPs and the Health Authority. Accountability at district level would be held by a Commissioning Executive Committee made up of democratically elected GPs working as peers with senior managers from the Health Authority. Thus the managers charged with a statutory responsibility for providing services for the local population would work in concert with the clinical generalists providing overall medical care to that population. Within this model the level of GP involvement in the day-to-day commissioning process would be at the discretion of the representative GP body, as discussed later.

The Commissioning Executive Committee would be the accountable body, on the one hand to the district population and on the other to the NHS Executive through the Health Authority Board. Nonetheless, accountability for the extent of available resources is clearly beyond the control of clinicians. This would remain with the Government, communicated through the Health Authority as its statutory authority.

The Commissioning Executive Committee would work with, and be informed by, any or all of local professional, voluntary and statutory agencies, including bodies representing users of the services. The irregular area in the figure that surrounds the Commissioning Executive represents this group of organisations. The Commissioning Executive would be accountable for deciding priorities and commissioning plans at both locality and district levels. It would be the 'top table' body for these decisions, and the expectation would be that the Health Authority board would only overrule its recommendations under exceptional circumstances.

Procurement and provision

GPs are self-employed, independent contractors to the NHS. The model avoids a difficulty inherent within many current arrangements, which allow or even encourage GPs to use public money to buy services from themselves or to invest in buildings they own. In contrast, Figure 14.5 incorporates a formal separation of procurement from provision. It achieves this by conforming to the concept of the purchaser–provider divide, and by ceding authority for the procurement of all services to the Health Authority.

Nonetheless, there may be circumstances in which a group of GPs wish to undertake a procurement role. Suitable arrangements would include the Health Authority allocating to the group a licence to purchase. The licence would require the group to work within a local and national framework reflecting the Secretary of State's seven guiding criteria. The licence would involve the equitable delivery of services within the broader local population. It would be concerned with public probity, in that savings from any budget could only be spent on direct clinical services for patients and not in ways that provided personal financial gain to the doctors concerned.

Whatever the vehicle chosen by a locality group for procurement, the commissioning of services for the locality and district would remain a collective endeavour involving all practices in one way or another. Overall, the model sees the main change in the emphasis of national policy to be an acceptance that the priority is widespread involvement in the effective planning of local services. Procurement is seen as a relatively mechanistic process that is subservient, as in most walks of life, to commissioning. Such an approach represents a complete reversal of emphasis from the period 1990–97.

A flexible approach to distinguishing commissioning from procurement

Figure 14.6 illustrates a generic, four-box model of locality commissioning and procurement. Each locality would be responsible for determining the level of its own involvement in commissioning and in procurement.

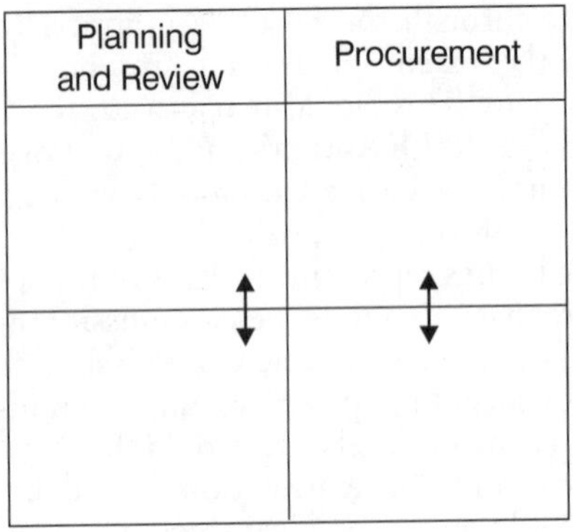

Figure 14.6

Figure 14.7 depicts an example where virtually all activity in both commissioning and procurement is conducted by the Health Authority, with the locality group adopting a largely reactive, advisory role. Such an arrangement might apply, for example, within some inner-city areas.

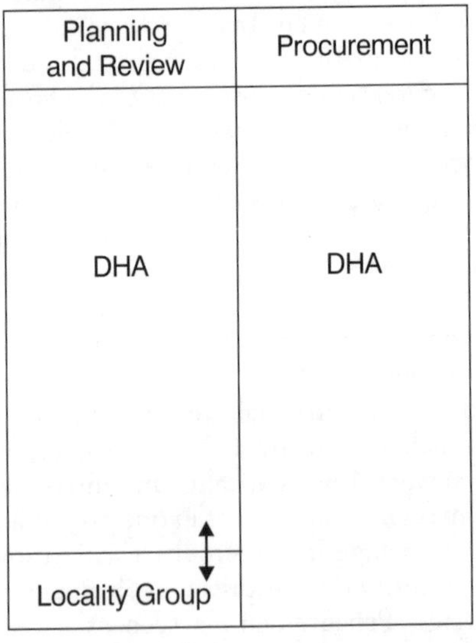

Figure 14.7

In Figure 14.8 the locality has elected to undertake most of the commissioning itself, as well as most of the procurement under licence from the Health Authority. This is in effect an evolution of a total purchasing project to locality size, but with a greater level of devolved budget than is possible within current regulations.

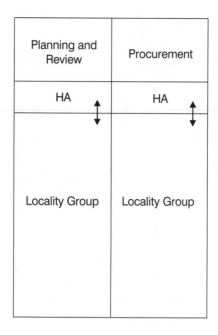

Figure 14.8

In Figure 14.9 the locality group elects to undertake most of the commissioning but delegates the procurement to the Health Authority, or indeed to some other agency acting on behalf of the locality. This is an evolution of the approach already undertaken by many existing GP Commissioning Groups and illustrates how models may emerge where the direct procurement of services is neither undertaken by the locality group nor by the Health Authority.

Each locality group would be able to alter its level of involvement in either area from year to year. Appropriate management funding would be attached to each, meaning that the financial support was proportional to the work undertaken. For example, a locality could pass the responsibility and funding for procurement to the Health Authority, or any other appropriate agency, if it so decided. The authority to make that decision would reside with the locality.

One effect would be to provide an incentive for the locality to undertake more of the commissioning and procurement itself. However, unlike previous arrangements, practices would no longer be materially disadvantaged if they decided not to do so. Thus the principles of equality of opportunity, plurality of approaches and equity of resource allocation are supported within a single generic model.

For locality commissioning to work effectively there is a need for a representative group of GPs to be selected by a democratic process. The group should receive a mandate from local GPs to work on their behalf,

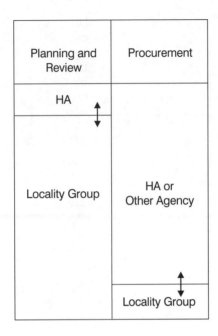

Figure 14.9

and it should have a peer-relationship with the Health Authority in matters relating to commissioning. It follows that there should be a written concordat, or working agreement, which defines the responsibilities of the representative group of GPs and the health authority (Singer 1997). Various approaches have already been developed to Locality Commissioning (Black *et al.* 1994, Edwards 1996, Jenner *et al.* 1997). In addition, the National Association of Commissioning GPs has made written recommendations to the Secretary of State concerning the structure of Commissioning Groups (NACGP 1996).

Ideally, a GP Commissioning Group will require the support and cooperation of all the practices in the locality or district. Measures that will help this include the collective development of an annual manifesto for service development; clear and timely communication between the Commissioning Groups and the practices they represent; the availability of reports detailing the resource usage of different practices; and the appropriate requests to practices for their opinion about the effect of initiatives.

Practice level commissioning

The principles apply within practices as they do at district and locality levels. Any provider of primary care will need to develop their service using the development cycle of Planning, Procurement, Provision and Review shown in Figure 14.2. This will either be an overt process or a covert one that takes place in a largely subjective and unstructured manner, but consciously or unconsciously any organisation follows this fundamental process. The following system is being developed by a Northampton practice with funding from the NHS Executive (KERS 1997) Here, commissioning entails combining and interpreting relevant information streams from three distinct areas in order to produce the practice's commissioning plan:

- the primary care team;
- the registered list of patients;
- the business focus of the practice.

The primary care team
Members of the primary care team are identifying priorities in the three areas of acute care, chronic dsease management and preventive care. Appropriate proposals will then be drawn up in the light of evidence from the literature and the practical experience of centres of good practice.

The patients
Various methods are being explored by a patient liaison officer to obtain the views of representative groups of patients concerning the services they want and need, and their priorities for service development.

National and local priorities
National and local directives and priorities form a third element of the strategic planning process and will be explored in joint working with the Health Authority. It is here that the practice is most clearly seen as a provider, and as a business concern in its own right.

The assessment of outcomes will occur through clinical and administrative audit for the primary care team, and through separate assessment by the patient liaison officer on behalf of patients.

Thus the business direction of the practice is driven forward by two separate but interlocking processes of planning and review; one investigated on behalf of the practice and the other on behalf of the patients. Both processes integrate with procurement, whether undertaken by the practice or through the locality, and both directly inform the work of the practice as a provider of primary medical services.

Resource implications for a national policy of locality commissioning

A co-ordinated information infrastructure is required to support multi-agency, multi-level planning and review across health and social care.

Management resources require allocation on an equitable basis according to relative need. The resource requirements of all general practices and all localities within a district should be appraised according to a common system. Areas of greater overall need would receive disproportionately large resource allocations.

The 1990 legislation concerning GP Fundholding is incompatible with equity, either for patients or practices, and requires replacement with a more sophisticated structure that supports the above model.

Conclusions

This chapter has considered the development of an equitable, population-focused NHS from the perspective of general practice. It has intentionally separated commissioning from procurement in order to develop a model that would:

- be acceptable to the great majority of clinicians and their patients.

- reduce bureaucracy by avoiding practice-based purchasing.

- support probity within a public service within which GPs are independent contractors.

- facilitate the cohesive planning of services that reflect local needs and priorities.

- encourage the effective use of resources to improve the health of the local community.

The models described have their roots in widespread experience throughout the country over the last seven years. They provide a platform for developing local health services based upon multi-level, multi-agency planning and review. Such a service would embrace social services and representative patient opinion in the pursuit of equity, efficiency and effectiveness of health care, while accommodating the inevitable need for cost-containment.

References

Allen, D (1989) *Lay Proposals for the development of General Practice: A review for the Royal College of General Practitioners Patient Liaison Group* Royal College of General Practitioners, London

Audit Commission (1996) *What the doctor ordered: A study of GP Fundholders in England and Wales* HMSO, London

Black, D, Birchall, A and Trimble, I (1994) Non-fundholding in Nottingham: a vision of the future *British Medical Journal* **309**, 930–932

BMA (1997) *Resolution 181* Minutes; British Medical Association ARM

BMJ (1965) Towards a New Contract *British Medical Journal* **5434**, 535–536

Buck, C, Fry, J and Irvine, D (1974) A framework for good Primary Care: The Measurement and Achievement of Quality *Journal of the Royal College of General Practitioners* **24**, 599–604

Buckley, EG (1989) Quality Assessment or Quality Control *Journal of the Royal College of General Practitioners* **39**, 309–312

Davis, SM (1988) 2001 Management: Managing the future now. Simon and Schuster

Department of Health (1989a) *Working for Patients* CMD 555, HMSO, London

Department of Health (1989b) *General Practice in the National Health Service: A new contract* Health Departments of Great Britain HMSO, London

Dobson, F (1997) *Speech by the Secretary of State to the NHS Confederation Conference* June 1997

Edwards, N (1996) *GP Commissioning – R&D or D&R* Report for NACGP by London Health Economics. Consortium, London School of Hygiene and Tropical Medicine, September 1996 (Unpublished)

Francome, and Marks, (1996) *Improving the Health of the Nation: The failure of the government's health reforms* Middlesex University Press, Enfield

Gilmour, I (1992) *Dancing with Dogma* Simon and Schuster, London, 150–161

Ham, C and Willis, A (1994) Think Globally, Act Locally *Health Service Journal* 13 January, 27–28

Irvine, D (1983) Quality: our outstanding problem *Journal of the Royal College of General Practitioners* **33**, 521–523

Jenner, D, Dixon, M and Morgan, G (1997) Commissioning Group at Work – the mid-Devon experience In Singer R (ed.), *GP Commissioning: an inevitable evolution* Radcliffe Medical Press, Abington, 160–161

KERS (1997) *Planning and Review Project Plan* King Edward Road Surgery, Northampton (Unpublished)

LMC (1997) *Resolution 81* Minutes; Local Medical Committees Conference

Merrison, Sir A (1979) *Royal Commission on the NHS* Cmnd 7615 HMSO, London

NACGP (1996) *Report to the Secretary of State on National Standards for GP Commissioning* NACGP 3 May 1996

NACGP (1997) *GP Commissioning: a Briefing Paper* National Association of Commissioning GPs, Nottingham

RCGP (1985) *What sort of doctor? Assessing quality of care in general practice Report from General Practice* **23**, Royal College of General Practitioners, London

Richards, C (1988) A car with flat batteries *Journal of the Royal College of General Practitioners* **38**, 535–538

Singer, R (1997) Suggested agreement between a Commissioning Group and its Health Authority Appendix A. *GP Commissioning: an inevitable evolution* Radcliffe Medical Press, Abingdon, 160–161

Smith, R (1997) Editorial *BMJ* **314**, 1495–1496

Webster, D and Willis, A (1993) *A Sense of Place: Co-ordinating the Commissioning of Appropriate Care by Different Agencies for Local Communities in Northamptonshire* Northampton District Health Authority, Northampton

Willis, A (1992) Who needs fundholding? *Health Service Journal* 30 April,
    24–26
Willis, A (1997) Developing the Health Service: Chaos or Cohesion?
    Community Care Management & Planning Review 5, 89–98

15 Care in the community
Stuart Cumella

Introduction

'Care in the community' is an ambiguous term, being simultaneously an activity, an aspiration and a policy. As an activity, it refers to the complex range of general and specialist health provision, social work and domiciliary care, housing, and leisure services, and public financial provisions which enable people with a severe disability to live outside hospital. The aspiration has been to close large long-stay hospitals, and enable people with disabilities to live a life that they wish and which corresponds to that lived by the rest of the population. As a policy, 'care in the community' refers to a series of laws and regulations by which central Government has sought to realise this aspiration while limiting its financial consequences.

Disability

The most comprehensive survey of the number and characteristics of disabled people in Great Britain was completed by the Office of Population Censuses and Statistics (OPCS) in the mid-1980s. This used the WHO definition of 'disability' as any 'restriction or lack . . . of ability to perform an activity in the manner or within the range considered normal for a human being' (World Health Organisation 1980). OPCS noted that disability is best viewed as forming part of a continuum of abilities, and that the choice of a threshold above which people are defined as 'disabled' is determined by the aims of the survey rather than any naturally occurring distinction between being disabled and able-bodied (Martin *et al.* 1988). This is confirmed by several surveys of psychiatric disorders, learning disability, and physical disabilities which have observed a continuum of symptoms rather than a clear discontinuity between 'disability' and 'nondisability' (Goldberg and Huxley 1992, Fryers 1997).

OPCS operationalised their definition by identifying 13 separate scales of disability, with points on each scale assigned according to respondents' ability to carry out a graduated range of day-to-day tasks with or without assistance. Panels were used to rate each scale point against a common severity scale. Table 15.1 shows the resulting OPCS estimates of the number of adults in Great Britain with a severity rating of one or more on each scale, and the rate per thousand adults in the general population. It indicates that over four million adults have problems with locomotion, and over two million with hearing loss and personal care. Approximately one million adults are disabled in terms of dexterity, vision, behaviour, intellectual functioning, continence, and/or communication. Taking account of people with multiple disabilities, OPCS estimated that over six million adults in Great Britain are disabled (Martin *et al.* 1988).

Table 15.1 OPCS estimates of the prevalence of disability among adults in Great Britain, by type of disability

Type of disability	Numbers	Rate/1,000
Locomotion	4,332,000	99
Hearing	2,589,000	59
Personal care	2,483,000	57
Dexterity	1,736,000	40
Seeing	1,668,000	38
Intellectual functioning	1,474,000	34
Behaviour	1,346,000	31
Reaching and stretching	1,230,000	28
Communication	1,202,000	27
Continence	1,144,000	26
Disfigurement*	>391,000	>9
Eating, drinking and digesting	276,000	6
Consciousness	230,000	5

* Data not available for population in institutions

There is a strong association between disability and age, and between severity of disability and age. Among younger age-groups, disability is uncommon (less than 3 per cent of those under the age of 30). About 10 per cent of those in later middle age have some form of disability, and this figure rises to about a quarter of those aged 60–69 years, 40 per cent of those aged 70–79, and over 70 per cent of those aged 80 and above. Severe disability is extremely rare among young adults, but prevalence rises rapidly after the age of 40, and almost two-thirds of people with the most severe disabilities are over the age of 70 (Martin *et al.* 1988). However, this pattern does not occur for all causes of disability. For instance, the prevalence of schizophrenia and other functional psychoses does not rise with age (Commander *et al.* 1997), while the peak incidence for traumatic brain injury occurs between the ages of 15 and 30 (Williams *et al.* 1997). The prevalence of severe learning disability declines with age, reflecting the combined effect of high death rates in the past, and improving survival rates among disabled children (Eyman *et al.* 1990, Fryers 1997).

Disability may have either a selective or a global impact on a person's life, and may have a substantial effect on income, occupation, social relationships, leisure and recreation, sexual relationships, and family roles. The extent to which a disability restricts opportunities and quality of life depends not just on the severity and nature of the disability itself, but also on a person's previous way of life, the availability of aids to daily living, the extent of services and support to compensate for loss of function, the income to pay for these, and the availability of day-to-day help from families, friends, and services. The acquisition of a disability often requires a person to develop new skills or re-learn old ones, to change their definition of the kind of person they are and their expectation of the kind of person they can become (Blaxter 1976).

The outcome of disability for many people is a move to institutional care (hospital, residential home or nursing home) or some other form of group living. There is a strong relationship between severity of disability and institutional care, and hence also between age and institutional care. OPCS estimated that 465,000 disabled people lived in institutional care at the time of their survey (equivalent to 7 per cent of the total), but that half of those with the most severe disabilities lived in institutional care (Martin *et al.* 1988). The proportion of the population in institutional care rises from one in 2,000 among those under 65, to one in four among those over 85 (House of Commons Health Committee 1996).

Domiciliary and day services for disabled people who live at home are implicitly based on the assumption that families will provide the bulk of care. About 1.5 million people in Britain spend 20 hours a week or more providing care for disabled family members (House of Commons Health Committee 1996). Few people severely disabled in early life marry, and most remain within their parental home. Their parents may continue to provide care and support, often at great personal cost, until they are themselves elderly and disabled. By contrast, people who become disabled in old age have family patterns similar to the general population and receive help primarily from partners and children (Wenger 1992). The term 'carer' is commonly used to refer to care staff employed in institutions, as well as to family members who either live in the same household as a disabled person or otherwise provide help to them. This latter sense of the term can be misleading because disabled people in some households may themselves act as a 'carer' for another disabled person (Walmsley 1996).

The diversity of characteristics and needs among the disabled population, and the complexity of services needed by individual disabled people to maintain an adequate quality of life and prevent admission to institutional care present three major organisational challenges for statutory services:

- Providing local access to an appropriate range of mainstream, sheltered, and compensatory services for different sections of the disabled population.

- Matching the needs of individual disabled people with appropriate services that respect their preferences and fall within available funding.

- Maintaining the quality and clinical effectiveness of services for disabled people.

Providing access to appropriate services

The key engines of change in community care policy have been the discrediting of hospitals as venues for the long-term care of disabled people, and therapeutic optimism about the treatment of people previously deemed beyond hope of change. A number of damning official reports in the 1960s and 1970s increasingly associated long-term hospital care with the neglect and abuse of the vulnerable (Means and Smith 1994), a view confirmed by persuasive sociological analyses of the character of institutional life (Goffman 1968, Morris 1969, Jones and Fowles 1984). Therapeutic optimism resulted from the effectiveness of new types of interventions such as psycho-active medication in psychiatry and special education and behavioural management in learning disability. Several demonstration projects showed how small community-based homes could provide an improved way of life for adults with a mental illness, and children and adults with a learning disability (Olsen 1979, Race 1995).

Yet there was a gap of a generation between the beginning of the decline in mental hospital beds in the 1950s, and the large-scale closure of hospitals for the mentally-ill, learning disabled, and elderly in the 1990s. The key reason was an unwillingness by Governments to commit themselves to what has probably always been an unpopular political move. Policy instead was to invest in alternative services which would minimise the accumulation of new long-stay ('continuing-care') patients. This was to be achieved in mental health by developing district general hospitals as the main centres for acute mental illness, in order to provide accessible services in a venue that would not deter patients from seeking early treatment (DHSS 1975). In learning disability, prevention of long-stay hospital care involved a major investment in educational provision following the 1970 Education (Handicapped Children) Act, and the closure of children's beds in mental handicap hospitals during the 1980s.

Poor cooperation between health and social services agencies was seen by Government as a key obstacle to the implementation of these policies. One response was the development and expansion of the joint finance system, which was a mechanism for the transfer of funds from Health Authorities to local authorities to facilitate NHS objectives (such as transfers of patients from hospital to community-based accommodation). Earmarked funds for joint finance were allocated for either short-term or tapering expenditure on community-based services, with allocations made by a system of local joint planning committees (Wistow 1990). Various other earmarked funds were also allocated by central Government for community care developments, of which the most important was the Care in the Community Initiative from 1983 (DHSS 1983).

In the absence of central direction, policies to replace long-stay hospitals were developed by the professionals providing specialist care of each group of disabled people, in dialogue with a range of non-governmental organisations (NGOs) which acted as advocates for a particular client group (eg Mencap, MIND, Age Concern). Initial attempts at non-hospital care mainly involved large hostels or boarding-out schemes, in which patients continued to use hospital-based day and treatment facilities. But there was a gradual shift towards an increasingly complex provision of autonomous community-based services to meet the needs of disabled people for access to recreation, friendship, occupation, educational opportunities, and primary health care. Hospital care became seen as peripheral rather than central, and appropriate only for the small number of people with the most severe disorders who could not be maintained in community-based accommodation.

Because debate about the most appropriate pattern of community-based services was dominated by specialist professionals and NGOs, quite separate discourses developed for each client group. For people with a learning disability, this involved a prolonged debate about the role of specialist services and the way of life they should promote for their clientele. The term 'normalisation' was used to denote how specialist services could compensate for skill deficits, to enable disabled people to exercise the same choice in everyday life as non-disabled people. Later writers changed the meaning of the term by placing greater emphasis on ending the social isolation of disabled people by minimising the external symbols of disability. This could result in opposing the use of specialist services themselves (Szivos 1992). In the UK, the most influential statement of objectives was in the report *An Ordinary Life*, which promoted the development of small (4–6 bed) staffed houses converted from ordinary domestic property, and emphasised the importance of enabling people with a learning disability to access the community services used by the general population (King's Fund Centre 1980).

By contrast, the discourse in care of the elderly has been concerned more with the means of maintaining income and hence quality of life, and the delivery of comprehensive and co-ordinated community health and social care services to enable people to continue to live in their own homes. There has been less debate about the type of institutional care for those who need it, than about its financial implications for residents and their families. The debate in mental health has been more fragmented. The emphasis among professionals on mental health problems as treatable illnesses resulted in diminishing attention being paid to the needs of people with long-term mental disabilities, and a neglect of the extent to which services which promote social inclusion are effective in reducing relapse (Warner 1994). NGOs were divided between those (like the National Schizophrenia Fellowship) which expressed the need of family carers for long-term support for mentally-ill people, and MIND which extended its opposition to mental hospitals into a general campaign against detention and involuntary treatment.

The professional domination of the debate about community care has been challenged by activists with physical and sensory disabilities, who have campaigned for rights of access to public facilities, services and employment (Finkelstein 1993). In common with other disadvantaged groups, disabled activists have sought to wrest control of terminology from professionals (eg Abberley 1993), but have sometimes diminished their effectiveness by engaging in boundary disputes rather than building broad coalitions, and by failing to articulate policies that can be implemented by Governments. The weakness of the disabled lobby is shown by the failure to achieve anti-discrimination legislation until the limited 1996 Disability Discrimination Act, and the continuing lack of any clear legal entitlement to services for disabled people.

The implementation of the new models of community care owed much to entrepreneurial activity by key individuals in Health Authorities and social services departments, and their equivalents in NGOs and the private sector. These were able to creatively exploit opportunities in the complex and ever-changing web of housing, social services, joint finance, and social security laws and regulations. The greatest single opportunity occurred when a small change in social security regulations in 1980 entitled claimants to receive payments to meet residential and nursing home care fees. This expenditure rose from £10 million in 1980 to over £2,000 million by 1991 (Lewis and Glennerster 1996), and funded a major expansion in residential and nursing homes managed by NGOs and private owners (Table 15.2). The bulk of this expansion involved care of the elderly, and enabled geriatric medical services to speed discharge to long-term institutional care. But social security funding was also exploited by resettlement teams responsible for moving long-stay patients from hospitals. Few of this group were able to return to their families or to independent living, and for them 'community care' meant transfer to a smaller staffed institution located among ordinary housing (Alaszewski and Wun 1994).

Table 15.2 Changes in long-stay places in institutional care 1983–1994

Long-term institutional care	1983	1994	Change
NHS	55,600	37,500	– 18,100
Private/voluntary nursing home	18,200	148,500	+ 130,300
Local authority residential home	115,900	68,900	– 47,000
Private/voluntary residential home	89,400	209,700	+ 120,300
Total	279,100	464,600	+ 185,500

Other funding opportunities were available. Regional Health Authorities were concerned to realise the site values of the old hospitals, and established schemes to develop the new community-based services by capital grants and transfers of revenue from the Health Authorities managing the hospitals. Regional Health Authorities were concerned to avoid increases in average cost per patient in all the long-stay hospitals, and therefore targeted particular hospitals for reduction. Nevertheless, the schemes were usually generous enough to fund the development of a range of community-based services for local users as well as resettled patients. Astute resettlement teams could supplement these funds by using joint finance, and (in the early 1980s) capital grants and hostel deficit grants from the Housing Corporation.

More complexity arose with the management of small staffed housing. Hospitals targeted for reduction faced major problems in redeploying staff. One solution was to set up their own staffed housing schemes which levied charges and thus also accessed Social Security funds. When this was eventually ruled illegal, several hospitals set up nominally-independent housing bodies which were able to charge residents, but contracted with the hospital for nursing staff who could thus remain NHS employees. These arrangements were closed down in the 1990s, as the new NHS trusts began to contract directly with social services departments for the provision of residential care services.

A tribute to entrepreneurial skill was the small staffed house for people resettled from mental handicap hospitals which emerged in the 1990s. Management of the home was usually split between a housing association which owned the property, and a care agency which employed and managed the staff. This provided security of tenure for the residents (as tenants of the housing agency), while enabling the social services department to change the care agency, should care standards prove inadequate. The house may have been purchased and converted with an input of NHS resettlement funding (paid via the local authority through the joint finance mechanism because Health Authorities are legally barred from directly funding housing), while revenue costs were met from Social Security, with Special Needs Management Allowance paid by the Housing Corporation and 'top up' funding from Health Authorities via the local authority.

Once effective local systems were in place to transfer patients and funds from hospitals to community-based services, they generated their own momentum. An increasing number of health districts began to extend reduction programmes into closure programmes. This offered the attraction of realising even more capital assets – particularly important after the introduction of capital charges in the NHS. Table 15.2 shows that the number of NHS long-stay beds fell by a third between 1983 and 1994, and formed a rapidly diminishing proportion of the total number of places in institutional care (House of Commons Health Committee 1996).

Central Government was slow in responding to the rapid growth in social security expenditure (Lewis and Glennerster 1996). The Audit Commission (1986) report *Making a Reality of Community Care* observed a perverse incentive in a system which made residential and nursing care free to claimants, while alternative and cheaper domiciliary services were means-tested and restricted by tight budgetary controls on local government services. The subsequent Griffiths Report recommended that social security payments to individuals for the care component of residential and nursing homes fees (but not the component attributable to personal and housing needs) should be transferred to social services departments. This sum would be cash-limited, with eligibility determined by an assessment of applicants' care needs and financial means. The report proposed that the primary role of social services departments should be to identify need and purchase social care services, thereby generating a 'mixed economy' of social care (DHSS 1988).

These proposals were accepted by the White Paper *Caring For People* (DHSS 1989), made law by the 1990 NHS and Community Care Act (NHSCCA), and implemented by April 1993. The new funding system only applied to new applicants for residential and nursing care, with existing residents continuing to receive social security payments for fees. As these died or moved to other residences, there would be a progressive transfer of funds from the social security to local authority budgets. The additional annual sum paid to local authorities to meet this increasing obligation was termed the 'Special Transitional Grant' (STG), and central Government specified that a minimum of 85 per cent was to be used for purchases of services from the independent sector. This gave a strong incentive to local authorities to transfer the provision of services to the independent sector, and in effect to shift from a mixed economy of social care to one with little or no local authority provision.

Social services departments reorganised in different ways to respond to the new funding system, and no consistent separation emerged in management structures between 'commissioning' and 'providing' functions (Lewis and Glennerster 1996). Most implemented contracting on a phased basis, initially restricted to new applicants for residential or nursing care, or clients for whom 'care packages' of domiciliary and day care were devised as alternatives to institutional admission. Remaining independent sector services were purchased using a large number of small block contracts. Some departments experimented with decentralised forms of commissioning, but the need to resolve multiple demands for funds within a fixed and very restrictive budget usually required decision-making at a senior level.

Centralisation of purchasing also made it easier to redeploy funds. Before the NHSCCA, responsibility for planning and development in community care services had been seen as a joint responsibility of local authorities and Health Authorities, exercised with limited effectiveness through joint planning procedures (Wistow 1990). The Act gave local authorities the lead role for community care services, and required them to produce an annual community care plan identifying local needs and priorities. Preparation of the plans usually involved a service mapping exercise for each client group, and an identification of local gaps in services. Social services departments gap-filled by commissioning existing providers to extend into new areas, or by tendering (Cumella *et al.* 1996). Joint commissioning with Health Authorities was also developed, to develop joint strategies for specific client groups and to police the boundaries between the separate health and social care markets (Wooley *et al.* 1995). This was necessary because the NHSCCA provided many opportunities for offloading, particularly in the field of continuing care.

After April 1993, the NHS retained responsibility for funding nursing care for all disabled people except those in nursing homes. This created an incentive for Health Authorities to discharge patients from hospital to nursing homes (and hence transfer the costs of their nursing care to the social services' budget), and a matching incentive for social services to place even the most disabled people in residential rather than nursing homes. Variations between health districts in the availability of NHS-funded continuing-care beds meant free care in one place, but means tests and substantial nursing home fees in another. Central Government responded with *NHS Responsibilities for Meeting Continuing Care Needs* (DoH 1995) which proposed that each Health Authority and social services department agree criteria for assessment for and access to NHS-funded continuing care. This resulted in a new *de facto* boundary within continuing nursing care between people with specialist nursing needs (defined as an NHS responsibility), and the remaining population in nursing homes (funded by local authorities or personal payment).

Matching needs and care

The rapid expansion of institutional care provided by the independent sector confirmed a trend towards the fragmentation of services for disabled people. The old long-stay hospitals aimed to provide a comprehensive range of services from a single site, under a centralised system of decision-making. The new pattern may involve a client attending several geographically-dispersed services, provided by different agencies, managerially responsible to no single person. Fragmentation requires effective networks between professionals in different provider agencies, and also some method for determining that disabled people access the most appropriate package of services. The main processes developed by professionals to achieve these objectives were the community-based multidisciplinary team (CMDT), and collaborative care planning.

CMDTs became standard provision in mental illness and learning disability services from the early 1990s, although there were considerable local variations in membership and organisation (Onyett *et al.* 1994, Grant *et al.* 1986). Teams characteristically grouped specialist staff from the NHS and social services, and provided domiciliary, outpatient, and day-care services to a defined geographical area. In mental health services, there was a trend towards basing each CMDT in a community mental health centre (CMHC), which would replace the mental hospital or district general hospital as the main access point for services. Following the NHSCCA, CMDTs began to respond to the increasing purchasing power of GP Fundholders by developing services for people with common mental disorders, and by changing from geographical to practice-based catchment populations (Cumella *et al.* 1996).

Collaborative care planning was initially developed and applied in learning disability services, where it was termed 'individual programme planning' (IPP). This involved a case conference including the client, appropriate family members, and relevant professionals, which would define a comprehensive assessment of the client's strengths and needs, set measurable targets for change, and identify the action needed to attain them. One professional might be nominated as 'keyworker', with responsibility for chasing progress. Such case conferences can be experienced as difficult and threatening by clients and their families, and tend to be dominated by the professionals. Alternative forms of collaborative care planning such as 'shared action plans' have been developed to enable clients to play a larger part in setting the agenda (Simons 1995).

Both CMDTs and collaborative care planning operate on a consensual basis, and are therefore vulnerable to inter-agency and inter-professional rivalries. They also tend to be unsuccessful in responding rapidly to changes in clients' needs, and in systematically prioritising resources (Galvin and McCarthy 1994). This can lead CMDTs in mental health to drift from providing services for people with a severe mental illness, towards more therapeutically-rewarding client groups (Patmore and Weaver 1991). A series of enquiries into suicides and killings by mentally-ill people (North East Thames Regional Health Authority 1994) showed poor transmission of information between mental health services, and a lack of effective clinical responsibility. Central Government responded by requiring mental health services to give priority to people with a severe mental illness, to maintain supervision registers to record people deemed at risk to themselves or others, and to adhere to a standard set of case management procedures for psychiatric patients termed the 'Care Programme Approach' (CPA) (NHS Executive 1996).

A second and rather different approach to case management appeared in the Griffiths Report. This introduced what was subsequently termed 'care management' as a means of prioritising expenditure on community care within a cash-limited budget. Social services departments would devolve responsibility for allocating funds to care managers, who would assess clients' needs, develop a care plan in collaboration with the client and significant family-members and carers, ensure access to the appropriate services, and monitor implementation. Access to services would be ensured by spot purchases of services from providers within the social care market. Information from individual care plans about unmet need could be aggregated as a means of identifying priorities for action in the Community Care Plan (Department of Health 1991).

Subsequent guidance by the Department of Health varied between proposing care management as a general means of allocating all funds in the social care market, and as a process that would focus on clients with complex needs or who may require high levels of expenditure (such as institutional care) (Lewis and Glennerster 1996). Case management in the latter sense already existed in private practice for disabled people who had received compensation payments. It also corresponded to the experiments completed at the University of Kent, which concluded that devolving purchasing responsibility to skilled social workers resulted in better and lower-cost outcomes for elderly people at the threshold of institutional care (Challis and Davies 1986, Challis *et al.* 1993).

Most social services departments applied care management in this restricted sense. The assessment phase was usually undertaken by the client's existing social worker acting as care manager, with decisions on spot purchasing made by more senior managers. Decisions on access to care management were usually determined by simple prioritising systems based on risks of harm or admission to institutional care. Local authorities became reluctant to complete formal care plans because of concerns about their legal status. A series of court decisions established that a local authority is obliged to provide a services identified as needed in a care plan. This was in conflict with the statutory requirement on local authorities to limit expenditure within centrally-determined cash-limits. A similar dilemma had occurred with statements of special educational needs, and the means of resolution were similar (Audit Commission 1992). Several local authorities attempted to restrict the use of written care plans, and to ensure that those that did exist used vague prescriptions that could not be interpreted as an entitlement to services.

Maintenance of quality and effectiveness

The increasing fragmentation and diversity of provision for disabled people has made it particularly difficult to ensure that a high quality of service is maintained and that vulnerable people are protected from exploitation and abuse. This appears to be confirmed by the shift in the location of reported cases of neglect and abuse from hospitals to community care services.

The response of central Government has been to intensify procedures for inspection and monitoring. The NHSCCA introduced local authority inspection units to register and monitor residential care homes (including those managed by the social services department as well as the independent sector). These usually report to the local authority's Chief Executive rather than the Director of Social Services, to avoid the conflict of interest involved in both managing and inspecting directly provided services. Local authority inspection units need to work closely with Health Authority registration officers (who are responsible for registering and inspecting nursing homes) because an increasing number of homes are 'dual registered' and the boundary between the two types of accommodation has become difficult to define.

The NHSCCA also introduced a further layer of inspection and quality monitoring, as Health Authorities and the commissioning sections of social services departments developed their own detailed quality standards, which were inserted into their contracts with provider agencies. Commissioners attempted to monitor local providers' conformance with these quality standards, relying on cooperation with other authorities to monitor the care received by patients and clients placed out-of-area. Residential and nursing care homes are also subject to inspection under other legislation, and need to meet the detailed requirements of fire officers and environmental health officers. As commercial organisations, they are also subject to fair trading legislation, and some homes have been referred to the Director of Trading Standards following disputes with residents about charges and quality of care.

There is therefore a paradox that the system for monitoring the quality of care is as fragmented as the services being monitored. This can place contradictory demands on providers, particularly in the case of small residential homes. Health and social services commissioners influenced by the principles of normalisation prefer these to be small in scale, resembling ordinary domestic housing. Fire officers and environmental health officers, however, tend to apply standard requirements on all residential homes, and may therefore specify fire escapes, boxed stair-wells, and double-sinks and multiple food preparation areas in kitchens. Local authority inspection units may view 'quality' more in terms of the achievement of hotel standards, requiring, for instance, sinks in each bedroom of a small adapted house.

One consequence of inspectorial fragmentation is that little attention is paid in most districts to monitoring the quality of community care services as a system, and its success in managing the characteristic 'care transitions' experienced by disabled people at the time of the first onset of the disability, when graduating from childhood to adulthood, being discharged from hospital, and being assessed for admission to long-term institutional care. There has also been little systematic monitoring by central Government of variations in the quality of community care services between different districts, reflecting the historic reluctance of central Government in England to define national standards for clinical services.

However, some information is available from a series of reports completed by the Clinical Standards Advisory Group (CSAG), the Audit Commission, and the NHS Health Advisory Service. These used observations by expert teams visiting small samples of health districts, to assess the quality of health and social care received by a defined group of disabled people. A consistent finding was that the effectiveness of community care services is impaired by poor liaison between specialist health, primary care, and social services, with a resulting failure to complete and implement holistic multi-disciplinary assessments. The reports also noted wide geographical variations in the amount, quality, and type of services available for disabled people, such that specialist services for some groups (such as people with head injuries or a learning disability and severe behaviour problems) were almost entirely absent in many districts. It was found that health and social services commissioners had often failed to clarify agency responsibilities, resulting in a lack of 'care pathways' from one service to another. The reports found that most districts had yet to establish effective joint commissioning procedures to remedy these defects (Audit Commission 1994, Clinical Standards Advisory Group 1995, Williams and Richardson 1995, Williams *et al*. 1997, Woodhouse *et al*. 1997).

The limited impact of community care planning and joint commissioning on the quality of community care services may have resulted in part from the multiple reorganisations of Health Authorities, NHS trusts, and social services departments which took place in the 1990s. But it also reflects more systemic problems, including the combined effect of the severe cash restrictions imposed by central Government and the perverse incentives introduced by the NHSCCA. These have encouraged commissioners to seek 'downwards substitution', ie developing less intensive (and less expensive) alternatives to existing types of care. This can result in the placement of people with severe disabilities (including some with a history of dangerousness) in facilities with low staffing levels and few professionally-qualified staff. Cost pressures on providers in the social care market are a disincentive to the recruitment of qualified staff or the provision of in-service training. It is not surprising that surveys have frequently identified high levels of stress among residential care staff (Rose 1995). Insufficient high-staffed accommodation, particularly for people with behavioural problems, has in turn placed severe pressure on inpatient services, and led to rising thresholds for admission and an increased tendency to discharge people with incomplete programmes of treatment into inappropriate community-based accommodation (Powell *et al*. 1995).

Conclusion

The system for delivering community care services introduced by the NHSCCA has proved effective in constraining expenditure, and in deflecting responsibility for inadequate provision from central to local Government. It has begun to stimulate a more systematic approach to priority-setting and social care planning, and has generated a more diverse range of provision. But it has not provided disabled people with an entitlement to health and social care services, nor any consistent access to treatment and care in different parts of the country. The imposition of cash limits on health and social care expenditure has also resulted in the loss of a key element of flexibility that enabled local entrepreneurs to develop new types of services, and facilitate transfers from hospital to other forms of care. This loss of flexibility is having an increasing impact on the NHS, in the form of blocked treatment beds, and re-admissions of patients discharged to inadequate or delayed domiciliary care. This suggests that the current pattern of community care services may have a limited duration.

Any new system will need to take account of changes in the pattern of demand, and opportunities for improving the organisational effectiveness of community care services. There has been considerable political debate about the impact of rising numbers of elderly people on the capacity of the health and social services to maintain current standards of community care services. However, the proportion of the population in Britain aged 65 and over is expected to rise by only a limited amount during the next quarter of a century (from 15.7 per cent in 1994 to 16.4 per cent in 2021). The increase is more marked among those aged 85 and over (from 1.7 per cent in 1994 to 2.3 per cent in 2021), although this is smaller in absolute numbers than that which occurred between 1971 and 1994 (House of Commons Health Committee 1996).

Changes in family structure and attitudes towards institutional care may have a greater impact. Higher rates of divorce and separation will probably increase the proportion of elderly people who are living alone, and reduce the amount of care they receive from families. The present generation of elderly people, with their experience of wartime and the regimentation of industrial work, may be the last to accept the routines of institutional life. As they are replaced, there will be increased demand for service packages which enable even the most disabled people to live in their own homes. This will require the development of more comprehensive domiciliary services to provide the 24-hour staff support essential to provide the sense of security required by people with impaired self-care skills, at risk of injury, or vulnerable to others. Supported living schemes of this kind are expanding, but are limited at present by the high cost of maintaining what are essentially one or two-person nursing homes, and by the organisational problems they present for health and social services.

The formal organisation of community care services at present reflects the basic assumptions of the 'Departmental Model', in which the productive process (treatment and care) is segmented into a series of specialist tasks, each provided by a distinct specialist team, each reporting to its own hierarchy or department. The inefficiencies of this model of organisation have been widely recognised in industry. In particular, the fragmentation of work tasks makes incremental improvement difficult to envisage or implement, while individual specialist teams manage their workload by developing idiosyncratic criteria for the acceptance and completion of tasks, leading to bottlenecks in production and an acceptance of poor quality work. In order to maintain the quality of output, management increasingly regulates each aspect of the productive process, with compliance monitored by specialist quality control teams (Womack *et al.* 1990).

To overcome these problems, many commercial enterprises have attempted to apply alternatives such as 'lean production', which involve the devolution of responsibility for a wide span of production to multiskill teams. Each such team groups together in one place the people who need to work together to complete a shared task, and thus facilitates the sharing of information and the innovation of simpler and more effective production processes. These techniques of process redesign have been applied in the hospital sector (Lathrop 1993), but less so in community care services. However, the increased influence of GP Fundholders has resulted in a shift towards multi-skill teams in primary care, including a number of experiments in which social workers have been based in GP practices (Cumella *et al.* 1996). Process redesign has often proved difficult to implement because it requires substantial organisational change and a shift in the management role from control to facilitation (Nelson and Coxhead 1997). But major changes in the organisation and ethos of the health and social services are probably an essential requirement if disabled people are to have the opportunity to truly fulfil their potential and lead the lives they wish.

References

Abberley, P (1993) The significance of the OPCS disability surveys In Oliver, M (ed) *Social work. Disabled people in disabling environments* Jessica Kingsley, London

Alaszewski, A and Wun, W-L (1994) Residential services In Malin, N (ed) *Implementing community care* Open University Press, Buckingham

Audit Commission (1986) *Making a reality of community care* HMSO, London

Audit Commission (1992) *Getting the act together: provision for pupils with special educational needs* HMSO, London

Audit Commission (1994) *Finding a place. A review of mental health services for adults* HMSO, London

Blaxter, M (1976) *The meaning of disability* Heinemann Educational Books, London

Challis, D, Chesterman, J, Darton, R and Traske, K (1993) Case management in care of the aged: the provision of care in different settings In Barnett, J, Pereira, C, Pilgrim, D and Williams, F (eds) *Community care: a reader* Macmillan, Basingstoke

Challis, D and Davies, B (1986) *Case management in community care* Gower, Aldershot

Clinical Standards Advisory Group (1995) *Schizophrenia* HMSO, London

Commander, M, Sashidharan, SP, Odell, SM and Surtees, PG (1997) Access to mental health care in an inner-city health district. II: association with demographic factors *British Journal of Psychiatry* **170**, 317–320

Cumella, S, LeMesurier, N and Tomlin, H (1996) *Social work in practice. An evaluation of the care management received by elderly people from social workers based in GP practices in South Worcestershire* The Martley Press, Worcester

Cumella, S, Williams, R and Sang, B (1996) How mental health services are commissioned In Thornicroft, G and Strathdee, G (eds) *Commissioning mental health services* HMSO, London

Department of Health (1991) *Care management and assessment: practitioners' guide* HMSO, London

Department of Health (1995) *NHS responsibilities for meeting continuing care needs* LAC(95)S/HSG(95)8 HMSO, London

Department of Health and Social Security (1975) *Better services for the mentally ill*, Cmnd 633 HMSO, London

Department of Health and Social Security (1983) *Care in the community and joint finance* HC(83)6/LAC(83)5 HMSO, London

Department of Health and Social Security (1988) *Community care: an agenda for action* HMSO, London

Department of Health and Social Security (1989) *Caring for people: community care in the next decade and beyond* Command paper 849, HMSO, London

Eyman, R, Grossman, H, Chaney, R and Call, T (1990) The life expectancy of profoundly handicapped people with mental retardation *New England Journal of Medicine* **323**, 584–589

Finkelstein, V (1993) Disability: an administrative challenge? (The Health and Welfare Heritage) In Oliver, M (ed) *Social work. disabled people in disabling environments*. Jessica Kingsley, London, 19–39

Fryers, T (1997) Impairment, disability and handicap: categories and classifications. In Russell, O (ed) *Seminars in the psychiatry of learning disabilities* Gaskell, London

Galvin, SW and McCarthy, S (1994) Multi-disciplinary community teams: clinging to the wreckage *Journal of Mental Health* **3**, 157–166

Goffman, E (1968) *Asylums. Essays on the social situation of mental patients and other inmates* Penguin, Harmondsworth

Goldberg, D and Huxley, P (1992) *Common mental disorders. A bio-social model* Tavistock-Routledge, London

Grant, G, Humphreys, S and McGrath, M (eds)(1986) *Community mental handicap teams: theory and practice* BIMH, Kidderminster

House of Commons Health Committee (1996) *Long-term care: future provision and funding. Health committee third report volume 1* HMSO, London

Jones, K and Fowles, A (1984) *Ideas on institutions. Analysing the literature on long-term care and custody* Routledge & Kegan Paul, London

King's Fund Centre (1980) *An ordinary life: comprehensive locally-based services for mentally handicapped people* King's Fund Project Paper 24, King's Fund Centre, London

Lathrop, JP (1993) *Restructuring health care. The patient focused paradigm* The Health care Forum Leadership Centre Publication Series, Maxwell Macmillan International, London

Lewis, J and Glennerster, H (1996) *Implementing the new community care* Open University Press, Buckingham

Martin, J, Melzer, H and Elliot, D (1988) *The prevalence of disability among adults* OPCS Surveys, HMSO, London

Means, R and Smith, R (1994) *Community care. Policy and practice* Macmillan, Basingstoke

Morris, P (1969) *Put away: a sociological study of institutions for the mentally-retarded* Routledge & Kegan Paul, London

Nelson, T and Coxhead, H (1997) Increasing the probability of re-engineering/culture change success through effective internal communication *Strategic Change* **6**, 29–48

NHS Executive (1996) *The spectrum of care – a summary of comprehensive local services for people with mental health problems. 24 hour nursed beds for people with severe and enduring mental illness. An audit pack for the care programme approach* LASSL(96)16 and HSG(96)6, Department of Health, London

North East Thames Regional Health Authority (1994) *The report of the inquiry into the care and treatment of Christopher Clunis* HMSO, London

Olsen, MR (ed.) (1979) *The care of the mentally disordered: an examination of some alternatives to hospital care* BASW Publications, Birmingham

Onyett, S, Heppleston, T and Bushnell, D (1994) A national survey of community mental health teams. Team structure and process *Journal of Mental Health* **3**, 175–194

Patmore, C and Weaver, T (1991) *Community mental health teams: lessons for planners and managers* Good Practices in Mental Health, London

Powell, RB, Hollander, DB and Tobiansky, RI (1995) Crisis in admission beds: a four-year study of the bed state of Greater London's acute psychiatric units *British Journal of Psychiatry* **167**, 765–769

Race, D (1995) Historical development of service provision. In Malin N (ed.) *Services for people with learning disabilities* Routledge, London, pp. 46–78

Rose, J (1995) Stress and residential staff: towards an integration of existing research. *Mental Handicap Research* **8**, 220–236

Simons, K (1995) Empowerment and advocacy In Malin, N (ed.) *Services for people with learning fisabilities* Routledge, London, 170–188

Szivos, S (1992) The limits to integration? In Brown, H and Ward, L (eds) *Normalisation. A reader for the nineties* Routledge, London

Walmsley, J (1996) Doing what mum wants me to do: looking at family relationships from the point of view of people with intellectual disabilities *Journal of Applied Research in Intellectual Disabilities* **9**, 324–341

Warner, R (1994) *Recovery from schizophrenia. Psychiatry and political economy* Routledge, London

Wenger, GC (1992) *Help in old age – facing up to change* Liverpool University Press, Liverpool

Williams, R, Barrett, K and Muth, Z (eds) (1997) *Heading for better care. Commissioning and providing mental health services for people with Huntingdon's disease, acquired brain injury and early onset dementia* NHS Health Advisory Service, HMSO, London

Williams, R and Richardson, G (eds) (1995) *Together we stand. The commissioning, role and management of child and adolescent mental health services* NHS Health Advisory Service, HMSO, London

Wistow, G (1990) *Community care planning. A review of past experience and future imperatives* Department of Health, London

Womack, JP, Jones, DT and Roos, D (1990) *The machine that changed the world* Rawson Associates, New York

Woodhouse, K, Williams, R, MacMahon, D, Archer-Jones, P, Kennedy, R and Main, A (eds) (1997) *Services for people who are elderly. Addressing the balance. The multi-disciplinary assessment of elderly people and the delivery of high quality continuing care* NHS Health Advisory Service, HMSO, London

Wooley, M, Ham, C, Harwood, A and Patchett, S (1995) *The route to total care: joint commissioning of community care* Institute of Health Services Management, London

World Health Organisation (1980) *International classification of impairment, disability, and handicap* Geneva, World Health Organisation

16 Evidence-based practice: a new era in health care?

Kieran Walshe

Introduction

In recent years, a new idea has taken hold in the health care systems of many countries with remarkable speed, gaining the attention of clinicians, managers, civil servants, policy analysts and politicians alike and gathering advocates and disciples across the world. It has led to the founding of major new institutions in several countries concerned with developing and applying the idea; the establishment of an international organisation to lead the new movement; and the creation of several new journals to prose-lytise, raise awareness and satisfy the growing demand for information about this new idea. In many, diverse health care systems the idea has started to influence the thinking of policy makers and to have an increas-ing impact on the organisation and funding of health services.

This new idea is, put simply, that the health services we provide should be based on the best available evidence of their effectiveness, drawing par-ticularly on the findings of rigorously conducted research – what has become labelled 'evidence-based health care'. It is argued that for far too long the patterns of clinical practice and the way in which we organise and deliver health care have been too influenced by professional opinion, his-torical practice and precedent, clinical fashion, and organisational and social culture. As a result, we have often persisted in using health care interventions which are demonstrably ineffective, failed to take up other interventions which are known to be effective, and tolerated huge varia-tions in practice which must mean some patients receive ineffective care. The advocates of evidence-based health care call for science and evidence to play a much greater role in decision making throughout health care, in the clinical practice of doctors, nurses and other professionals, in the actions of managers and health care funders or purchasers, and in the health care policies adopted by Governments.

This chapter provides an overview of the origins and development of the evidence-based health care movement, outlines the changes it has already started to bring about in health services research and health care provision, and explores its likely future directions and impact. In so doing, it attempts to offer a balanced, critical analysis of the growing role of evidence-based health care which recognises both the powerfully persuasive nature of the concept and some of the potential problems and pitfalls which face those charged with translating the ideas into the realities of health care.

The origins of evidence-based health care

Some clinicians would argue that there is little new in the ideas of evidence-based health care, and that they have been practising in accordance with the available evidence on the effectiveness of health care interventions for many years, doing their best to offer patients the most effective therapies and treatments. Indeed, the suggestion that ineffective and outdated clinical practices are widespread is seen by some as a slight on their profession. However, the evidence seems to suggest that, despite clinicians' best intentions and genuine endeavours, there is real cause for concern about the effectiveness of many commonly used health care interventions.

A quarter of a century ago, an influential epidemiologist named Archie Cochrane published a book entitled *Effectiveness and efficiency: random reflections on health services* which set out, arguably for the first time, the idea of evidence-based health care (Cochrane 1972). Cochrane, whose working life had been spent evaluating the effectiveness of health services and exploring the epidemiology of various diseases, argued strongly that many commonly used and widely provided health services were of dubious effectiveness, and he criticised the medical profession in particular for failing to take proper account of the evidence from clinical and health services research, and instead basing their clinical practice on personal clinical experience, expert opinion, precedent and fashion. He advocated the establishment of a register of all randomised controlled trials (RCTs), which he regarded as the best source of evidence on the effectiveness of health care interventions. This register, which would be continually updated to take account of new findings from RCTs as they became available, would be organised in such a way that clinicians could easily identify the findings of relevance to their own areas of practice and so improve the effectiveness of the health services they provided.

Cochrane had been particularly critical of some practices of obstetricians and gynaecologists, and his book spurred a group of clinicians to take up his challenge and to start producing just such a register of RCTs in the field of pregnancy and childbirth (Chalmers *et al.* 1993). They began by using databases and manual searching of relevant journals to identify all RCTs undertaken of relevance to these areas, and then started, in collaboration with a growing number of other interested clinicians, to produce systematic reviews on particular themes or topics. The task was a massive undertaking, which eventually led to the publication in 1989 of a collection of hundreds of systematic reviews drawing on thousands of RCTs in a book entitled *Effective Care in Pregnancy and Childbirth* (Chalmers *et al.* 1989). This publication was then made available in a more condensed form, designed for everyday use by clinicians, and was also published on CD ROM so that it could be easily updated. The authors put in place arrangements to ensure that each systematic review in the collection continued to be revised and updated by one or more authors as new RCTs became available, so that the conclusions and recommendations for practice would be continually updated to take account of technological advances. For the first time, Cochrane's proposals for a register of RCTs had been realised, in one specialty at least. The book was received at first with some suspicion because it challenged many widespread clinical practices in obstetrics. However, it soon met with growing enthusiasm from obstetricians, midwives and health professionals in other specialties as its groundbreaking nature was realised. As the value of this collection of systematic reviews to those working in obstetrics was realised, many health professionals began to think about how it might be replicated in other clinical areas.

The science of undertaking systematic reviews developed in tandem with the work in obstetrics described above. Traditionally, reviews of the literature on clinical topics tended to present rather personal views of their subjects, often written by experts in the field but open to accusations of bias and subjectivity. In particular, the way in which studies in the area were identified was often unclear; the process for selecting which studies to include in the review and which to exclude was rarely specified; the quality of studies reviewed was very variable and sometimes rather poor; and the approaches used to combine the findings of multiple studies on the same research issue, especially when they produced differing results, were rather limited. While some reviews were undoubtedly very good, it was often difficult to establish which were rigorous and systematic analyses of the literature and which really represented a personal view on the topic, supported by a selective and partial scattering of references.

Gradually, a more systematic and objective approach to reviewing the literature on a topic began to emerge, in which explicit standards were set out for identifying relevant studies, deciding whether to include or exclude them, and presenting or combining their results (NHSCRD 1996). Statistical approaches to combining the quantitative results from a series of RCTs were developed. The meta-analysis of RCTs, though subject to some debate about its merits and meaning, provided a new tool for synthesising literature and offering simpler conclusions and recommendations to clinicians. In short, the process of producing systematic reviews of the literature on the effectiveness of health care interventions became more scientific, rigorous and credible. The ability of systematic reviews to combine the findings from several research studies and so offer more authoritative, certain and generalisable conclusions than any single study could give, began to demonstrate that such reviews were an important source of evidence in themselves (Chalmers and Altman 1995).

While the necessary tools and methods of evidence-based health care were being developed, a growing body of literature was accumulating to demonstrate the need for greater adherence to evidence on effectiveness. In many areas of clinical practice, there was quantitative data available to show that three forms of problem existed: first, that ineffective practices persisted long after they had been demonstrated to be ineffective; second, that effective treatments were taken up slowly, or not at all, despite the availability of evidence of their effectiveness; and third, that substantial and unjustifiable variations in clinical practice existed between countries, regions, hospitals, and even between clinicians in the same department or team. Some examples of each problem may help to illustrate the need for evidence-based health care:

- It has been known since the publication of some very large RCTs in the late 1980s (ISIS-2 1988) that if people who have a myocardial infarction (heart attack) are given thrombolytic therapy (drugs which help to prevent blood clots forming and to break up blood clots) promptly their chances of survival are increased significantly. In fact, a meta-analysis of RCTs on this topic showed that this was first demonstrated to be unequivocally effective in 19xx (Antman *et al.* 1992). However, clinical audits of practice (Ketley and Woods 1993) have found that up to 65 per cent of patients with myocardial infarctions who should be given thrombolytic therapy continue not to get it. Some must be dying as a result.

- Dilatation and curettage (D&C – the scraping of the lining of the womb) has long been a procedure used in the management of menorrhagia (heavy bleeding). It has been employed both in diagnosis, to exclude the possibility that the heavy bleeding results from some form of cancer of the uterus, and therapeutically, with the aim of reducing future bleeding. There has never been much evidence that D&C had any therapeutic benefit, and it has been described, to general agreement, as 'therapeutically useless and diagnostically inaccurate' (Lewis 1993). However, it continues to be one of the commonest operative procedures performed in the NHS, even though rates have fallen in recent years (Coulter 1993). Not only does this represent a massive waste of resources, in performing unnecessary procedures on thousands of women, it subjects those patients to the risks of anaesthesia and surgery, and also means that they have not been offered other, more effective medical and surgical interventions to treat their mennorhagia.

- Venous leg ulceration is a significant cause of chronic ill-health, particularly in the elderly. For many years, venous leg ulcers have been treated with a variety of dressings and topic preparations, with little success. Surgical debridement and skin grafting have also been used, again with relatively disappointing results. However, research in the 1980s showed that a particular form of compression bandaging, designed to apply graduated compression to the leg and so prevent the fluid accumulations which cause venous leg ulcers, was markedly more effective both in curing existing leg ulcers and in preventing recurrence

(NHSCRD 1997). Nevertheless, studies of actual practice demonstrate that up to 60 per cent of patients with leg ulcers still do not receive compression bandaging from the community nurses who care for this group of patients (Freak *et al.* 1995). Not only does this result in avoidable pain and suffering for these patients, it means that they require expensive continuing treatment for their condition.

- People who have had a cerebrovascular accident (CVA, or stroke) consume about 5 per cent of health care spending in the UK, partly in managing the immediate aftermath of the stroke but also in providing long-term care to patients who may be severely mentally and physically impaired by their stroke. However, the arrangements for managing stroke patients vary widely across the country. For example, in some places stroke patients are much more likely not to be admitted at all, but to be cared for at home, than in others. Some hospitals have specially designated stroke units, while others do not. The provision of speech therapy, physiotherapy and other rehabilitation is similarly haphazard (Wade 1994). Our current understanding of the effectiveness of stroke care and rehabilitation is rather limited, though there is evidence to suggest that specialised stroke units achieve better outcomes (NHSCRD 1993). Nevertheless, the current huge variations in patterns of care and clinical practice cannot be justified, and must mean that some patients receive ineffective care.

These examples of ineffective health care are unarguable, but there is much debate about how representative they are of wider clinical practice. While it has often been said that there is only good research evidence to demonstrate the effectiveness of 15 per cent of health care interventions (Smith 1991), other studies have suggested that in actual clinical practice up to 82 per cent of what clinicians do is well supported by the evidence (Ellis *et al.* 1995). It seems, however, that whatever specialty or profession one chooses, it is far from difficult to identify areas like those cited above, in which current practice and the recommendations of research are at odds. In some clinical areas, such as psychiatry, community nursing, or physiotherapy, there is a real dearth of evidence to support much of current clinical practice.

The term 'evidence-based health care' first started to be used in the 1990s to describe the greater use of research findings and other appropriate sources of evidence in health care decision-making. Sackett, one of the gurus of the EBH movement, defines evidence-based medicine from a clinician's perspective as consisting of five linked ideas (Sackett 1995). First, clinical decision-making should be based on the best available information about effectiveness, from individual patients and from epidemiological, research and laboratory sources. Second, the clinical situation facing the professional should determine the nature and source of evidence used to make decisions, rather than habits, precedent or tradition. Third, clinicians should be more willing to use epidemiological and statistical ways of thinking, and more able to integrate such evidence with their own personal experience. Fourth, the evidence must be translated into actions which improve the effectiveness and quality of care for patients. Fifth, clinicians should continually evaluate their own performance against these ideas. Sackett argues that practising evidence-based health care requires clinicians both to learn to find and use evidence of clinical effectiveness for themselves, and to make use of tools like guidelines and protocols which others have produced and based on the best available information on the effectiveness of interventions.

From a wider perspective, Appleby *et al.* (1995) suggest that evidence-based health care can be defined as the rigorous evaluation of the effectiveness of health care interventions; the dissemination of the results of those evaluations to those who need them; and the application of those results to influence clinical practice. They argue that each of these stages in the process (Figure 16.1) needs to be in place for evidence-based health care to work, and that there have been important shortcomings in all three.

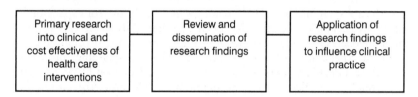

Figure 16.1 The evidence-based healthcare process

Later in this chapter, each of these stages in the process of evidence-based health care is examined in turn, and some of the current developments in the NHS aimed at making the process work better are examined.

The rise of the evidence-based health care movement

Cochrane first wrote about the need for evidence-based health care in 1972 (though many of his earlier writings might also be seen as advocating the ideas he brought together in his book on effectiveness in health care). Chalmers and his colleagues struggled to obtain funding and support for the development of their work on effective care in pregnancy and childbirth during the late 1970s and 1980s. Yet in the 1990s, and particularly over the last five years, evidence-based health care has seemed to be an idea whose time has come. In the UK, it now figures high on the national health care policy agenda and is explicitly part of the vocabulary of politicians of all parties. We have seen substantial resources invested in research and development and in promoting evidence-based health care, and increasing importance attached to issues of effectiveness and evidence by health care purchasers and providers. In the Netherlands, Sweden, France and other European countries, the USA, Canada and elsewhere there are similar developments in train, though the UK can probably claim to have done most to place evidence-based health care on the agenda to date (Walshe and Ham 1997).

We can only speculate about the reasons for this sudden and unprecedented rush towards evidence-based health care. It is tempting to attribute the current enthusiasm to the undoubted persuasive power of the concept – after all, who would argue that health services should not make good use of evidence on effectiveness? But we have to recognise that the idea was around for some years before it attracted such widespread attention and interest, so its current prominence cannot be ascribed simply to its intellectual appeal.

It might also be argued that the continuing cost pressures on health services that afflict most health care systems, resulting from rising consumer expectations, technological advance, demographic change and so on, are also a factor in the new focus on evidence-based health care. It is certainly true that in the UK some have attributed the Government's enthusiasm for evidence-based health care to a belief that there are swathes of ineffective health care interventions which could be eliminated, so reducing health care spending or at least creating some headroom for expansion in other areas. This expectation has been encouraged by some very prominent advocates of evidence-based health care, predicting it could save 2.5 per cent, 5 per cent or even 19 per cent of health care spending (Professor Sir Michael Peckham, quoted by Timmins 1996, Professor David Sackett, reported by the Office of Health Economics 1996, and Professor Colin Roberts 1995), though in fact there is little evidence that any real savings will result, and plenty of examples of areas where evidence-based practice is likely to cost more, not less. In any case, these cost pressures, though now greater than ever, are hardly new, so they cannot be the sole reason for evidence-based health care's new popularity.

Other causes for the rise of evidence-based health care seem somewhat likelier. First, the body of clinical knowledge which individual clinicians need to marshal and put to use has become increasingly large and complex, as the pace of technological advance has quickened and the volume of published material has mushroomed. It has been estimated that in order to stay up to date, doctors need to read 19 journal papers a day (Davidoff *et al.* 1995) – and not just read them, but understand and digest them, and be able to recall their findings when needed. The days are gone when clinicians could rely on what they were taught during their training, or could keep on top of things by reading one or two key professional journals. In a sense, the growing complexity of clinical knowledge has created an urgent need for systematic reviews, guidelines and the other tools of evidence-based health care.

Second, many of the tools and techniques used to support evidence-based decision making have only been developed recently. Cochrane's proposals for a register of all RCTs predated the development of some of the technologies which would make such a register feasible and usable – such as meta-analysis, systematic reviews, and particularly the widespread use of computerised bibliographic databases of journal publications. Information technology has also made it far more possible for clinicians to access evidence (in the form of guidelines, databases, on-line textbooks, and other sources) in the course of clinical practice at the locations where care is actually delivered. Realising the ambitious vision of evidence-based health care is more feasible now than it ever was in the past.

Third, it is now far easier than it used to be to question clinical behaviour and performance, and to raise issues of clinical effectiveness. In the UK, the last two decades have seen fundamental shifts in the power balance and accountability of clinicians and managers. Through a series of health care reforms, managers have become more able and more willing to engage clinicians in a discussion of issues of clinical performance and to seek to understand clinical decisions. Clinicians, particularly doctors, are generally more willing to recognise the need to account for their actions to others outside their own profession. Moreover, a new breed of clinical managers has been created, with both the clinical knowledge and the managerial remit to address problems of clinical performance or behaviour. Some years ago, it would have been difficult or even impossible to question the effectiveness of the clinical practices of clinicians, especially doctors. Now that kind of enquiry is more legitimate and is increasingly seen as a central task for health care purchasers and provider managers.

Fourth, the health care reforms which the British NHS underwent in the late 1980s and early 1990s made many of the decisions which used to be taken in rather hidden and implicit ways in the old NHS much more explicit and visible to the general public. The splitting of responsibility for purchasing and providing health care, and the creation of an internal market, left health care purchasers with new responsibilities for prioritising health care needs and ensuring the quality and effectiveness of the service they purchased. Both tasks require evidence on the effectiveness of health care interventions, and the visibility of the process; and the opportunity for both health care providers and members of the general public to challenge the decisions that health care purchasers take, created a real need for strong evidence to back up those decisions.

The rapid rise to prominence of the evidence-based health care movement has had two less positive effects. First, it has left some groups of health professionals with serious reservations about the likely impact on their own areas of work, and some legitimate objections to the proselytising tone of some of the strongest advocates of evidence-based health care (Lancet 1995). Some feel that the opportunity for careful debate and critical analysis of the ideas of evidence-based health care has been lost. Second, it has created unrealistically high expectations in some quarters of the degree of change that is likely to result from a greater adherence to the evidence. If the substantial investment of resources and policy makers' attention in evidence-based health care does not bring concomitant benefits in the short term, there is a risk that the issue will slip down the policy agenda and be seen, rather unfairly, to have failed to some degree.

Researching health care: the need for evidence

Unless the right research studies are undertaken, using appropriate and rigorously applied methods to address important and relevant research questions, the rest of the evidence-based health care process lacks the information on which is it crucially reliant. So in order to promote a more evidence-based approach to health care, the first step is to examine the way in which health care research is organised, funded and undertaken.

In the past, clinical and health services research in the UK has been funded by a variety of sponsors including the Government, publicly funded research councils, major medical research charities, universities, pharmaceutical companies, NHS organisations, and other charitable bodies. With a mosaic of funders, each with their own research agenda, it was difficult to discern much strategic direction. Apart from the inevitable problems of duplication and fragmentation, the financing of research tended to favour particular clinical areas and types of interventions (such as pharmaceutical research, and medical interventions) and not others (for example, physiotherapy interventions, or research into the care of people with learning disabilities). It was far from clear how the priorities were determined, but it seemed that researchers themselves and research funders were not necessarily responsive to the actual research needs of the NHS.

In 1991, the Department of Health established, for the first time in the history of the NHS, a research and development strategy for the health service (Box 16.1) whose aims were centred around the promotion of evidence-based health care (NHS Executive 1995).

Box 16.1 The NHS research and development strategy

Aim is 'to secure a knowledge-based health service in which clinical, managerial and policy decisions are based on sound and pertinent information about research findings and scientific and technological advance . . . maximising the effectiveness, efficiency and appropriateness of patient services'.

Key research and development functions, which did not generally exist before, include:

- Identifying NHS requirements for research and science-based knowledge
- Ensuring that knowledge is forthcoming through research commissioning etc
- Making knowledge available to decision makers through dissemination
- Promoting the use of research and development findings
- Promoting an evaluative culture in the NHS
- Developing and evaluating the NHS research and development strategy

Source: NHS Executive. Research and development in the new NHS: functions and responsibilities. Leeds: NHS Executive, 1995.

Since this strategy was established, some fundamental changes to the organisation and funding of research in the NHS have taken effect. An infrastructure for R&D has been created, headed by a Director of R&D for the NHS who sits on the NHS Executive Board and is supported by R&D directorates in each NHS Executive regional office. A number of commissioned programmes of research have been launched, developed from a systematic analysis of the research needs of the NHS. In some key areas, such as health technology assessment, a standing programme of work has been established, led by a new national centre. The research spending of Health Authorities and NHS trusts has been identified, and brought together into a new single central budget for research which will be used more strategically and accounted for more carefully in future. Overall, the NHS is believed to be investing about £400 million each year (or about 1 per cent of total spending) in research and development. Of course, much of the investment in health care research (and especially in clinical research) still lies outside the control of the NHS, in the Medical Research Council, medical research charities and pharmaceutical companies, but the more corporate and strategic approach being taken by the NHS is certainly beginning to influence their funding decisions too. While the new NHS approach to R&D is not without its problems, its achievements in a relatively short space of time are impressive.

Disseminating knowledge: a new industry in health care

Traditionally, the main channel for the dissemination of new knowledge resulting from research was publication in academic journals. For researchers (whose performance has sometimes been measured in terms of their publication rates), the publication of findings in journal papers was often seen as the completion of their task. Apart from presentations at conferences, there was really no other route for them to get the findings of their research to the clinicians and others who might need to know about them and apply them. Indeed, many researchers simply did not see the dissemination and implementation of their findings as their concern at all.

In practice, many clinicians do not read the academic journals in which research findings are published; it is simply unfeasible for some to keep up with the volume of publications in their specialty or clinical area; academic journals papers can be dense, demanding and even more or less unreadable at times; and clinicians often have neither the time nor the skills to appraise the quality of the papers they read and so decide what weight to give their conclusions and recommendations. Instead, clinicians rely on informal advice from colleagues, popular publications, information from drug companies and other lobbies, text books and other sources, so it is hardly surprising that it can take years before research findings published in journals become commonplace in clinical practice.

The second stage in evidence based health care – managing, reviewing and disseminating the findings from research studies to those who need to use them – demands a more organised, systematic and proactive approach. There have been a number of developments in recent years which provide the foundation for such an approach.

First, a number of journals of secondary publication have been established which specialise in abstracting the contents of academic journals, critically appraising the quality of papers, and publishing summaries of their subjects, methods and findings in a standardised format. The first such journal was the *American College of Physicians Journal Club* which was established in the early 1990s to provide general physicians with a single source of data on studies published in over 20 clinical journals. More recently it has been joined by *Evidence Based Medicine*, produced by the British Medical Journal, which includes some material from *ACP Journal Club* but also covers a number of journals in other specialties (surgery, obstetrics and gynaecology, paediatrics) – in total, over 50 journals. Most recently, the *Journal of Evidence Based Policy and Management* has been established with the ambitious aim of abstracting papers from a wide range of journals concerned with public health, health policy and planning, health services research, health economics and similar areas.

Second, the publication of *Effective Care in Pregnancy and Childbirth* (Chalmers *et al.* 1989) led to the establishment of an international collaborative effort to replicate this achievement in other clinical areas. Named after the epidemiologist who is credited with inspiring this movement, the Cochrane Collaboration is made up of teams in Cochrane Centres in the USA, Canada, Australia, and Europe – including a UK Cochrane Centre in Oxford. Each centre supports and co-ordinates review groups in various specialties who are undertaking systematic reviews on a range of research questions. The results of this enormous collective effort are published in the *Cochrane Library*, a CD ROM database of systematic reviews. The Cochrane Collaboration is a very new organisation, with a structure that is probably unique. The task it has set itself is hugely challenging, especially since most of those undertaking reviews do so as volunteers and are not recompensed for their efforts. If it can establish a database of systematic reviews throughout health care to parallel that already in place in obstetrics, the *Cochrane Library* will be an invaluable resource.

As well as supporting the UK Cochrane Centre, the British Government has also funded the establishment of a national centre to lead the review, management and dissemination of research findings in the UK. The NHS Centre for Reviews and Dissemination (NHSCRD), based in York, has started to compile a database of systematic reviews published in journals (the *Database of Abstracts of Reviews of Effectiveness* or *DARE*, published as part of the *Cochrane Library*), has produced guidance on the production of systematic reviews, and has commissioned reviews on behalf of the NHS. In particular, it has published a series of *Effective Health Care* bulletins, containing a review of the evidence and recommendations to clinicians, managers, purchasers and policy makers on a range of topics (Box 16.2).

Box 16.2 List of *Effective Health Care* bulletins published by the NHS Centre for Reviews and Dissemination

Volume 1.
1. Screening for Osteoporosis to Prevent Fractures
2. Stroke Rehabilitation
3. The Management of Subfertility
4. The Treatment of Persistent Glue Ear in Children
5. The Treatment of Depression in Primary Care
6. Cholesterol: Screening and Treatment
7. Brief Interventions and Alcohol Abuse
8. Implementing Clinical Practice Guidelines
9. Management of Menorrhagia

Volume 2.
1. The Prevention and Treatment of Pressure Sores
2. Benign Prostatic Hyperplasia: Treatment for Lower Urinary Tract Symptoms in Older Men
3. Management of Cataract
4. Preventing Falls and Subsequent Injury in Older People
5. Preventing Unintentional Injuries in Children and Young Adolescents
6. Management of Primary Breast Cancer
7. Total Hip Replacement
8. Hospital Volume and Health Care Outcomes, Costs and Patient Access

Volume 3.
1. Preventing and Reducing the Adverse Effects of Unintended Teenage Pregnancies
2. The Prevention and Treatment of Obesity
3. Mental Health Promotion in High Risk Groups
4. Compression Therapy for Venous Leg Ulcers

In addition to these facilities, there is now a growing range of other resources available in the UK to support the practice of evidence-based health care. The Centre for Evidence Based Medicine, based in Oxford and led by David Sackett, provides training, networking and resources for professionals to use. A number of regionally based units in the South and West, Midlands and Trent NHS regions have been set up to help health service staff and health care organisations to access available information about the effectiveness of health care interventions. A programme of critical appraisal training designed to help clinicians to read and interpret publications of research findings has been established in the Oxford and Anglia region and used nationally.

It is perhaps in this second stage in the evidence-based health care process – the review, management and dissemination of research findings – that the most dramatic changes have taken place so far. Where a decade ago there was almost nothing but an array of academic journals available to those who made the considerable effort needed to access their contents,

now there is a series of resources and facilities which can help those working in the health service to access the evidence they need, when and where
they need it. Of course, the task before us, in making clinical professionals
aware of these resources, enabling them to use them, and managing the
resulting demand, is daunting. Moreover, there are still weaknesses in
these new resources – their coverage of clinical topics and areas is far from
complete, and the evidence they contain tends to be focused on RCTs to
the exclusion of other equally important and valid quantitative and qualitative research methods. Nevertheless, it seems certain that the importance of reviewing, managing and disseminating research findings has, at
last, been recognised.

Changing practice: the greatest challenge of all

All the worthwhile improvements to the research process and innovations
in the review, management and dissemination of research findings
described above are of little real value if there are not effective mechanisms
for then applying that evidence to change clinical practice.

In the past, the task of changing clinical practice has largely been left to
the health care professions in the NHS. It has not been a corporate objective, figuring in strategies and business plans. Rather, it has happened
gradually, piecemeal, and sometimes rather invisibly as individual clinicians or clinical teams have adopted new practices – or not, as the case may
be. When new health care interventions have required additional
resources, or new equipment or facilities, then managers will usually
(though not always) have known about them. But when, for example, a
new drug has been substituted for an old one, or a new surgical technique
has replaced an existing procedure, managers and even clinical colleagues
or members of other professions have often been unaware of the change.
Similarly, when clinicians or clinical teams have continued to use outdated
or ineffective health care interventions, no-one has had the remit, the
authority (or, perhaps, the willingness) to encourage, promote and even
direct the necessary changes in practice. The NHS has lacked what
Berwick (1996) has called a 'system for improvement'.

Somewhat paradoxically, although the task of changing clinical practice
may be the most challenging and difficult stage in the evidence based
health care process, it seems to be the area in which there has been the least
investment of resources and effort to date. Researchers examining the
process have concluded that while there are many approaches to promoting and facilitating change – educational interventions, guidelines, financial incentives, feedback on performance, and so on – none seem to work
markedly better or worse than others (Oxman 1994). Moreover, whether
or not a particular approach works appears to depend crucially on how it is
employed; who uses it, and with whom; in what setting or context it is
used; and what form of change it is used to bring about. In other words, it
is extremely difficult to draw generalised conclusions about the effectiveness of different strategies for bringing about changes in clinical practice.

However, it is undeniable that in order to bring about changes in clinical practice, some form of systematic approach to identifying deficiencies in the quality and effectiveness of care, analysing their causes, and putting in place solutions which improve quality and effectiveness is needed. And such mechanisms need to exist in every clinical department, specialty or health care organisation which is expected to apply the evidence on effectiveness to change clinical practice. Without them, the pace of change is likely to be disappointingly slow and frustratingly uneven.

In fact, since 1989 doctors and other health care professionals working in the NHS in the UK have been required to take part in some form of clinical audit – the 'systematic critical analysis of the quality of clinical care' (NHS Executive 1996). Health care organisations have been expected to set up organisational structures and arrangements for clinical audit, and have received additional resources to enable them to do so. In theory, these clinical audit committees and groups which now exist in almost all hospitals and health care organisations should provide an ideal channel for the implementation of evidence-based health care. However, in practice a number of evaluations have indicated that the progress made in establishing clinical audit has been rather uneven, and while some health care organisations now have quite well organised systems for clinical audit in place, others have little or nothing to show for their efforts and investments in clinical audit to date (Walshe 1995).

Voices of dissent: problems with the new paradigm

The rapid rise of evidence based health care and the preaching tenor of publications and presentations from some of those involved in its development have, as was noted earlier, created some concerns and suspicions among clinicians, who view the evidence-based health care 'bandwagon' with a degree of cynicism. However, there have also been a number of serious and important reservations raised about the direction and implications of evidence-based health care which deserve serious consideration.

The feasibility of creating and maintaining systematic reviews across the whole health care arena, and marshalling and disseminating new evidence on effectiveness to all health care professionals, has yet to be demonstrated. Whether the sheer volume of information and pace of technological advance will defeat the reviewers and disseminators remains to be seen. It has been suggested that the advocates of evidence-based health care have underestimated the complexity of clinical practice and the inevitable ambiguity and subjectivity of much clinical decision making (Naylor 1995), and that they seek to impose a 'spurious rationality' on a process which cannot be analysed quite so simplistically (McKee and Clarke 1995)

The impact of evidence-based health care on the professions has also been questioned (Rees 1995). There is a legitimate fear that the greater use of guidelines and the recommendations of systematic reviews will deskill the professions, creating a body of clinicians who are less analytical and critical and who have much less clinical freedom than they have at present. Not everyone is convinced that evidence-based health care will bring unalloyed benefits for patients either. There is a rather paternalistic, technocratic feel to the logic of evidence-based health care, especially since the evidence on which is it based is largely drawn from a professionally driven, rather biomedical view of what constitutes effective care. Where patients' desired outcomes or valuations of health care risks and benefits differ from those embedded in the evidence, there may be rather less room in future for patient choice.

Some clinicians involved in research have questioned the impact of evidence-based health care on the processes by which health care advances and new knowledge is created. In particular, the broad limits placed on clinical practice have traditionally allowed considerable scope for diversity and experimentation. If there are, in future, rather more stringent evidence-based constraints on practice, some of the advances which might have come from such diversity and experimentation could be delayed or lost. Moreover, some health care technologies are apparently ineffective when first developed but become more effective as they are refined (transplant surgery being an obvious case in point). The timing of the evaluation of effectiveness may be crucial, and early evaluations could lead to potentially valuable therapies being prematurely labelled as ineffective.

The development of evidence-based health care also has some wider, health policy implications. Taken to its logical extreme, the evidence-based health care movement might presage the end of health policy as we know it – since we should be able to evaluate the effectiveness of the policy alternatives before us and opt for the most effective, rather than making the decision on political or social grounds. In reality, health policy making will remain a complex and subjective business, formed as much by the cultural, social and political environment in which it takes place as it is by the evidence on effectiveness.

Finally, we should acknowledge that the evidence-based health care movement is not the first attempt to sort out the way that health care or other areas of human endeavour use scientific knowledge and evidence. Klein and colleagues (1996), in expressing doubts about the objectivity and feasibility of evidence-based health care have labelled the movement the 'new scientism' – drawing implicit parallels with previous rationalist movements who have believed they can solve the problems of the world through the application of the scientific method. For example, advocates of evidence-based health care might see some welcome and unwelcome parallels in the rise and fall of 'scientific management' earlier this century.

The future of evidence-based health care

Evidence-based health care has certainly been oversold – and there will, unfortunately but inevitably, be a reaction of disappointment and disillusion when the reality fails to live up to the hyped expectations of some.

Having said that, it would be churlish in the extreme not to acknowledge the improvements to the research and development process which have already been brought about, and to support the ambitious and highly worthwhile aims of endeavours like the Cochrane Collaboration and other centres striving to get the evidence on the effectiveness of health care interventions into clinical practice. It is unarguably true that in the past, for a number of reasons, we failed to use this evidence properly and as a result ineffective practices were perpetuated and effective practices were introduced slowly or not at all. It is important to remember that, as a result, some patients will have lost their lives and others will have suffered unnecessary morbidity. But it is still to be proven that the new focus on evidence-based health care, and particularly the strategies and approaches which are now being implemented, will change this situation for the better.

References

Antman, EM, Lau, J, Kupelnick, B et al. (1992) A comparison of results of meta-analyses of randomised control trials and recommendations of clinical experts: treatments for myocardial infarction *Journal of the American Medical Association* **268**, 240–248

Appleby, J, Walshe, K and Ham, C (1995) *Acting on the evidence* NAHAT, Birmingham

Berwick, D (1996) A primer on leading the improvement of systems *British Medical Journal* **312**, 619–622

Chalmers, I and Altman, D (eds) (1995) *Systematic reviews* BMJ Publishing Group, London

Chalmers, I, Enkin, M and Keirse, M (1989) *Effective care in pregnancy and childbirth* Oxford University Press, Oxford

Chalmers, I, Enkin, M and Keirse, M (1993) Preparing and updating systematic reviews of randomised controlled trials of health care *Milbank Quarterly* **71**, 411–438

Cochrane, AL (1972) *Effectiveness and efficiency: random reflections on health services* Nuffield Provincial Hospitals Trust, Leeds

Coulter, A, Klassen, A, MacKenzie, I et al. (1993) Diagnostic dilatation and curettage: is it used appropriately? *British Medical Journal* **306**, 236–239

Davidoff, F, Haynes, B, Sackett, D et al. (1995) Evidence based medicine. A new journal to help doctors identify the information they need *British Medical Journal* **310**, 1085–1086

Ellis, J, Mulligan, I, Rowe, J et al. (1995) Inpatient general medicine is evidence based *Lancet* **346**, 407–409

Freak, L, Simon, D and Kinsella, A (1995) Leg ulcer care: an audit of cost effectiveness *Health Trends* **27**, 133–136

ISIS-2 (Second International Study of Infarct Survival) Collaborative Group (1988). Randomised trial of intravenous streptokinase, oral aspirin, both or neither among 17,187 cases of suspected myocardial infarction: ISIS-2 *Lancet* **ii**, 349–360

Ketley, D and Woods, KL (1993). Impact of clinical trials on clinical practice: example of thrombolysis for acute myocardial infarction *Lancet* **342,** 891–894

Klein, R, Day, P and Redmayne, S (1996). *Managing scarcity: priority setting and rationing in the National Health Service* Open University Press, Buckingham

Lancet (1995) Evidence based medicine, in its place *Lancet* **346,** 785

Lewis, BV (1993). Diagnostic dilatation and curettage in young women should be replaced by outpatient endometrial biopsy *British Medical Journal* **306,** 225–226

McKee, M and Clarke, A (1995) Guidelines, enthusiasms, uncertainty and the limits to purchasing *British Medical Journal* **310,** 101–104

Naylor, CD (1995) Grey zones of clinical practice: some limits to evidence-based medicine *Lancet* **345,** 840–842

NHS Centre for Reviews and Dissemination (1993) Stroke rehabilitation *Effective Health Care Bulletin* **2**

NHS Centre for Reviews and Dissemination (1996) *Undertaking systematic reviews of research on effectiveness* NHSCRD, University of York, York

NHS Centre for Reviews and Dissemination (1997) Compression therapy for venous leg ulcers *Effective Health Care Bulletin* **3**

NHS Executive (1995) *Research and development in the new NHS: functions and responsibilities* NHS Executive, Leeds

NHS Executive (1996) Clinical audit in the NHS NHS Executive, Leeds

Office of Health Economics (1996) *OHE News No 3* Office of Health Economics, London

Oxman, A (1994) *No magic bullets: report prepared for North East Thames Regional Health Authority* McMaster University, McMaster, Canada

Rees, J (1995) Where medical science and human behaviour meet *British Medical Journal* **310,** 850–853

Roberts, C *et al.* (1995) Rationing is a desperate measure *Health Service Journal* **12 Jan,** 15

Sackett, D (1995) The need for evidence based medicine *Journal of the Royal Society of Medicine* **88,** 620–624

Smith, R (1991) Where is the wisdom . . . ? The poverty of medical evidence *British Medical Journal* **303,** 798–799

Timmins, N (1996) NHS 'wastes £1 billion on ineffective treatment'. *Independent* Jan 2 1996 5

Wade, DT (1994) Stroke (acute cerebrovascular disease) In Stevens, A and Raftery, J (eds) *Health care needs assessment (vol 1)* Radcliffe Medical Press, Oxford

Walshe, K (ed.) (1995) *Evaluating clinical audit: past lessons, future directions* Royal Society of Medicine Press, London

Walshe, K and Ham, C (1997) *Acting on the evidence: progress in the NHS* NHS Confederation, Birmingham

17 Public involvement in the NHS

Shirley McIver

Introduction

The debate about whether or not public involvement in health service decisions should be increased has flowed in and out of the limelight since the inception of the NHS. In the 1960s and 1970s, the subject attracted a great deal of attention. In the 1980s it received less publicity, but in the 1990s it has returned to a prominent position.

The structure of the NHS has changed significantly over the intervening years but little has been done to alter the relationship between the NHS and its public. The parameters of the debate about public involvement remain essentially the same. There have been changes, particularly in guidance from the NHS Executive, and in methods for involving the public, but many of the issues raised in earlier analyses remain relevant.

This chapter will examine public involvement in three main sections. The first will provide a brief historical overview of the subject, looking particularly at the implications of recent structural change and at government documents, such as *Local Voices* (NHS Management Executive 1992) and *Patient Partnership: Building a Collaborative Strategy* (NHS Executive 1996). The second will examine some of the key issues in the debate about increasing public involvement, such as who should be involved and what decisions they should be involved in. The third section will look at methods for involving the public, especially recent innovations such as health panels and citizens' juries.

Historical overview

The NHS was set up with an indirect rather than direct form of public involvement. Health services were to be accountable to the public through the democratic system, the line of accountability being upwards to parliament and the elected members of the House of Commons.

The only significant structural change was made during the 1974 reorganisation of the NHS, when Community Health Councils were introduced to represent the views of the public to Health Authorities.

Subsequent changes to the NHS have had implications for the relationship between the public and the NHS, rather than any direct effect on that relationship. This has meant that although changes have occurred, these have not been dramatic.

The 1983 NHS Management Inquiry, led by Sir Roy Griffiths (The Griffiths Report 1983) was responsible for encouraging a change in the relationship between professionals and patients into one more closely modelled on that between service providers and customers in the business sector. The Griffiths Report made a series of recommendations for overcoming what it identified as weaknesses in the management of the NHS, and encouraged the introduction of business innovations such as quality management, market research and a consumer focus. Comments made in the Report included:

> *Businessmen have a keen sense of how well they are looking after their customers. Whether the NHS is meeting the needs of the patient, and the community, and can prove that it is doing so, is open to question.* (p. 10)

The NHS largely responded to this recommendation by carrying out surveys of patients, a practice which has continued, and by the appointment of various personnel with responsibilities for overseeing developments in this area, such as quality managers and consumer relations officers, many of which were short-lived posts.

Initiatives stimulated by the Griffiths Report were mainly directed at patients rather than the public, although the Report had included responsiveness to the needs of 'the community' within its scope. It was not until the 1989 White Paper *Working for Patients* (Secretary of State 1989) and the subsequent 1990 NHS and Community Care Act which introduced an internal market into the NHS that a focus on the public was introduced.

The internal market separated service providers from purchasers of services. District Health Authorities were given the job of purchasing health services according to the needs of their local communities. A guidance document *Local Voices* issued by the NHS Management Executive in 1992 made it clear that the Government expected Health Authorities to take into account the needs and preferences of local people when purchasing services.

Local Voices introduced the notion that Health Authorities should be 'champions of the people' in that:

> ... *their decisions should reflect, so far as practical, what people want, their preferences, concerns and values.* (p. 3)

The 'champions of the people' role can be seen as an extension to the local community of the emphasis on consumerism introduced by the Griffiths Report, but it also begins to suggest a changing relationship with the public of a different kind. This is illustrated by the emphasis in *Local Voices* on involving local people in health service decision-making, and by the identification of a need to enhance NHS credibility with the public.

The advice given by the NHS Management Executive encourages a closer relationship between the Health Authorities and the public. For example:

> ... *as Health Authorities seek to bring about changes in services and make explicit decisions about priorities they are likely to be more persuasive and successful in their negotiations with providers if they secure public support.* (p. 3)

Although in some places *Local Voices* appears to be doing no more than encouraging better public relations in Health Authorities, in others it is clearly advocating greater public influence over purchasing decisions:

> *The aim should be to give local people the opportunity to influence the debate at critical stages of the (purchasing) cycle.* (p. 5)

The emphasis in *Local Voices* on gaining public support for decisions is perhaps not surprising given that the 1989 White Paper appeared to remove some degree of local accountability to the public by abolishing local authorities' right to nominate Health Authority members. When this is combined with the fact that the internal market also created self-governing NHS trusts as the principal providers of health services, allowing them greater freedom to change services without consultation and without the requirement to hold their meetings in public, attempts to address what was perceived by some as a growing democratic deficit in the new arrangements, were not unexpected.

Another strand of what came to be known as the 1989 NHS reforms was the introduction of fundholding for general practitioners. This meant that some GPs became purchasers of services as well as service providers. Many fundholders joined together into large commissioning groups, creating new organisations which did not have clearly worked out relationships with either Health Authority purchasers or the local community on behalf of whom they purchased services.

Historically, GPs were professionally accountable for the clinical decisions they made regarding patients, but lines of accountability for purchasing decisions were unclear. The reforms created a new relationship between many GPs and their local communities.

Apart from these changes which had implications for the relationship between the NHS and the public, there were also a few which had implications for the relationship between the NHS and service users, or patients. Changes in community care policy required health and local authorities to work together to produce joint community care plans and there was a statutory requirement that these should be developed after consultation with service users. This meant that for the first time it was obligatory for service users to be consulted over the development of services.

The Patient's Charter was introduced in 1991 along with over 40 other national public service charters under the umbrella of the Citizen's Charter (Prime Minister 1991). The stated aims of these public service charters were to raise quality standards and make these explicit to service users, hence the six Charter principles which were listed as:

- publish standards of service;
- be more open and provide more information;
- provide choice and consult you where possible;
- be polite and helpful at all times;
- put things right when they go wrong;
- give value for money.

The Patient's Charter (DoH 1991) gave details of established rights and standards in the NHS, and an updated version published in 1995 introduced three new rights and some new standards. Of the rights and standards contained in the Charter, only one has fairly radical implications for the relationship between the patient and the professional. This is the right:

> *To be given a clear explanation of any treatment proposed, including any risks and any alternatives, before you decide whether you will agree to the treatment.*

This legitimises patients' continuing appeal for better information to be made available when they use services, and makes it clear that there should be some discussion about treatment before a course of action is agreed upon. In other words, it raises patients' expectations that they should have some say in decisions that are made about their treatment and care.

The NHS Executive guidance document *Patient Partnership: Building a Collaborative Strategy* published in 1996 (NHS Executive 1996) reinforced messages about greater public and patient involvement in decision-making. The document was intended

> *. . . to stimulate further debate, discussion and local action, rather than as a single definitive policy statement.* (p. 1)

It backed up one of the NHS Executive's medium term priorities for 1996/7 to:

> *Give greater voice and influence to users of NHS services and their carers in their own care, the development and definition of standards set for NHS services locally and the development of NHS policy both locally and nationally.* (DoH 1995/6)

The *Patient Partnership* document proposed a strategy for addressing four main aims. These were stated as:

- to promote user involvement in their own care, as active partners with professionals;
- to enable patients to become informed about their treatment and care and to make informed decisions and choices about it if they wish;
- to contribute to the quality of health services by making them more responsive to the needs and preferences of users;
- to ensure that users have the knowledge, skills and support to enable them to influence NHS service policy and planning.

To meet these aims, the document proposed that work needed to be undertaken in four main areas:

- production and dissemination of information for health service users and their representatives;
- structural, organisational and resourcing requirements for patient partnership and involvement including skill development and support for users;
- supporting all staff in achieving active partnership and user involvement in service development;
- research and evaluation of effective mechanisms for patient partnership and involvement.

At the time of writing it was too early to track how the aims would be worked through into practice, apart from the fact that a Patient Partnership Strategy Co-ordinator had been appointed, a national conference on Patient Partnership had taken place in 1997, and a national Centre for Health Information Quality established with a launch date of November 1997.

In sum, there have been no major statutory changes to alter the relationship between the NHS and the public since Community Health Councils were introduced in 1974. The 1989 White Paper introduced changes, such as the abolition of local authorities' right to nominate Health Authority members, the creation of self-governing trusts, and the establishment of GP Fundholders which could be interpreted as weakening local accountability to the public, although accountability has always been primarily upwards to parliament.

Any changes have been in the form of increased guidance from the centre on the issue of public and patient involvement in the NHS. In documents such as *Local Voices* and *Patient Partnership*, the NHS Executive has encouraged health professionals and managers to involve the public and patients in health service decisions at all levels.

Key public involvement issues

Like much guidance from the NHS Executive, that concerning public and patient involvement has been fairly general and non-prescriptive. This has left plenty of room for local interpretation around issues such as which aspects of the considerable agenda should be prioritised, to what extent it should be resourced, who should be involved, what decisions should be open for public involvement, and what methods should be used.

Taking the issue of the breadth of the agenda first, it is worth clarifying what types of public and patient involvement are being encouraged by the Centre. There are three main types:

1. Patient and user involvement in decisions about their treatment and care

If patients are to have more say in decisions about their treatment and care, health professionals will have to learn how to provide better information and be more explicit about the way they make decisions. Whereas in the past, health professionals have tended to wait for the patient to ask for information, they will now have to offer information and the opportunity to discuss treatment and care. Professional training will need to change to take this into account, service providers will have to include this aim in their standards of care, and purchasers will be expected to monitor progress.

Despite the apparent straightforwardness of this type of patient involvement in decisions, it is not without controversy. Many clinicians state that a large number of patients expect the health professional to make the decision because they are the expert. They claim that patients do not want to be laden with technical information, frightened by statistics about the side effects or consequences of treatment or burdened by difficult decisions. The law upholds the clinicians' view in this respect. Legal rulings promote the view that the imparting of information to patients is a matter of clinical judgement (Gilbert 1995).

Whilst surveys of patients' views of care since the 1960s have shown that patients would like better information (McIver 1993), there has not been a great deal of research on the extent to which different types of patients want to be involved in treatment decisions. What few studies there have been have shown that although many patients want to participate in the decision-making process, the extent can vary. For example, Savage and Armstrong reported a study which randomly allocated patients to a 'directing style' or a 'sharing style' of consultation and then measured patient satisfaction. They found that patients who received the directing style were more satisfied except in cases of longer consultations; consultations in which advice was the main treatment; patients whom the doctor judged to have a chronic illness; and patients who judged themselves to have a psychological illness. In other words, the 'directing style' was beneficial to those patients whom the GP thought had mainly physical problems and those who received a prescription. This led the researchers to suggest that patients with a simple physical illness may benefit from a directing style, whereas those with a more complex illness may respond better to an interactive approach (Savage and Armstrong 1990).

Some of the most interesting and significant research findings in terms of the implications for shared decision-making have emerged from studies which examine patients' views of risk. For example, O'Meara *et al.* (1994) found that patients who had suffered a deep vein thrombosis were unwilling to accept even the very small short-term risk of intracranial haemorrhage and death associated with experts' preferred treatment, while McNeil *et al.* (1978) found that many lung cancer patients were not prepared to take the risk of death associated with surgery even though long term survival rates were better for surgery than radiotherapy.

If a patient's view of risk may well be different from that of the health professional, should the professional make the decision 'in the best interests of the patient', or should they discuss the treatment with the patient and let them make the final decision, even though they may disagree with it?

The extent to which health professionals can act paternalistically 'in the best interests of the patient' is being eroded culturally, if not legally in the UK and, if nothing else, this means that they will need to find out from the patient their expectations of the relationship. The task will become easier as materials are developed which promote shared decision-making. The interactive video *Shared Decision-Making Programmes* produced in the USA and being piloted in the UK by the King's Fund are an example (Kasper *et al.* 1992).

2. User involvement in service development, monitoring and evaluation

What started in the 1980s as increased market research activity in the form of patient satisfaction surveys has been extended to an expectation that service users will be involved in other aspects of service planning and evaluation. This development is probably due to a combination of the perceived failure of patient satisfaction surveys and a realisation that it is probably more cost effective to design a service in a way that suits users, than to correct the design at a later stage. Patient satisfaction surveys are carried out by most trusts, and an increasing number of general practitioners, but they have been the subject of both academic and practitioner criticism. Academics have questioned the validity of the concept of 'patient satisfaction' (Williams 1994) and the lack of technical skill with which most practitioners design and carry out surveys (Carr-Hill 1992).

When expertly designed standard questionnaires have been developed, such as those for assessing patients' views of surgery (Meredith *et al.* 1993) and for inpatients (Bruster *et al.* 1994), there has been very limited interest. There appears to be a great demand for good quality questionnaires to gather users' views of service quality and yet little uptake when these are produced nationally. This is puzzling but may be due to the need for locally tailored questionnaires, or the high cost of purchasing and using national instruments. Providers may also be suspicious of joining national surveys because the data could be used for comparison purposes, and whilst benchmarking is often considered useful, 'league tables' are not generally popular.

Practitioners have questioned the usefulness of surveys compared with qualitative methods for obtaining patients' views of service quality and many have replaced surveys with focus group discussions and similar techniques designed to explore user views rather than measure the extent of their satisfaction with services. There is a place for both qualitative methods which explore users views, and quantitative methods which establish the extent to which users are happy with different aspects of a service. Both types of research method are useful in monitoring and evaluating services.

Research methods are less useful during the design and planning stages of services and when service standards are being set. This is because planning is a complex activity and user views may be required at several stages of the process as new information is received and the boundaries shift. An interactive model is likely to be more productive in these circumstances than the information collection model epitomised by most research methods.

One of the problems with involving users in the planning and design of services is that it is not always clear who should be responsible for carrying it out. Should it be the service provider, or the purchaser? And who else should be involved – social services, general practitioners? If duplication is to be avoided, collaboration is necessary.

3. Involving the public

The area where most uncertainties exist is that of public involvement. Where service development is concerned, it is clear that those who have used the service will have a role to play in saying how it could be improved, but how can people who have never used a service and who may not be particularly interested, legitimately be involved?

There are two main justifications for the involvement of the public in service development issues. The first is that, as taxpayers, they have a right to have a say in how their money is spent. This justification rests upon a broader argument about the need for greater public accountability in the NHS and for a more participative democracy generally (Coote 1996). The second, which is often linked to the first, is that lay people who have no vested interest in a service bring a unique and valuable perspective which is needed alongside those of professionals and users (Barnes 1997). Even if these arguments are accepted, there are still a range of issues which need to be addressed before the public can be involved.

First, for many services there is a fairly clearly defined body of users from whom it is relatively easy to recruit a representative sample. Quite large numbers of people may be involved in some cases, but by a combination of research methods and consultation it will usually be possible to gather details of how services may be improved and to work with a small number of users to implement changes. However, if the wider public is to be involved, there is no such easily defined target population. Who among the local people should be involved ? A representative sample would be enormous.

Not only that, but unlike users, they cannot be expected to know very much about the service, so they will need information to prepare them. This means that the method used to involve them will have to take this into account. Research methods such as surveys may be able to gather the views of hundreds of people but this will be an uninformed view unless information is supplied at the same time. Service development issues are complex and so it is unlikely that even if information is supplied, this type of method will be satisfactory. A second issue, then, is how the public can be involved, given that they will need information.

Third, the range of issues the public could potentially be involved in is limitless. Once it is accepted that the public have a right to have a say in how their taxes are spent to provide NHS services, where does this end? Apart from service development issues, there are related issues about service change and reconfiguration, and there are decisions that are made about how money should be spent, both that allocated between different services, and the way it is spent within a particular service area.

To increase the involvement of patients, service users, and the public, in the way described above is a formidable task and one which the Government apparently expects to be carried out with little extra funding and probably no new legislation. Many Health Authorities and trusts are already doing work, particularly in the area of service user involvement. The statutory requirement that health and local authorities consult service users on joint community care plans has resulted in an upsurge of activity in this area, and it is likely that this will continue. The DoH investment of several hundred thousand pounds in the Centre for Health Information Quality and a co-ordinator to help promote the *Patient Partnership Strategy* means that the area of patient involvement in treatment and care is also likely to proceed steadily.

The area of most uncertainly is that of public involvement. Developments in this area rest on whether or not the Government decides to make any statutory changes to increase the level of public accountability in the NHS. If changes are made then this should clarify the issue for service providers and purchasers. If they make no change but the DoH continues to expect greater public involvement then there will have to be discussion between the NHS and the public to provide some guidance on what level of public involvement is acceptable. To avoid expensive duplication of effort, it would be best if this were to take place at a national level.

In the meantime it may be worth pointing out that the Codes of Conduct and Accountability in the NHS which took effect from April 1994 confirmed that Health Authorities and trusts were accountable to the Secretary of State, but emphasised the need for openness with the public. To reinforce the latter, the new codes included an obligation for Health Authorities (as well as trusts) to publish an annual report on their performance and stewardship of public finances. Most of the emphasis in the codes was on the need for openness about financial matters but the codes also mentioned the need for openness about the need for service change, stating that the reasons for changes should be fully explained to the public before decisions are reached (DoH 1994).

It would appear from this document that accountability in relation to the public, is largely considered to be about transparency in decision-making rather than public involvement in decisions. If that is the case then Health Authorities and trusts need to be more concerned about devising ways of explaining and justifying their decisions to the public than involving them in those decisions. Of course, one way of justifying a decision may be by demonstrating that the public made a contribution.

In sum, the public involvement agenda has a number of different aspects which entail a considerable amount of development work. A paternalistic culture where health professionals make decisions in the best interests of patients is no longer acceptable to many people. There is a demand for better information and more opportunity to take part in decisions about treatment and care. This is being supported by a DoH funded Centre for Health Information Quality.

User involvement in service development has since the 1980s mainly comprised market research on users' views of services, through the use of 'patient satisfaction' surveys and focus groups. The 1990 NHS and Community Care Act required health and local authorities to consult with users over community care plans and this has set a precedent for user involvement in service design and may mean that activity in this area increases.

There is considerable confusion over the extent to which the public should be involved in health care decisions. Although some Health Authorities are experimenting with methods which ask groups of the public to produce recommendations, others are concentrating on explaining their decisions to the public through public meetings, newspapers or annual reports.

Methods for public and user involvement

Community Health Councils (CHCs), introduced in 1974, are the statutory mechanism for involving users and the public, but since their inception the effectiveness with which they carry out this task has been questioned.

The main criticism is over their ability to act as an intermediary between service providers and the public, given that most of the public do not seem to know of their existence, a fact acknowledged by CHCs themselves. As recently as 1997, the national CHC organisation, the Association of Community Health Councils for England and Wales (ACHCEW) was, at its Annual General Meeting, deploring the

> lack of public awareness of CHCs, even after 23 years, despite considerable efforts on the part of the CHCs themselves (ACHCEW 1997).

Critics have also questioned the extent to which CHCs are able to represent the views of a wide range of people given that their members are frequently drawn from the pool of typical volunteers – white, elderly and middle class. This would not be such a problem were they able to canvass the views of a wider range of people, but they are not often skilled in research methods and the finance at their disposal is very limited – the total CHC budget being less than 0.1 per cent of the total NHS budget.

One of the problems for CHCs is that their original brief was not very explicit and so it is difficult for them to use their limited budgets in an effective way. ACHCEW has attempted to address this by issuing guidance on performance standards (ACHCEW 1994) and objective setting (ACHCEW 1992), but some of the problem lies with NHS managers and professionals who are not clear about how they should relate to the CHC. They are aware that they must consult CHCs over major service change, but the mechanisms of consultation have largely been left in their hands and may not be satisfactory from the CHC point of view.

In 1996, when Regional Health Authorities were abolished, responsibility for establishing CHCs moved to the Regional Offices of the NHS

Executive and new resource allocation arrangements were developed. At the same time, the NHS Executive commissioned a review of CHC resourcing and performance management. The subsequent Insight Report proved to be controversial in that it recommended the phasing out of several of the major activities carried out by CHCs, including information provision and advice to the public, and support for complainants (ACHCEW 1996/7).

One positive aspect of the review is that it has encouraged ACHCEW to try to clarify the terms of its working relationship with different areas of the NHS, including NHS trusts, GP Fundholders, and the NHS Executive, and this may result in a clearer understanding of their role.

A range of methods have been used by CHCs and health professionals and managers for gathering the views of users and the public. These methods have different aims and objectives. There are two broad categories of method: those deriving from social science research, and a range of informal methods which have been developed largely by practitioners. The range of informal methods has been extended recently and more formal ways of involving users and the public have been piloted.

User and public views have been sought using both qualitative research methods, such as in-depth interviews and group discussions, and quantitative methods, such as large scale postal questionnaires or interview surveys (McIver 1991). These methods are designed to collect information which is reliable and valid. The information, when analysed, can then be used to inform decision-making.

Most research methods are not designed to involve the research subjects in the process of research, nor are they intended as a way of involving people in service design or decision-making. A range of more informal methods has emerged to cope with these aims and to complement research methods.

The informal methods range from those designed to help individuals to give their views, such as patient advocates and representatives (McIver 1994), to those aimed at facilitating groups of users to express their collective views, such as patients' councils and health fora (McIver 1991). During the 1980s, innovations in these informal methods were mainly concerned with involving service users, and consultation with the public was confined to contact with the CHC or public meetings. In the 1990s greater pressure on Health Authorities and trusts to consult with the public combined with the apparent weakness of public meetings, led to experimentation with new methods.

Two new methods have attracted most interest in the NHS. The first comprises groups or panels of the public and these are based on the consumer panels and group discussions which have been run by commercial organisations for many years for market research purposes.

For example, Somerset Health Authority runs eight groups of 12 people which meet three times a year to discuss health service priorities. The groups represent as far as possible a cross-section of the population and each group member is recruited for a year. The groups are asked about 'live' issues for the Health Authority and are given background information before and during the meeting. The discussions are tape recorded and analysed, and there are also scoring exercises for group members to carry out (Bowie *et al.* 1995).

The second new method is the citizens' jury which has been piloted in Health Authorities and local authorities by the Institute for Public Policy Research, and in Health Authorities by the King's Fund. The concept originated in the USA and Germany where it has been developed and applied over approximately 20 years. A citizens' jury comprises a group of between 12 and 20 people who have been recruited to represent a cross-section of the population. They are given a question to address and over a four-day period they receive information, hear evidence from witnesses, discuss the issue and produce recommendations (Stewart *et al.* 1994).

Most of the pilot juries which have taken place have involved important local service planning or policy issues, such as the priorities for palliative care development, how gynaecological cancer services should be provided, or the provision of back pain services.

The recommendations produced by the jury, although not binding on the Health Authority, must be taken seriously because the juries receive a large amount of local publicity. This makes it necessary to explain how they are implementing the recommendations or the reasons why they are unable to do so.

Both citizens' juries and health panels offer advantages over the public meeting because they build in the opportunity for the public who attend to become informed about the issue under consideration. This happens through the allocation of time for questions as well as facilitated discussion and deliberation. Citizens' juries are more time intensive and also more expensive than group discussions and panels because the jurors are paid for the four days work, but they enable the participants to tackle an issue in an extremely thorough way.

The high cost – approximately £17,000 plus staff time – of a citizens' jury means that it is likely to be a method which is only used occasionally for certain kinds of issues, but it should be possible to adapt aspects of the process to enhance other methods or devise new ones. For example, public meetings could be greatly improved by including more accessible information and time for small group discussion of issues. One day public workshops on issues could be organised with local people being recruited to represent a cross-section of the local population. They could be given an issue to address and asked to produce recommendations.

In sum, Community Health Councils are the statutory mechanism for involving the public in the NHS but the limited role of the CHC combined with a growing expectation that the public will be consulted over a range of issues, has generated experimentation with a number of methods. Research methods generally collect the existing views of the public, whilst new methods such as citizens' juries enable the public to become informed before giving their views. Where the issues they are being asked to comment on are complex, this can be useful.

Conclusions

The 1990 NHS and Community Care Act introduced changes such as the abolition of local authorities' right to nominate Health Authority members, the creation of self-governing trusts, and the establishment of GP Fundholders which have been seen as weakening local accountability to the public. These changes have been accompanied by increased guidance from the NHS Executive on the issue of patient and public involvement but this covers a broad spectrum and leaves room for local interpretation.

A number of initiatives are being centrally driven to support the guidance, such as the establishment of a Centre for Health Information Quality, but as yet these have related to patient involvement in treatment and care and user involvement in service development. Public involvement is a relatively undeveloped area.

Little research has been carried out to assess the merits of different user and public involvement methods or to evaluate what is achieved from greater involvement. In this respect the situation is not that radically different from the early 1980s when one researcher commented:

Little consensus has been reached about what participation actually does, for the new participants or for anyone else (Richardson 1983)

Until the NHS and its public are clear about the mutual benefits obtained by working together and until compatible expectations are achieved, progress in this area will continue to feel like an uphill struggle to those who are trying to create change.

References

Association of Community Health Councils for England and Wales (1992) *Self Reviews in Community Health Councils*

Association of Community Health Councils for England and Wales (1994) *Performance Standards for CHCs – developing the framework*

Association of Community Health Councils for England and Wales (1996/7) *Annual Report*

Association of Community Health Councils for England and Wales (1997) *Resolutions of the Annual General Meeting*

Barnes, M (1997) *The People's Health Service* The NHS Confederation, Research paper No. 2

Bowie, C, Richardson, A and Sykes, W (1995) Consulting the public about health service priorities *British Medical Journal* **311,** 1155–1158

Bruster, S, Jarman, B, Bosanquet, N *et al.* (1994) National survey of hospital patients *British Medical Journal* **309,** 1542–1549

Carr-Hill, RA (1992) The measurement of patient satisfaction *Journal of Public Health Medicine* **14,** 236–249

Coote, A (1996) The democratic deficit In Marshall Marinker (ed.) *Sense and sensibility in health care* BMJ Publishing Group, London

Department of Health (1991) *The patient's charter* HMSO, London

Department of Health (1994) *Code of Conduct, Code of Accountability* Corporate Governance Task Force, April 1994, HMSO, London

Department of Health (1995/6) *Priorities and planning guidance* HMSO, London

DHSS (1983) *NHS management inquiry report* (The Griffiths Report) HMSO, London

Gilbert, H (1995) *Redressing the balance: a brief survey of literature on patient empowerment* King's Fund, London

Kasper, JF, Mulley, AG and Wennberg, JE (1992) Developing shared decision-making programs to improve the quality of health care *Quality Review Bulletin* **18**, 182–190

McIver, S (1993) *Obtaining the views of health service users about quality of information* King's Fund Centre, London

McIver, S (1991) *Obtaining the views of users of health services* King's Fund Centre, London

McIver, S (1994) *Establishing Patient's Representatives* National Association of Health Authorities and Trusts, Birmingham

McNeil, BJ, Weichselbaum, R and Pauker, SG (1978) The fallacy of the five year survival in lung cancer *New England Journal of Medicine* **299**, 1397–1401

Meredith, P, Emberton, M and Devlin, BH (1993) What value is the patient's experience of surgery to surgeons? The merits and demerits of patient satisfaction surveys *Annals of the Royal College of Surgeons Bulletin* **75**, May 1993

NHS Management Executive (1992) *Local voices: the views of local people in purchasing for health* January 1992, NHS Executive, Leeds

NHS Executive (1996) *Patient partnership: building a collaborative strategy* NHS Executive, Leeds

O'Meara, JJ *et al.* (1994) A decision analysis of streptokinase plus heparin as compared with heparin alone for deep vein thrombosis *New England Journal of Medicine* **330**, 1864–1869

Prime Minister (1991) *Citizen's charter: raising the standard* HMSO, London

Richardson, A (1983) *Participation* Routlege & Kegan Paul, London

Savage, R and Armstrong, D (1990) Effect of a general practitioner's consulting style on patients' satisfaction: a controlled study *British Medical Journal* **301**, 968–970

Secretary of State for Health (1989) *Working for patients* HMSO, London

Stewart, J, Kendall, E and Coote, A, (eds) (1994) *Citizens' Juries* Institute for Public Policy Research, London

Williams, B (1994) Patient satisfaction: a valid concept? *Social Science and Medicine* **38**, 509–516

Index